NCLEX-RN® 101:

How to Pass! Sixth Edition

Sylvia Rayfield, MN, RN, CS
Executive Officer
ICAN Publishing, Inc.
Bossier City, LA
Board Chairwoman
Sylvia Rayfield & Associates, Inc.
Pensacola, FL

Loretta Manning, MSN, RN, CS, GNP
Executive Officer
ICAN Publishing, Inc.
Bossier City, LA
Regional Director
Sylvia Rayfield & Associates, Inc.
Pensacola, FL

D1537904

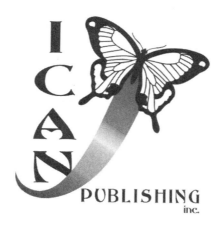

PUBLISHING
inc.

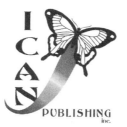

ICAN Publishing, Inc. ◆ **Bossier City, LA**
www.icanpublishing.com

Editorial Assistance: Jackie Lobo, Sacramento, CA; Teresa Davidson, Greensboro, NC
Cartoon Illustrations: C.J. Miller, RN, Washington, IA
Production Manager: Alisha Call, Winfield, KS
Cover Design: Teresa Davidson, Greensboro, NC

Quotes from Michael Dooley or tut are from Totally Unique Thoughts. You can visit their web page at **http://www.tut.com** where all the latest, totally-unique graphics and thoughts can be found.

◆

Printed in the United States of America
ISBN 0-9761029-2-7
Library of Congress Control Number: 2006935031

◆

Nursing procedures and/or practice described in this book should be applied by the nurse, or health-care practitioner, under appropriate supervision according to established professional standards of care. These standards should be used with regard to the unique circumstances that apply in each practice situation. Every effort has been taken to validate and confirm the accuracy of information presented and to describe generally accepted practices. However, the authors, editors, and publisher cannot accept any responsibility for errors or omissions or for consequences from application of the information in this book and make no warranty, express or implied, with respect to the contents of this book.

Every effort has been exerted by the authors and publisher to ensure that drug selection and dosage set forth in this text are in accord with current recommendations and practice at the time of publication. However, in view of ongoing research, the constant flow of information relating to government regulations, drug therapy, and drug reactions, the reader is urged to check the manufacturer's information on the package insert of each drug for any change in indications and dosage and for added warnings and precautions. This is particularly important when the recommended agent is a new or infrequently used drug.

This book is written to be used as a test question review book for the NCLEX-RN® and the CGFNS™ examination. It is not intended for use as a primary resource for procedures, treatments, medications, or to serve as a complete textbook for nursing care.

Copies of this book may be obtained directly from:

ICAN Publishing, Inc.
P.O. Box 6192
Bossier City, LA
1-866-428-5589
Web Site: www.icanpublishing.com

Contributors

Ester Acree, MSN, RNC, FNP
Family Nurse Practitioner
Indiana State University
Terre Haute, Indiana

Marie Bremner, DSN, RN, CS
Adult Health Nursing
Kennesaw State University
Kennesaw, Georgia

Marianne M. Call, MN, RN
Regional Director
Sylvia Rayfield & Associates
New Orleans, Louisiana

Jo Carol Claborn, MS, RN
Executive Director
Nursing Education Consultants
Dallas, Texas

Katherine Crawford, MSN, RN
Case Manager, Quality Management
Schumpert Medical Center
Shreveport, Louisiana

Linda Delunas, PhD, RN
Assistant Professor
Indiana University Northwest
Gary Indiana

Mary Rose Drigger, MSN, RN
Davidson County Community College
Davidson, North Carolina

Linda Fisher, MN, RN
Management–Maternal Child Nursing
Gwinnett Medical Center
Lawrenceville, Georgia

Sandra Galura, RN, MSN, CCRN
Assistant Professor, Dept. of Nursing
Florida Hospital College of
  Health Sciences
Orlando, Florida

Lynette Jack, PhD. RN, CARN
Psychiatric Nursing Addictions
University of Pittsburgh
  School of Nursing
Pittsburgh, Pennsylvania

Patricia A. Jones, RN, MSN
Assistant Prof. of Nursing
Pensacola Junior College
Pensacola, Florida

Sharon Shook Kallam, RN, BSN, MSN
Nursing Education Consultant
RN Supervisor
Hugh Chatham Nursing Center
Elkin, North Carolina

Eileen Kohlenberg, PhD, RN, CNAA
Adult Health Nursing
University of North Carolina
  at Greensboro
Greensboro, North Carolina

Susan L.W. Krupnick, MSN, RN,
  CARN, CS
Psychiatric Nursing
University of Pennsylvania
Philadelphia, Pennsylvania

Jana Lyner, BSN, RN
Faculty
Pensacola Junior College
Pensacola, Florida

Sylvia McDonald, RN, MEd, MSN
Director
Athens Technical College
Athens, Georgia

Mary Alice Middlebrooks, MSN, RN
Adult Health, Critical Care
  Nursing
Northwestern State University
Shreveport, Louisiana

C.J. Miller, RN
School Nurse, Nurse Illustrator
Washington Community Schools
Washington, Iowa

Kathy O'Leary Oller, MSN, RN
Maternal Child Nursing
Professor of Nursing
Florida Community College
Jacksonville, Florida

Bruce A. Scott, MSN, APRN, BC
San Joaquin Delta College
Stockton, California
Clinical Nurse, Orthopedics
University of California
Davis Medical Center
Sacramento, California

Martha Sherman, MSN, MA, RN
Consultant
Sylvia Rayfield & Associates
Burnsville, North Carolina

Charlotte Taylor, MSN, RN
Psychiatric Nursing
University of Arkansas
Monticello, Arkansas

Libby Turnipseed, MSN, RN,
LNCC, NLCP, CNP
Turnipseed & Associates, LLC
Rainbow City, Alabama

Mayola L. Villarruel, RN, MSN, ANP
VA Chicago Health Care System
ABJOPC
Crown Point, Indiana

Jo Ann Zerwekh, EdD, RN, FNP
Executive Director
Nursing Education Consultants
Dallas, Texas

Acknowledgments

We would like to acknowledge and thank our families, associates and good friends who have offered their support during the preparation of this book.

Our sincere appreciation to:

Dr. Phoebe K. Helm, past President, Truman College, Chicago, IL, who developed some of the test-taking strategies we have included in this book.

THE BIG DIFFERENCE

*C*omparable to NCLEX® and CGFNS™

*A*ddresses the nursing activities in the New NCLEX-RN® Test Plan

*R*ationales for correct and incorrect answers

*E*asy ways to pinpoint your needs

WE CARE!!

NCLEX-RN® 101: HOW TO PASS
Sixth Edition

This sixth edition is current, updated and streamlined. The items are written succinctly to mimic the computer adaptive test. Plus, we have made a distinct effort to save as much paper (and consequently as many trees) as possible.

Our objective is to help you PASS by providing the latest information on the NCLEX-RN® exam. The exam as reflected by the test plan published by the National Council of State Boards of Nursing was updated in April, 2007. The chapter titles and items in this edition reflect these changes.

We will help you replace FEAR (False Expectations Appearing Real!) with FAITH in your ability to be successful by helping you focus on the appropriate nursing activities as reflected on the exam. We want to help you fulfill your dream to be a registered nurse!

F   feel more confident
A   activities on current Test Plan
I   I CAN DO IT!
T   thinking skills
H   help identify your study needs

Remember, FOCUS on questions regarding the nursing activities and you will PASS!

Loretta Manning and Sylvia Rayfield

TABLE OF CONTENTS

Prelude

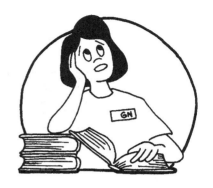

✳   *What if you've just graduated from nursing school?*

✳   *What if you've just applied to take the NCLEX® or CGFNS™ exam?*

✳   *What if you have 50,000 pages of notes, tape recordings and nursing books and you don't have a clue as to where to start?*

✳   *What if you just need help?*

Then…

Read on..

What if you knew —

*How to focus—not freak out

*Proven NCLEX® test-taking strategies

*How the NCLEX® is organized

*How to determine your own study needs

*What the questions look like on the computer exam

*That test questions in this book are organized around the most current NCLEX-RN® Test Plan

The priority for the NCLEX® is always safety. This acronym is organized around the priority NCLEX-RN® activities.

S *system-specific, focused assessment*

A *accuracy of orders/assignments*

F *firsts—prioritize, especially in emergencies*

E *evaluate pharmacology*

T *teach and practice infection control*

Y *cYa—cover your assets—license, identification, confidentiality, falls, suicide, drugs, electrical hazards, malfunctioning equipment, malfunctioning staff*

Interpreted from *Report of Findings from the 2005 RN Practice Analysis Linking the NCLEX-RN® to Practice*. Anne Wendt and Thomas O'Neill–National Council of State Boards of Nursing Research Brief, 2006.

All gray boxes at the beginning of Chapters 2–9 are interpreted from this Brief. Our appreciation to the NCSBN for their hard work in compiling this data.

*B*locks to Critical Thinking

P   *"Poor me" attitude (shut off your negative tape recorder and remember <u>The Little Engine That Could</u>, **I CAN, I CAN, I CAN!!**)*

I   *Inappropriate preparation (don't worry about old notes and tapes; use questions to determine your needs)*

T   *"Too much work, too little time" (passing this exam is an investment in your future; **PRIORITIZE**)*

S   *Spending too much time griping (use your time to practice questions)*

———— ◆ ————

How to Be A Critical Thinker

T *Take time to think! (especially on the first few questions; they will get you headed in the right direction).*

H *Help yourself by answering all questions (practice, practice, practice makes you better, better, and best).*

I *Integrate all the situation tells you (look at age, symptoms, lab values, sex, culture, etc.).*

N *Notice the healthcare setting (hospital, clinic, or home answers may differ depending on location).*

K *Keep the mind clear and nerves calm (take a deep breath and slowly let air out all the way).*

———— ◆ ————

*S*urround yourself with people who respect you and treat you well.

—Claudia Black

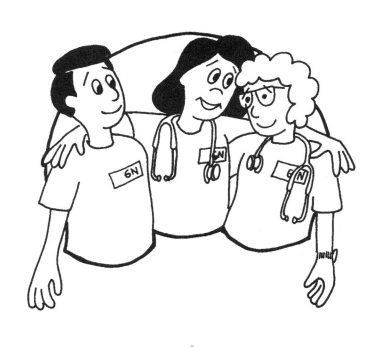

Supportive people give you strength. It's hard to think with people putting you down.

Remember...

If you think you can do it—you can!

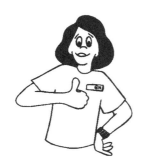

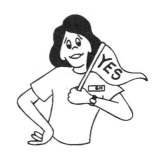

Yes! You can do it!

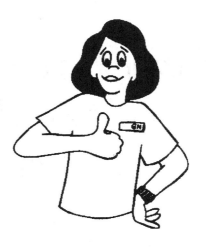

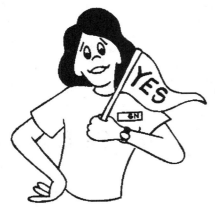

Now let's get started on how you can be successful on the NCLEX-RN®!

*T*est-taking strategies...

Our passion is to make you successful at passing this exam. We have conducted hundreds of NCLEX® reviews and have more than 50 years total experience in helping new graduates.

PASS THE NCLEX®!

Let's look at how this exam is organized. Here's the "bottom line."

➤ The National Council of State Boards of Nursing (NCSBN) (the organization that provides the exam to the local state board office), conducts periodic research on new graduates to determine what kinds of "nursing activities and roles" the new graduates perform most frequently in their work setting and which of these activities have the highest priority for client safety.

➤ After the research is completed, the "nursing activities" become the "backbone" of the NCLEX-RN® exam. These nursing activities are divided into four areas of client needs which are:

☑ Safe, Effective Care Environment—approximately 21-33% of the exam

☑ Health Promotion and Maintenance—approximately 6-12% of the exam

☑ Psycho-Social Integrity—approximately 6-12% of the exam

☑ Physiological Integrity—approximately 43-67% of the exam

YOU MAY RECOGNIZE THIS TERMINOLOGY—particularly if you have taken some sort of diagnostic pretest for NCLEX®. Many of the pretests use these words to indicate your strong and weak areas. The CGFNS™ certification exam is organized around the NCLEX-RN®.

The Nursing Process is also used as a way to approach the exam. If you are like most new grads, you KNOW the nursing process because you've been trying to figure out which instructor wants which thing in which column of your care plans for at least the last two years.

You will find a list of our interpretation of the nursing activities at the beginning of each chapter, except the Pretest, Posttest and Practice Exam. These nursing activities were interpreted from *Report of Findings from the 2005 RN Practice Analysis Linking the NCLEX-RN® to Practice.* Wendt & O'Neill.

First let's look at techniques that will improve your pass rate!

New Question Types:

The NCSBN has operationalized the use of "alternative item formatted" questions. These items will be in addition to the multiple choice format that has been used in the past. These questions may include:

* Fill in the blank.
* Check all that apply with more than 5 and less than 6 possibilities.
* Point and click.
* Prioritize in order of importance.

* Charts
* Tables
* Graphics

The *NCLEX-RN® 101: How to Pass* includes some of these types of items for your practice. Since this book is in a paper/pencil format, the practice will be similar to the CAT. The Computer Adaptive Test has many more ways of allowing the test taker to complete point and click and prioritize.

PRACTICE ANSWERING TEST QUESTIONS

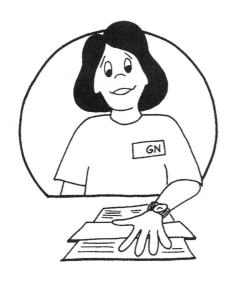

Step 1

Cover the Distracters.

➤ Did you know that in educational jargon, the question part of a multiple choice question is called the stem and the answers are called—DISTRACTERS????

➤ Did you know that instructors stay up nights—WRITING DISTRACTERS????

➤ We do not want you to be DISTRACTED—so cover the DISTRACTERS with your hand, a 5x7 card, a left-over Lotto ticket, your shirt tail or anything!!!

➤ YOU CAN'T BE DISTRACTED IF THEY ARE COVERED.

➤ Answer the question in your head. USE YOUR BRAIN. IT'S THE ONLY THING YOU CAN TRUST!!!

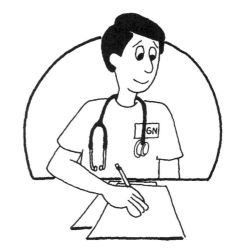

Step 2

Create a pool of answers.

*W*here were you on September 1, 1997?

Did you raise your palms to heaven and say, "How am I supposed to know that?"

That's exactly what some people do when they see an NCLEX-RN® question.

The brain thinks first in large clumps of material, then smaller clumps. Like this…

*T*hink—how old was I in 1997? Married, single, in school???

Most of you at least know where you were in September 1997.

First of school year? Near an anniversary, birthday, or holiday?

*D*on't worry about what you don't know. Think about what you do know.

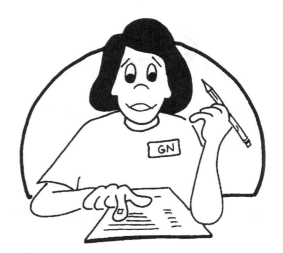

Step 3

Uncover the distracters and make your decisions— one by one.

➢ After creating a pool of answers, uncover the first distracter.

Is it a yes or no?

MAKE A DECISION.

➢ Next, uncover the second distracter. *Is it a yes or no?* GET THE DRIFT?

➢ Uncover Distracter 3. *Yes or No?* BE SURE, and uncover Distracter 4. Even though you may have found a good answer in 1, 2, or 3, the last one might be the highest priority!

➢ Remember—these options are written to **distract**—so make a decision on **each** before continuing.

Step 4

Commit one hour per day to answering questions.

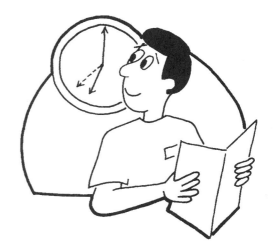

Our experience has documented that the more questions practiced, the better success rate on NCLEX®!!!

The people who wrote this book have over 50 years of collective successful experience in preparing graduates to PASS the state board exam. We have put together a team of experts in item writing and have given them specific guidelines that reflect the NCLEX-RN® Test Plan and the "nursing activities" that are the basis of the NCLEX-RN® exam.

This book has been divided into sections of 60 items. WHY?

We believe you should be able to answer approximately one (1) question per minute. Practicing at this pace will give you enough time to complete your exam in plenty of time. Besides, you'll probably want a break after an hour of practice!

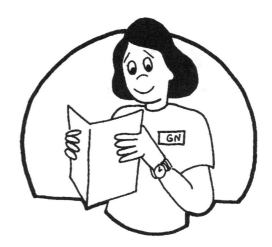

***D**on't major in a minor activity.*

***E**ach question is worth one minute of your time.*

DO NOT—repeat—**DO NOT** look at the end of the chapter for the answers.

Forget "instant gratification" until the entire hour is completed. Then determine which questions were missed and why.

Looking at the answers after each question encourages memorization, and **WE DON'T WANT YOU TO MEMORIZE!** Why? Because we doubt if any question in this book or any other question/review book on the market will be exactly as it is on NCLEX®.

I thought we'd never take a break!!!!

TAKE A BREAK BETWEEN STEPS 4 AND 5!!!!

YOU DESERVE IT!

ALL WORK AND NO PLAY IS NO FUN!

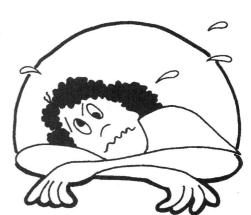

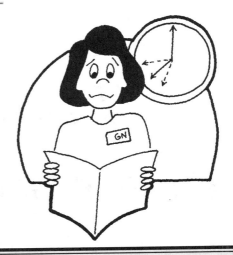

Step 5

Commit your second hour per day to studying what you don't know!

Our experience has taught us that new graduates like to study the material with which they are most comfortable. They want to forget the stuff that they don't know because it gives them butterflies.

Here are some ways to use this book:

- ☑ Figure out which questions you got correct. FORGET THEM! Don't say, "Oh, that was just a lucky guess." You had some basis for choosing the correct answer. Let them go!

- ☑ Now, WHICH ONES DID YOU MISS?
  Were they on safe effective care, health promotion, psycho-social-integrity, fluid-gas transport, elimination, nutrition, sensory-perception-mobility? Use the Test Worksheet, Content Analysis page and Table of Contents to help.

- ☑ Once you've determined your study needs, use a good review book to refresh your memory on the facts. To help you with easy, fun ways to remember, we recommend ***Nursing Made Insanely Easy, Fourth Edition*** and ***Pharmacology Made Insanely Easy, Second Edition*** by Sylvia Rayfield and Loretta Manning, ICAN Publishing, Inc. (1-866-428-5589). We also recommend ***Illustrated Study Guide for the NCLEX-RN®, Sixth Edition*** by JoAnn Zerwekh and Jo Carol Claborn, Publisher Elsevier. www.elsevierhealth.com

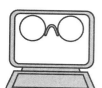

Advantages To Computer Adaptive Testing

You can take the test in any state and practice in the state where you have applied for license. You will have choices of dates, times, and test centers. You will be FINISHED WITHIN HOURS!

HOT TIPS to Decrease Stress and Improve Scores!

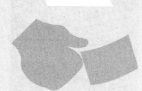

- ❤ You will get an authorization to test from your state board office. It's like American Express—"Don't leave home without it!"

- ❤ Don't leave home without your thumb either because you may be thumbprinted and have your picture taken.

- ❤ You may be provided with lockers for your "stuff."

- ❤ You will be given a computer practice period with help on the equipment. There will be someone to help you get started on your computer—a warm-up time.

❤ There will be a drop-down calculator for math calculations and a mouse for your use.

❤ There are a minimum of 75 questions and a maximum of 265. About 60% of test takers complete the exam in about 75 questions. DO NOT PANIC if you hit question #76! It means you have more time to demonstrate your intelligence.

75 to 265 questions

❤ You will have six (6) hours from start to finish including "warm-up."

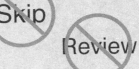

❤ You will not be able to skip a question or go back and review questions once they have left the screen. This is an advantage since many "changed" answers are wrong.

No more than 2 minutes per question

❤ There is no time limit per question, BUT DO NOT SIT ON A QUESTION FOR MORE THAN TWO (2) MINUTES or you may not have enough time in the six-hour limitation to answer enough questions to pass.

❤ If you don't have a clue as to the answer, pick any one.

Which response represents the best guess?
1. *Alright!*
2. *Boy Howdy!*
3. *Cool!*
4. *Delightful!*

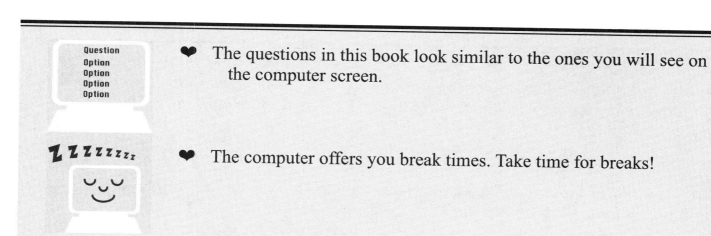

❤ The questions in this book look similar to the ones you will see on the computer screen.

❤ The computer offers you break times. Take time for breaks!

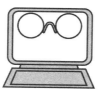

YES!

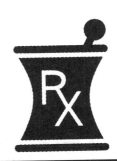

Tips For Answering Questions On Medications

Medications are a "biggie" on NCLEX®—in fact, they are integrated throughout the test. We have included medications that go with the concepts included in each chapter. Because graduates asked for more medication questions, we have included an entire chapter on Pharmacology.

C   *Check why the client is receiving medication. (Is it an antibiotic for pneumonia, or a vasodilator for anginal pain?)*

H   *How do you know the medication is working? (If the medication is Lasix, someone had better be emptying the bedpans!)*

E   *Exactly what time and how should you give it? (Is it before meals, at bedtime, or on an empty stomach, by mouth, IV, intracath, with a 25 ga or 18 ga needle?)*

C   *Client teaching tip. (If they are taking Lasix, they had better be eating their bananas!)*

K   *Keys to giving it safely. (These are the nursing implications—like checking the client's identification bracelet and the apical pulse before giving the Lanoxin.)*

S   *Seek information on other food the client is using. (We don't want to give them something that is incompatible with a previous prescription or over-the-counter product.)*

The Pretest

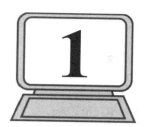

In pursuit, even of the best things,
we ought to be calm and tranquil.
— Cicero

✔ **About this test...**

This 60-item test will help you begin to pinpoint your study needs.

FOR BEST RESULTS:

☛ Complete the entire Pretest. Do NOT look in the back of the book for the answers until you have completed the exam.

☛ Spend a few minutes analyzing the questions you have missed. Use the test worksheet and Category Analysis to help determine your study needs. Once you determine your weak area(s), spend the next hour studying this content using a good review book as a guide.

REMEMBER THAT MISTAKES ARE A WAY OF GROWING—BE GENTLE WITH YOURSELF!
" The reason that angels can fly is that they take themselves so lightly."
—G. K. Chesterson

These activities are taken from the *Report of Findings from the 2005 RN Practice Analysis : Linking the NCLEX-RN® Examination to Practice. Wendt and O'Neill*

TOMORROW —

☛ Skip to the chapter in this book that asks questions on the area of your biggest identified weakness.

☛ Take the test from this chapter and note the questions that you missed. Spend the next hour studying this content. ETC! ETC! ETC!

As NIKE says, **"Just do it!"** *You are the only one who can pinpoint your own study needs. This is an excellent way to begin.*

1.1 Select the rights to medication administration. (Select all correct answers.)

 ① Right organism.
 ② Right diagnosis.
 ③ Right client.
 ④ Right dose.
 ⑤ Right time.
 ⑥ Right medication.

1.2 Select the correct procedures when following standard precautions. (Select all correct answers.)

 ① Wear a face shield whenever entering the room.
 ② Wear gloves when coming in contact with any body fluid.
 ③ Place the client in a private room that has negative air pressure in relation to surrounding area.
 ④ Discard used needles immediately in the trash can.
 ⑤ Wear gloves when entering the room.
 ⑥ Avoid contact with client if nurse has an exudative lesion.

1.3 Which statement made by the 70-year-old client indicates he understands how to take his steroid and bronchodilator inhalers?

 ① "I will take my steroid first and follow it with my bronchodilator."
 ② "I will take 2 puffs very quickly and then hold my breath."
 ③ "I will take my bronchodilator first and follow it with my steroid."
 ④ "I will separate the inhalers and rotate when I take them."

1.4 Which nursing action has the highest priority following a cardiac catheterization procedure?

 ① Place a warm pack to increase the temperature of the left foot.
 ② Evaluate the vital signs every 2 hours.
 ③ Compare the quality of the pulses on the right and left legs.
 ④ Determine the presence of pulses above the catheterization site.

1.5 Which nursing action has the highest priority in preparing the client the evening prior to an intravenous pyelogram procedure?

 ① Administer a cathartic enema to cleanse the bowel.
 ② Identify through a history any client allergies to iodine or food.
 ③ Instruct the client to be NPO after midnight.
 ④ Teach the client that x-rays will be taken at multiple intervals.

1.6 Which equipment is more important for the nurse to have available at the bedside of a client with a history of seizures?

 ① Pump for IV solution.
 ② Suction equipment.
 ③ Defibrillator.
 ④ IV cutdown tray.

1.7 A 2-year-old is admitted to the Pediatric Unit with numerous bruises, fractured left humerus and several lacerations of unexplained origin. Which nursing action is a priority?

 ① Report the findings to the Child Protection Agency.
 ② Share this information only with other health care professionals.
 ③ Document this information in the chart only.
 ④ Share the information with the Pediatric Social Worker.

1.8 Which documentation would be the most accurate when an error has been made on the flow sheet?

 ① Make the record look neat by using correction fluid.
 ② Draw several lines through the entry so it is not readable.
 ③ Write the word "error" above or beside the original words with your initials and draw a single line through the entry.
 ④ Cross through the error with correction fluid and write over the entry.

1.9 One hour to discharge, a postpartum client requests more peripads, diapers, tucks, and Americaine spray. Which response made by the nurse would be most appropriate and demonstrate an understanding of cost effectiveness?

① "I will be glad to get these supplies for you."
② "It would be much better if you would just stop and pick them up on your way home."
③ "I will be happy to get them for you and pull some extras for you to take home."
④ "What items do you need until you leave to go home?"

1.10 In a 7-month-old infant, which is the best way to detect fluid retention?

① Weigh the child daily.
② Test the urine for hematuria.
③ Measure abdominal girth weekly.
④ Count the number of wet diapers.

1.11 Which nursing approach would be most appropriate for obtaining a specimen from a retention catheter?

① Disconnect the drain at the bottom of the draining bag and drain urine into a sterile container.
② Disconnect the tubing between the catheter and the drainage bag and drain urine into sterile container.
③ Clamp the drainage tube. When fresh urine collects, open the tubing and drain into a sterile container.
④ Use a sterile syringe and needle to obtain urine from the porthole.

1.12 Which evaluation would best determine if fluid is amniotic versus urine?

① Digital evaluation.
② pH determination of fluid.
③ Urinalysis by lab.
④ Glucose determination.

1.13 The nurse would determine the client understands the collection of urine specimen for culture and sensitivity when he states:

① "I will call the lab before I collect my urine."
② "I will drink several glasses of water before the urine is collected."
③ "I will call the nurse to help me with aseptic technique."
④ "I will discard my first voiding in the morning."

1.14 Which nursing observation would most likely indicate an early side effect of the elderly client taking digoxin (Lanoxin)?

① Confusion.
② Bradycardia.
③ Constipation.
④ Hyperkalemia.

1.15 Which assessment of the lungs by auscultation would the nurse expect to evaluate if a client has a left lower lobe consolidation?

① Absent breath sounds
② Bronchophony
③ Vesicular breath sounds
④ Wheezes

1.16 Which statement by a client would indicate an understanding of when to take the medication, cromolyn sodium (Intal)?

① "I will take the medicine with my meals."
② "It is important that I take the medication before going to bed."
③ "If I experience respiratory distress, I will take the medicine."
④ "I will take the medication before I begin any vigorous exercise."

1.17 Which neonatal assessment finding should the nurse report to the physician 1 hour after delivery?

① A caput succedaneum that crosses the suture lines.
② A resting heart rate of 140 and a respiratory rate of 40.
③ Head circumference—34 cm. Chest circumference—30 cm.
④ The umbilical cord has 2 arteries and 1 vein.

1.18 Which assessment indicates a neonate with an infection is not fully recovered?

   ① Heart rate of 150.
   ② Axillary temperature of 98.6°F.
   ③ Weight increase of 4 oz.
   ④ Resting respiratory rate of 65.

1.19 Which order should be questioned on a client in vaso-occlusive crisis due to sickle cell anemia?

   ① Place client on bed rest with bathroom privileges.
   ② Administer 2 liters oxygen via nasal cannula.
   ③ Maintain IV rate at keep open.
   ④ Administer analgesics as ordered.

1.20 Which symptom is indicative of an increase in respiratory distress in a 4-year-old client with drooling and an inflamed epiglottis?

   ① Bradycardia.
   ② Tachypnea.
   ③ General pallor.
   ④ Irritability.

1.21 A patient has had profuse vomiting for 6 hours. Arterial blood gases note a pH 7.50, $PaCO_2$ 40 mm Hg and HCO_3 40mEq/L. Which additional physical assessment findings would the nurse anticipate?

   ① Muscular twitching.
   ② Kussmaul's respirations.
   ③ Anuria.
   ④ Irregular pulse.

1.22 A client has a history of oliguria, hypertension, and peripheral edema. Current lab values include BUN-25, K-5.0. Which nutrients should be restricted in this client's diet?

   ① Protein.
   ② Fats.
   ③ Carbohydrates.
   ④ Magnesium.

1.23 An older client with diabetes is being managed with insulin in the AM and PM. Which observation is the best for indicating the overall therapeutic response to the management?

   ① Glycosylated hemoglobin (HgbAlc)%.
   ② Fasting blood sugar 128 mg/dl.
   ③ Blood pressure is maintained at 130/82.
   ④ Serum amylase is normal.

1.24 Which assessment finding would indicate an increase in the intracranial pressure in a 4-month-old infant?

   ① A positive Babinski.
   ② High pitched cry.
   ③ Bulging posterior fontanel.
   ④ Pinpoint pupils.

1.25 The client shares some very confidential information with her nurse. The nurse demonstrates appropriate management with this information when he:

   ① openly discusses this information with all of his colleagues.
   ② documents the information only on the client's flow sheet.
   ③ reviews the information with those staff involved in the plan of care.
   ④ shares the information with nobody.

1.26 The nurse demonstrates an appropriate understanding of safely prioritizing the workload when she assesses which client initially?

   ① A client who had a lobectomy 24 hours ago with a chest tube inserted.
   ② A postoperative larnygectomy client.
   ③ A client with headaches of unknown origin.
   ④ A client who is in Buck's traction.

1.27 Which food should the client be taught to avoid if they are taking a MAO inhibitor?

   ① Roast beef, slice of white bread
   ② Fried chicken, green beans
   ③ Boiled fish, milk
   ④ Grilled cheddar cheese sandwich

1.28 Which of these clients would be the highest risk for acquiring pneumonia during hospitalization?

   ① A postoperative client who is ambulating.
   ② An infant in Bryant's traction who is frequently crying and screaming.
   ③ A school-age child with diabetes mellitus.
   ④ An immobile client with a spinal cord injury.

1.29 A hospitalized client has been vomiting for three days with a low grade temperature, and feels lethargic. Which nursing action is most appropriate in evaluating for fluid volume deficit?

   ① Obtain a urinalysis for casts and specific gravity.
   ② Determine client's weight and assess gain or loss.
   ③ Ask client to provide a 24-hour intake and output record.
   ④ Determine the quality of the skin turgor.

1.30 A client is placed on bed rest with an order to immobilize the right leg due to tenderness, increased warmth, and diffuse swelling. Which nursing action is most appropriate to maintain skin integrity?

   ① Apply a trapeze to client's bed.
   ② Assess bony prominence every 12 hours.
   ③ Apply granular spray to the bony prominence.
   ④ Turn client every 2 hours.

1.31 During the first 24 hours after a below-the-knee amputation, which nursing action would be most important?

   ① Notify the physician for a small amount of sero sanguineous drainage.
   ② Elevate the stump on a pillow to decrease edema.
   ③ Maintain the stump flat on the bed by placing the client in the prone position.
   ④ Do passive range of motion TID to the unaffected leg.

1.32 Which measure should the nurse take in reducing the discomfort of gas pains in a client?

   ① Encourage a diet high in fiber.
   ② Assist with early ambulation.
   ③ Teach how to splint the abdomen with activity.
   ④ Position on right side.

1.33 The nurse receives a call that a piece of glass is imbedded in an 8-year-old child's eye. The nurse instructs the mother that it would be most important to:

   ① put an eye patch over both eyes and have the child taken to an emergency room immediately.
   ② place pressure dressing to the injured eye and have the child taken to an emergency room.
   ③ remove the broken glass immediately from the eye to reduce the possibility of further trauma and apply Vaseline on the eyelid.
   ④ irrigate the injured eye with warm normal saline and apply a dressing to the eye.

1.34 Which emergency medication should the nurse administer to a client with ventricular tachycardia?

   ① Nitroglycerin (Nitrostat).
   ② Morphine sulfate.
   ③ Lidocaine (Xylocaine).
   ④ Dopamine (Intropin).

1.35 In which position would a nurse place a client who is in respiratory distress, extremely anxious, edematous, and cyanotic?

   ① Lithotomy position.
   ② Low-Fowler's position.
   ③ Sim's position.
   ④ High-Fowler's position.

1.36 Your patient has just been intubated in preparation for mechanical ventilation. In evaluating the effectiveness of this intervention, your first action will be to:

   ① assess lung sounds.
   ② call for a stat chest x-ray.
   ③ call for stat arterial blood gasses.
   ④ suction the endotracheal tube.

1.37 A client has been complaining of sharp pain in the epigastric area and has an order for an antacid. Which statement made by the client indicates a correct understanding of when to take the antacid?

① "It is important to only take my medicine prior to bedtime."
② "By taking the medication before meals, I will decrease the side effects."
③ "I will take the medication one hour after meals."
④ "As I start to feel uncomfortable, I will take the medication."

1.38 The client needs an infusion of IV fluid at 40ml/hr. If the tubing set is calibrated at 15 gtt/ml, what is the drip rate?

Answer:

_____

1.39 Which selection indicates compliance for a client with cardiac disease?

① Baked chicken, green vegetables, and fresh fruit.
② Hot dog, cup of canned soup, and lettuce salad.
③ Baked fish, baked apples, and avocado salad.
④ Baked ham, rice, and fruit cup.

1.40 An RN assigns the care of a new post-operative mastectomy client to an LPN. At the time of the assignment, the RN reminds the LPN not to take the blood pressure on the operative side. Later in the shift, the RN discovers the blood pressure cuff deflated, but still on the arm of the client's affected side. How should the RN handle the situation?

① Make a note to talk with the LPN in private after the shift is over.
② Call the LPN in for counseling to determine why she did not follow directions.
③ Find the LPN and review with her the importance of not taking the blood pressure on the affected side.
④ Write up a report regarding the incident and place it in the LPN's personnel folder.

1.41 The staff nurse of an acute pulmonary unit is preparing notes that will be necessary for a shift report on her assigned clients. What information is critical to communicate in a shift report on this unit?

① Laboratory work drawn on the client, arterial blood gas reports, nutritional intake, and vital signs for the shift.
② Any respiratory difficulty client experienced, tolerance to activity, sputum production, and significant variances in vital signs during the shift.
③ Name of the client's doctor, date client was admitted, dietary intake and his general condition.
④ Urinary output, PO and IV fluid intake, visits by attending doctor, vital signs each time evaluated, any respiratory problems encountered.

1.42 An LPN is anchoring a Foley catheter on a female client. As the nurse walks in the room, the Foley drops on the floor. Which action would be the highest priority?

① Review aseptic technique with the LPN.
② Complete an incident report.
③ Get a new Foley catheter and assist LPN with the procedure.
④ Report the incident in the continuous quality improvement (CQI) report.

1.43 A provider has ordered timolol (Timoptic) 1 gtt OU bid. Point to the location of the eye where the medication will be placed.

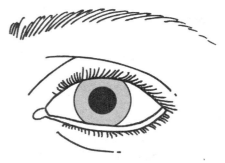

1.44 An elderly client is admitted to an inpatient psychiatric unit with an initial diagnosis of psychotic depression. The initial nursing priority is to:

① clarify perceptual distortions.
② establish reality orientation.
③ ensure client and milieu safety.
④ increase self-esteem.

1.45 Which clinical findings would confirm the suspicion of elder abuse?

① Poor nutrition and hygiene.
② Disorientation and problems with short-term memory.
③ Dirty laundry in the kitchen.
④ Recent fractured leg.

1.46 A client diagnosed with a lower GI bleed has an order for 1 unit of packed red blood cells. What information is most important to be documented during this procedure?

① Vital signs prior to procedure
② Confirmation that the nurse alone verified the blood label information
③ The total volume that is to be infused
④ Vital signs before, during, and after procedure, date and time started and completed

1.47 Prior to developing a nursing care plan for a hospitalized 3-year-old, which activity would be a priority?

① Assess the child's rituals and routines at home.
② Introduce child to the other personnel.
③ Explain to parents the importance of limiting visiting hours.
④ Identify the child's favorite foods.

1.48 What would be the plan of care for a client who has a blood sugar of 200 at 7:00 AM?

① Increase the PM dose of NPH insulin.
② Increase the AM dose of regular insulin.
③ Have the client wake up at 3:00 AM and evaluate the blood sugar.
④ Decrease the PM dose of NPH insulin.

1.49 Which nursing action represents the best technique to set up a sterile field?

① Place all supplies as close to the edge as possible.
② Wear gown and gloves at all times.
③ Set up the field above waist level.
④ Open supplies with sterile gloves.

1.50 During the shift report, a client's ventilator alarm is activated. Which action would the nurse implement first?

① Notify the respiratory therapist.
② Check the ventilator tubing for excess fluid.
③ Deactivate the alarm and check the spirometer.
④ Assess the client for adequate oxygenation.

1.51 Nursing interventions implemented within an hour prior to any major surgery would include:

① administering an enema.
② checking for signed consent form.
③ performing preoperative shave and scrub.
④ evaluating for food or medication allergies.

1.52 What would be the priority assessment for a client who is taking a sulfonylurea and prednisone?

① Monitor hemoglobin.
② Monitor platelets.
③ Monitor photosensitivity.
④ Monitor serum glucose.

1.53 Which response by the client indicates an understanding of how to collect a 24-hour urine specimen? "I will:

① discard my first morning voided specimen, and then collect my urine for 24 hours into one container."
② start collecting all of my urine into one container after 8:00 a.m. and continue until 8:00 p.m. tonight."
③ place each of my urine specimens in a separate container."
④ notify the nurse so she/he can call the lab to start this test."

1.54 Which fluid would be the most appropriate for a client receiving furosemide (Lasix) and digoxin (Lanoxin)?

① Milk
② Gatorade
③ Orange juice
④ Water

1.55 One hour after a bronchoscopy is completed on a client, which nursing observation would indicate a complication?

① Depressed gag reflex
② Sputum streaked with blood
③ Tachypnea
④ Widening pulse pressure

1.56 Which instruction would be included in the teaching plan for a client on oral steroids regarding when and how the medication should be taken?

① With 8 oz. of orange juice once each morning.
② With meals.
③ Between meals.
④ On an empty stomach.

1.57 Which instruction would be included in planning care for a client with signs of increased intracranial pressure?

① Encourage coughing and deep-breathing to prevent pneumonia.
② Suction airway every 2 hours to remove secretions.
③ Position the client in the prone position to promote venous return.
④ Determine cough reflex and ability to swallow prior to administering PO fluids.

1.58 The nurse is assessing the emotional support available to an adolescent client who is starving herself. Which question would be most important for the nurse to ask in the assessment interview?

① "What do you consider your ideal weight?"
② "How does your eating habit change when you are around other people?"
③ "What happens at home when you express opinions that are different from those of your parents?"
④ "What do you think about your present weight?"

1.59 Which symptoms might alert the nurse to an alcohol problem in a client hospitalized for a physical illness?

① Depression, difficulty falling asleep, decreased concentration.
② Elevated liver enzymes, cirrhosis, decreased platelets.
③ Tremors, elevated temperature, complaints of nocturnal leg cramps, complaints of pain symptoms.
④ Flu-like symptoms, diarrhea, night sweats, elevated temperature, decreased deep tendon reflexes.

1.60 Which client would be the highest risk for injury?

① A 3-month-old in an infant seat sitting on a coffee table.
② A 2-year-old playing in the living room unattended by an adult.
③ A 2-1/2-year-old with a tracheostomy playing outside in the backyard.
④ A 7-year-old who goes to after school care in a 38-year-old home.

Category Analysis – Pretest

1. Pharmacology
2. Safe Effective Care
3. Pharmacology
4. Fluid Gas
5. Safe Effective Care
6. Sensory-Perception-Mobility
7. Safe Effective Care
8. Safe Effective Care
9. Safe Effective Care
10. Fluid-Gas
11. Elimination
12. Elimination
13. Elimination
14. Pharmacology
15. Fluid-Gas
16. Pharmacology
17. Health Promotion
18. Health Promotion
19. Safe Effective Care
20. Fluid-Gas

21. Fluid-Gas
22. Nutrition
23. Pharmacology
24. Sensory-Perception-Mobility
25. Safe Effective Care
26. Safe Effective Care
27. Pharmacology
28. Health Promotion
29. Fluid-Gas
30. Safe Effective Care
31. Sensory-Perception-Mobility
32. Elimination
33. Sensory-Perception-Mobility
34. Pharmacology
35. Fluid-Gas
36. Fluid-Gas
37. Pharmacology
38. Pharmacology
39. Nutrition
40. Safe Effective Care

41. Safe Effective Care
42. Safe Effective Care
43. Pharmacology
44. Psycho-Social
45. Psycho-Social
46. Safe Effective Care
47. Health Promotion
48. Nutrition
49. Safe Effective Care
50. Fluid-Gas
51. Safe Effective Care
52. Pharmacology
53. Elimination
54. Pharmacology
55. Fluid-Gas
56. Pharmacology
57. Sensory-Perception-Mobility
58. Psycho-Social
59. Psycho-Social
60. Safe Effective Care

Directions

1. Determine questions missed by checking answers.
2. Write the number of the questions missed across the top line marked "item missed."
3. Check category analysis page to determine category of question.
4. Put a check mark under item missed and beside content.
5. Count check marks in each row and write the number in totals column.
6. Use this information to:
   - identify areas for further study.
   - determine which content test to take next.

We recommend studying content where most items are missed—then taking that content test.

Number of the Questions Incorrectly Answered

Pretest		Items Missed																								Totals
C	Safe Effective Care																									
O	Health Promotion and Maintenance																									
N	Psycho-Social Integrity																									
T	Physiological Adaptation: Fluid Gas																									
E	Reduction of Risk Potential: Sensory-Perception-Mobility																									
N	Basic Care and Comfort: Elimination																									
T	Physiological Adaptation: Nutrition																									
	Pharmacology and Parenteral Therapies																									

Answers & Rationales

1.1 ③ Options #3, #4, #5, and #6 are correct. The
④ 5 rights to medication administration include
⑤ the right patient, medication, time, dose, and
⑥ route. Options #1 and #2 are not included in the
5 rights.

1.2 ② Options #2 and #6 are correct for this infection
⑥ control procedure. Options #1 and #3 are correct
for airborne transmission-based precautions.
Option #4 should read "discard needles intact
immediately after use into an impervious dis-
posal box." Option #5 isn't necessary. This
would be appropriate for contact transmission-
based precautions.

1.3 ③ The bronchodilator inhaler will open up the
bronchioles so the steroid can be effective.
Option #1 is incorrect. Option #2 is incorrect
because the client needs time between the 2 puffs.
Option #4 is incorrect.

1.4 ③ The two extremities should be compared in
relation to the pain, pulse, pallor, temperature,
and capillary filling time. Option #1 makes
no comparison to effectively evaluate the circulation. Option #2 is incorrect because vital
signs are usually evaluated every 15 minutes
after the procedure to identify hypotension and
dysrhythmia. Option #4 should be evaluated
distal to the site for equality between the two
extremities.

1.5 ② Clients who are sensitive to iodine can develop
anaphylaxis. The client should be asked specifically regarding allergy to iodine. Iodine is present
in the radiopaque material which is injected
intravenously. Options #1, #3, and #4 contain
correct information but are not priorities. The
test may be canceled if the client is allergic to
iodine.

1.6 ② The suction equipment should be available to
facilitate removing the nasal and pharyngeal
secretions which could lead to airway obstruction.
Options #1 and #4 are not specific to providing
safety after a seizure. Option #3 is unnecessary
for the disorder.

1.7 ① Any suspicion of child abuse should be reported
to the Child Protection Agency. Options #2, #3,
and #4 do not provide nor plan for protection of
the child.

1.8 ③ Out of the options, this is the best answer.
Options #1 and #4 — A breach in the nursing
standards of care is alteration of records. The
use of correction fluid cannot be used on
medical records because it denotes alteration
of records. Words covered by correction fluid
have been deciphered with x-ray equipment.
Insurance companies will not cover nurses who
use correction fluid on patient records. Option
#2 is incorrect. Errors should never be obliter-
ated or covered up.

1.9 ④ This option is the most diplomatic response and
considers cost effectiveness. Many insurance
companies view extra supplies on the day of
discharge as stockpiling, and the client may be
stuck with the bill. While some companies may
still pay the entire bill as presented, many are
becoming dollar-wise and view each bill with a
critical eye. Options #1 and #3 do not consider
cost effectiveness. Option #2 is an inappropriate
response.

1.10 ① Fluid retention is best detected by weighing
daily and noting a gaining trend. Options #2
and #3 are incorrect and will not provide information regarding fluid retention. Option #4 can
provide an estimation of the amount of urine
output but not about fluid retention.

1.11 ④ This represents the appropriate process in collecting a "sterile" urine specimen. Options #1
and #2 open a closed system which allows
bacteria to be introduced. Option #3 is incorrect
information.

1.12 ② Amniotic fluid is alkaline; test with phenaph-
thazine (nitrazine) paper which turns blue if
it is amniotic fluid. Normal vaginal and urinary
secretions are acidic. Option #1 will assist in
evaluating a prolapsed cord or dilation. Options
#3 and #4 are incorrect.

1.13 ③ Aseptic techniques decrease the possibility of contamination with organisms. Options #1, #2, and #4 are incorrect.

1.14 ① The elderly are particularly prone to digoxin-induced confused states which can occur in the presence of subtoxic digoxin levels and without other signs of toxicity. Option #2 occurs as a late side effect. Option #3 and #4 are incorrect.

1.15 ② Option #2 is correct. Bronchophony may be auscultated with a consolidation. Option #1 would be present with a prolapsed lung. Option #3 would be auscultated over the majority of the lung fields. Option #4 would be auscultated with conditions such as asthma due to swollen alveoli.

1.16 ④ Cromolyn sodium (Intal) is used to prevent the release of histamine and other allergy-triggering substances. Options #1 and #2 contain inappropriate information. Option #3 is incorrect because it is ineffective.

1.17 ③ Option #3 should be reported. The head circumference should be 2 cm larger than the chest circumference. 4 cm larger is not normal and requires further assessment. Options #1, #2, and #4 are normal clinical findings.

1.18 ④ The normal respiratory rate of a neonate is 30–50. Tachypnea is a sign of sepsis or hypoxia with a neonate. Option #1 is incorrect because it is within the normal range. Option #2 is not significant. Option #3 is incorrect. Neonates normally experience between a 5–10 percent loss of weight within the first few days of life.

1.19 ③ The keep-open rate is too slow. Adequate hydration must be maintained to prevent sickling and clumping of the affected cells. Options #1, #2, and #4 are appropriate orders for this client.

1.20 ② An increase in the respiratory rate is an early sign of hypoxia. Another early assessment of hypoxia would be tachycardia. Option #1 is incorrect because tachycardia occurs early in hypoxia. Option #3 is a general symptom and not measurable for hypoxia. Option #4 is incorrect because the client may be anxious and restless but is generally not described as irritable.

1.21 ① Metabolic alkalosis results in neuromuscular excitability. Alkalosis causes calcium to bind with albumin making less available for contraction of smooth skeletal muscle leading to muscle cramps and twitching.

1.22 ① A decreased production of urea nitrogen can be achieved by restricting protein. These metabolic wastes cannot be excreted by the kidneys. Options #2 and #3 decrease the non-protein nitrogen production; therefore, these foods are encouraged. Option #4 is incorrect.

1.23 ① The glycosylated hemoglobin will indicate the overall glucose control for approximately the past 120 days. This allows evaluation of control of the blood sugar regardless of increases or decreases in blood sugar immediately prior to drawing the sample. Option #2 is not a priority to #1. Option #3 would be evaluating the response to an antihypertensive medication. Option #4 is evaluating for pancreatitis.

1.24 ② A high-pitched cry is one of the first signs of an increase in intracranial pressure in infants. Option #1 is normal for the first year of life. Option #3 is incorrect because the fontanel should be closed by the third month. Option #4 is incorrect because with increased pressure, the pupils may respond to light slowly rather than with the usual brisk response.

1.25 ③ This information must be respected and remain confidential. Under the Invasion of Privacy it states that the client has the constitutional right to be free from publicity and exposure to public view. Option #4 does not benefit the client in any constructive way.

1.26 ② The maintenance of a patent airway for a post-operative larnygectomy client would be a priority. Options #1, #3, and #4 would not be a priority to a potential airway issue.

1.27 ④ MAO inhibitors and aged cheese may cause hypertensive crisis. Options #1, #2, and #3 should be safe foods.

1.28 ④ Clients who are immobilized from a spinal cord injury are high risk for developing pneumonia. Options #1 and #2 are not high risk. A postoperative client who is ambulating and has no direct insult to the respiratory system is not high risk. The infant is in traction, but is frequently expanding the lungs with the crying. Option #3 is a concern, but not a priority to Option #4.

1.29 ② The daily weight is the best way to evaluate for fluid volume deficit. Options #1, #3, and #4 provide information regarding the fluid volume level, but are not the best actions for evaluation.

1.30 ④ Turning client at frequent intervals is one of the most effective methods of preventing the development of skin breakdown caused by pressure, friction, or shearing forces. Option #1 encourages independent moving but does not relieve pressure. Option #2 is an incorrect standard of practice. Skin inspection should be carried out at least once every 8 hours. Option #3 does not offer any prevention.

1.31 ② Elevation after surgery will minimize edema and optimize venous return. This would not be done for more than 24 hours due to the potential development of contracture. Option #1 is not correct because some bloody drainage is expected. The nurse should outline the drainage and assess again in 5 minutes. Options #3 and #4 contain incorrect information.

1.32 ② Ambulation increases the return of peristalsis and facilitates the expulsion of flatus. Option #1 should not be encouraged until the bowel sounds have returned. Option #3 does nothing to increase peristalsis, but may make the client more comfortable. Option #4 doesn't provide anything.

1.33 ① The objective is to minimize eye movement in order to prevent further injury. Options #2, #3, and #4 would lead to further injury.

1.34 ③ Lidocaine is the anti-arrhythmic drug of choice for ventricular arrhythmias. Option #1 is a coronary vasodilator. Option #2 will be given to decrease pain. Option #4 augments the cardiac output by increasing myocardial con tractibility and stroke volume.

1.35 ④ This allows optimum pulmonary expansion. Sitting decreases the venous return to the heart which assists in lowering the ventricle's output and pulmonary congestion. Options #1, #2, and #3 do not enhance ventilation.

1.36 ① Option #1 helps establish equal, bilateral lung expansion. Intubation of the right mainstem bronchus would cause decreased or absent sounds in the left lung. Option #2 is not the appropriate first action. Option #3 will cause a delay in adjusting tube placement. Option #4 is not diagnostic. Waiting for this result will cause a delay in adjusting tube placement.

1.37 ③ Antacids are the most effective after digestion has started but prior to the emptying of the stomach. Option #1 will not be beneficial because they must be taken several times a day to be effective. Option #2 contains incorrect information. Option #4 is incorrect because antacids are used to prevent pain through protecting the gastric mucosa.

1.38 Answer: 10 gtts/min.

First convert 1 hour to 60 minutes to fit the formula.

Then set up a fraction. Place the volume of the infusion in the numerator. Place the number of minutes in which the volume is to be infused as the denominator.

$$\frac{40ml}{60\ min}$$

To determine X, or the number of drops per minute to be infused, multiply the fraction by the drip factor. Cancel units that appear in both the numerator and denominator.

$$X = \frac{40\ ml}{60\ min.} \times \frac{15\ gtt}{ml}$$

$$X = \frac{40 \times 15}{60\ min.}$$

$$X = \frac{60}{6} \quad X = 10\ gtts/min.$$

On the NCLEX®, you may have a box for your answer. Put only the number in the box.

1.39 ① This option is low both in sodium and fat. Option #2 contains selections (hot dog and canned soup) high in sodium. Option #3 is incorrect due to the avocado salad which is high in fat. Option #4 includes baked ham which is high in sodium.

1.40 ③ The problem needs to be taken care of now. If the LPN continues to make mistakes in client care, then a counseling report should be done. An LPN is expected to understand the importance of this requested procedure. Options #1, #2, and #4 are not appropriate at this time.

1.41 ② This option lists critical information that is significant to the safety and quality of the client's care. Other items are important, but not a priority to #2.

1.42 ③ This indicates the action of a client advocate and dealing with the immediate situation. Option #1 would not be done in front of a client. Options #2 and #4 are not addressing the immediate problem.

1.43

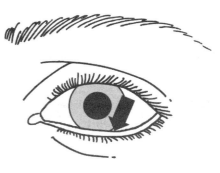

1.44 ③ The initial nursing priority for all psychiatric patients is to ensure their safety and the safety of all members of the milieu. Options #1, #2, and #4 are extremely important but secondary to safety issues.

1.45 ① Clinical findings which indicate elder abuse may include: poor nutrition, hygiene, poor skin integrity, dehydration, missed physician appointments, etc. Option #2 may be associated with several factors. Disorientation may be a result of delirium or dementia (need for information for clarification). A decrease in the short-term memory may be a normal change with aging. Option #3 may be a result of lack of time or part of the home routine. Option #4 may be secondary to osteoporosis.

1.46 ④ Option #4 is correct. Option #1 is not as inclusive as #4. Option #2—blood should be verified with another nurse. Option #3 should be actual volume versus projected amount since the infusion may need to be discontinued prior to total amount being infused.

1.47 ① Encourage exploration of home routines so this can be incorporated into care plan. A toddler's sense of security comes through consistency. Options #2 and #4 are not priorities with a 3-year-old. Option #3 is incorrect since "rooming in" is encouraged with this developmental state.

1.48 ③ It is important to evaluate the 3:00 AM blood sugar to determine if the hyperglycemia is from the somoygi effect. Options #1 and #4 will be adjusted after knowing if the AM blood sugar is the accurate reading or a rebound response to a low blood sugar at 3:00 AM. Option #2 is incorrect.

1.49 ③ Sterile fields should be set up above the waist. Option #1 will not maintain sterility. Option #2 is incorrect because gowns are not always necessary. Option #4 is incorrect because supplies can be opened with bare hands, but touched inside the package with sterile gloves.

1.50 ④ The priority intervention is to assess the client's airway. Option #1 is done only if the nurse is unable to determine the problem. Option #2 would be appropriate after the client assessment. Option #3 contains inappropriate information. The alarm may be silenced but not deactivated.

1.51 ② The surgical consent should be rechecked prior to going to surgery. Options #1, #3, and #4 should be done prior to one hour before surgery.

1.52 ④ An undesirable effect of prednisone may be hyperglycemia. It is important to monitor the glucose since prednisone is working in direct opposition to the action of sulfonlyureas. Sulfonylureas stimulate insulin release from the beta cells in the pancreas resulting in a lower serum glucose. Options #1, #2, and #3 are incorrect.

1.53 ① The initial specimen is to remove the residual urine prior to the collection. Options #2, #3, and #4 contain incorrect information.

1.54 ③ This will assist in restoring potassium which is depleted through diuresing. Option #1 is inappropriate since it does not have any potassium to assist in correcting the depletion. Option #2 is too high in sodium, and it counteracts the effectiveness of giving Lasix. Option #4 is ineffective in restoring the potassium.

1.55 ③ After a bronchoscopy, the client should be assessed for symptoms of respiratory distress from swelling due to the procedure. Signs of respiratory distress include tachypnea, tachycardia, respiratory stridor, and retractions. Option #1 does occur and could become a complication if the client is given fluids before reflex has returned. Option #2 is common for a few days after a biopsy. Option #4 is not associated with the procedure, but is a sign of intracranial pressure.

1.56 ② Oral steroids have ulcerogenic properties and need to be administered with meals. Options #1, #3, and #4 contain incorrect information for the administration of steroids.

1.57 ④ A cough or gag reflex and swallowing reflex may be affected by the increased pressure, increasing the incidence of aspiration. Options #1 and #2 increase intracranial pressure. Option #3 is incorrect because the head of the bed should be elevated 15 to 30 degrees to promote venous drainage.

1.58 ③ This is the question that identifies the ability of parents to support the emotional needs of their children as separate human beings. Options #1, #2, and #4 are important questions to ask during the assessment, but are not directly related to the issue of emotional support.

1.59 ③ When a client is admitted to a general medical, surgical, or critical care unit for another physical problem, the nurse may become the case finder and must be alert for subtle symptoms of an alcohol-related problem. The client who has several complaints of pain that do not appear related to the admissions problem requires a further investigation. Tremors, elevated temperature, and pain may be indicative of an alcohol-related problem. Option #1 is more indicative of a dysphoric or depressed, medically ill client. Option #2 could warrant further exploration of alcohol use. Option #4 is more indicative of withdrawal from narcotics or an infective problem such as tuberculosis.

1.60 ③ This age of child puts everything in their mouth, so they could put an object in the tracheostomy. This creates a risk for airway obstruction. Option #1 is not a priority to #3 due to the possibility of airway obstruction. Option #2 is a concern, but not a priority. Option #4 is incorrect because while this home may have older paint, which would present a risk with lead poisoning, this age of child does not have a tendency to put objects in the mouth.

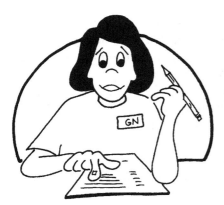

This page is for your notes!

Safe Effective Care:
Management of Care,
Safety and Infection Control

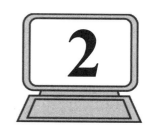

All our dreams can come true
if we have the courage to pursue them
—Walt Disney

✔ **Clarification of this test...**

The minimum standard includes performing and directing activities that manage client care. Activities that may be tested in this chapter include:

☛ Apply principles of infection control (hand-washing, room assignment, isolation, aseptic/sterile technique, universal/standard precautions).

☛ Ensure proper identification of client when providing care.

☛ Maintain client confidentiality/privacy.

☛ Ensure appropriate and safe use of equipment in performing client care procedures and treatments.

☛ Protectect client from injury (falls, electrical hazards, malfunctioning equipment).

☛ Evaluate and document responses to procedures and treatments.

☛ Collaborate with health care members in other disciplines when providing care.

☛ Receive and/or transcribe primary health care provider orders.

☛ Provide and receive report on assigned clients.

☛ Plan safe, cost effective care for the client.

☛ Initiate and update plan of care, care map, clinical pathway used to guide and evaluate client care.

☛ Recognize tasks/assignments you are not prepared to perform and seek assistance.

☛ Ensure that client has given informed consent for treatment.

☛ Educate client and family about client's rights and responsibilities.

☛ Follow procedures for handling biohazardous materials.

☛ Perform procedures necessary for admitting, transferring or discharging a client.

☛ Supervise care provided by others (LPN, VN, assistive personnel, other RNs).

☛ Initiate and update plan of care, care map, clinical pathway used to guide and evaluate client care.

☛ Assess/triage client(s) to prioritize the order of care delivery.

2.1 The physician's order reads: "100cc D_5W with 80 mEQ of KCL to infuse in 1/2 hour." Your first action will be to:

  ①   assess urine output.
  ②   ensure the patency of the IV line.
  ③   request an order for Lidocaine to be added to the IV.
  ④   check the accuracy of the order.

2.2 A client diagnosed with acquired immunodeficiency syndrome (AIDS) is admitted to a medical unit for treatment of dehydration secondary to diarrhea. Which nursing action is necessary to prevent nosocomial infection?

  ①   Provide room with an intercom.
  ②   Use sterile sheet whenever possible.
  ③   Use chux to prevent skin irritation.
  ④   Use a doughnut foam ring on coccyx.

2.3 The nurse is changing a dressing on an infected abdominal wound with Penrose drains and a large amount of purulent drainage. What is the best way to perform this procedure?

  ①   Obtain clean gloves and dressings, remove the soiled dressing, and use another pair of clean gloves to dress the wound.
  ②   Use clean gloves to remove the soiled dressings, change to sterile gloves and use sterile dressings to cover the wound.
  ③   Use the sterile gloves to remove the dressing, obtain clean gloves and sterile dressing to reapply to the wound.
  ④   Initiate protective isolation, utilize only sterile gloves when removing the dressing, and reapply using sterile technique.

2.4 A client with a history of cardiac disease is admitted to the hospital with a diagnosis of congestive heart failure. The doctor's orders are: continue all previous medications which include digoxin (Lanoxin) .25 mg po each AM, and propranolol (Inderal) 20 mg po tid; oxygen at 4L/minute via nasal cannula, establish an IV and give furosemide (Lasix) 40 mg IV now, bathroom privileges, full liquid diet. Which part of the order would be a priority for the nurse to discuss with the doctor?

  ①   Digoxin (Lanoxin) 0.25 mg PO in AM.
  ②   Level of oxygen concentration.
  ③   Propranolol (Inderal) 20 mg tid.
  ④   How fast should the IV infuse?

2.5 Which assignment is the most appropriate for a client in the burn unit who has a cytomegalovirus (CMV) infection? A nurse who:

  ①   has an upper respiratory infection.
  ②   is eight weeks pregnant.
  ③   is CMV negative.
  ④   has thirty years experience.

2.6 Which measure should a nurse take to prevent the spread of active pulmonary tuberculosis?

  ①   Restrict visitors to immediate family only.
  ②   Wear gown and gloves at all times.
  ③   Wear mask and gloves when in direct contact.
  ④   Dispose of waste articles more frequently.

2.7 The nurse observes that a fire has started in the client's room. Which action should the nurse take first?

  ①   Confine the fire to the client's room.
  ②   Extinguish the fire.
  ③   Pull the fire alarm.
  ④   Rescue the client.

2.8 A 54-year-old client with tertiary syphilis is admitted to a nursing unit exhibiting signs of marked dementia and disorientation. Which nursing action should be done initially?

  ①   Place the nurse call bell within reach.
  ②   Frequently observe client behavior.
  ③   Apply a vest-type restraint.
  ④   Provide an around-the-clock sitter.

2.9 A client with a necrotizing spider bite is to perform dressing changes at home. Which statement made by the client indicates a correct understanding of aseptic technique?

  ①   "I need to buy sterile gloves to redress this wound."
  ②   "I should wash my hands before redressing my wound."
  ③   "I should not expose the wound to air at all."
  ④   "I should use an over-the-counter antimicrobial ointment."

2.10 Which room assignment is most appropriate for an adult male client who has sustained a second degree burn over 10% of the body?

   ① A semi-private room with a male client undergoing chemotherapy.
   ② A semi-private room with a male client who is three days post abdominal surgery.
   ③ A semi-private room with a male pediatric client.
   ④ A semi-private room with a male client admitted for chest pain.

2.11 Which observation indicates the need for a nurse to stay with a client admitted to the emergency room following a car wreck?

   ① Disorientation and irregular vital signs.
   ② Irregular vital signs and hostility.
   ③ Rapid respirations and agitation.
   ④ Elevated vital signs and apprehension.

2.12 In planning the debridment of a burn, a nurse would give priority to which action?

   ① Assemble all necessary supplies and medications.
   ② Organize time for dressing change and provide emotional support.
   ③ Prepare the client and family for the pain the client will experience during and after the procedure.
   ④ Limit visitation prior to procedure to reduce client stress.

2.13 A city council person is admitted to the hospital after experiencing chest pain at a ribbon-cutting ceremony. A journalist from the newspaper contacts the hospital's nursing supervisor and asks her for a report on the client's status. Prior to giving information to the journalist, it is most important for the supervisor to:

   ① Advise the journalist of HIPAA guidelines.
   ② Contact the hospital's chief executive officer.
   ③ Ensure the journalist is authorized to receive such information.
   ④ Obtain signed authorization from the client.

2.14 During the insertion of a central venous pressure monitor, the tip of the monitor device brushes the underside of the sterile field. Which nursing action is most appropriate?

   ① Wipe the tip with alcohol before connecting to system.
   ② Notify the physician of the occurrence so an antibiotic can be given.
   ③ Back-flush catheter for several seconds before connecting.
   ④ Obtain a new monitor device, and prepare for a second attempt.

2.15 Which postoperative nursing goal will assist in preventing deep vein thrombosis?

   ① Decrease the flow of the venous blood.
   ② Increase the coagulation of the blood.
   ③ Increase the flow of the venous blood.
   ④ Improve the oxygen capacity of the blood.

2.16 During the history, a client reports a previous allergic reaction to penicillin. The provider of care orders Cefaclor (Ceclor). What is the highest priority of care?

   ① Immediately start an IV.
   ② Identify wrist bracelet for correct client identity.
   ③ Verify accuracy of order.
   ④ Monitor BUN and creatinine prior to administering the medication.

2.17 A client with chronic lung disease is admitted to the acute pulmonary unit with: respiratory rate of 50; pulse of 140 and irregular; skin pale and cool to touch; client confused as to place and time. Orders are: oxygen per nasal cannula at 4L/minute, bed rest, soft diet and pulmonary function tests in the AM. What is the best sequence of nursing activities?

   ① Place in semi-Fowler's position, begin the oxygen, have someone stay with the client, then notify the doctor regarding the current status of the client.
   ② Begin the oxygen, call the nursing supervisor, keep the bed flat to maintain blood pressure, and stimulate client to take deep breaths.
   ③ Call the nursing supervisor, discuss with the family if the client has experienced this problem before, offer the client sips of clear liquids.
   ④ Advise respiratory therapy of the client's problem, place the client in semi-Fowler's position, and begin the oxygen.

2.18 The nurse arrives for the day shift and receives her assignments around 7:30 a.m. The assignment includes:

- a man with a diagnosis of rule-out an MI. He is on a monitor and having 4-6 premature beats per hour.
- an elderly lady who is confused and has constant urinary dribbling.
- a pneumonia client with increasing confusion and a temperature of 104° at 6:30 a.m.
- a diabetic client who experienced a restless night and 7:00 a.m. blood sugar was 170mg%.

Which client is a priority and how should the nurse plan the care?

① The pneumonia client has priority; his condition should be assessed immediately.
② The elderly lady is probably wet and uncomfortable and should be taken care of first. Then obtain a stat blood glucose to determine the diabetic client's current blood sugar level.
③ The cardiac client should be assessed immediately as the monitor indicates cardiac irritability. Then the temperature on the pneumonia client should be reassessed.
④ The diabetic client should be seen immediately to assess for evidence of hyperglycemia. Then the pneumonia client should be assessed for patency of airway.

2.19 Which nursing observation is most important to report to the physician on a client with a second-degree thermal injury to right arm?

① Pain around the periphery of injury.
② Gastric pH less than 6.0.
③ Increased edema of right arm.
④ An elevated hematocrit.

2.20 What action is the most important before administering any medication?

① verifying orders with another nurse.
② counting medication in the medication cart drawers.
③ documenting the medication given.
④ checking the client's identification and allergies.

2.21 A postoperative client is receiving bupivacain hydrochloride (Marcaine) for pain through an epidural catheter. Which response should the nurse recognize as desirable for this pain management technique?

① Decreased respirations.
② Somnolence.
③ Decreased restlessness.
④ Decreased blood pressure.

2.22 At 5:00 p.m., the nurse on the evening shift opens the nurses' notes and discovers that the last entry was at 9:00 a.m. The day nurse did not complete the charting and did not sign the nurses' notes. The best action for the evening nurse is to:

① leave a note on the front of the chart for the day nurse to make a late entry and begin charting on the line below the last entry on the nurse's notes.
② leave enough space for the day nurse to complete her charting when she comes in the next morning.
③ not chart anything until the day nurse returns to complete the charting for her care delivered that morning.
④ call the day nurse and ask her about the care she gave that morning so the evening nurse can complete the chart.

2.23 Which assignment would be appropriate for the Labor and Delivery (L&D) nurse who will be working for one shift on the Medical Surgical unit?

① A 3-year-old with croup
② A 30-year-old with malignant hypertension
③ A 40-year-old with unstable angina
④ A 50-year-old with congestive heart failure

2.24 A client has returned from surgery with a fine reddened rash noted around the area where Betadine prep had been applied prior to surgery. Nursing documentation in the chart should include:

① the time and circumstances in which the rash was noted.
② explanation to client and family the reason for rash.
③ notation on an allergy list and notification of the physician.
④ application of corticosteroid cream to decrease inflammation.

2.25 The nurse is changing the dressing on a client with a large abdominal wound. There are two Penrose drains in place. What is the priority information for the nurse to include when recording this procedure?

① Condition of the surrounding tissue, time necessary to change the dressing, the type of dressing used.

② Client's tolerance of the procedure, time the dressing was changed, amount of wound drainage.

③ Client's response to the dressing change, status of Penrose drains, type of drainage from Penrose drains.

④ Time dressing was changed, description of the wound, color and amount of drainage from Penrose drains.

2.26 A client is admitted to the emergency room after a motor vehicle accident. He does not remember the accident. He is awake, oriented to person, but does not know what city he is in. He is confused regarding the day and month. Pupils are equal in size and equally reactive to direct light reflex. He is complaining of a severe headache and is becoming restless. The priority of care for this client is to:

① continue to stimulate the client to keep him oriented to his surroundings.

② restrain the client to prevent him from injuring himself.

③ perform bedside neuro checks every fifteen minutes.

④ administer Meperidine hydrochloride (Demerol) for pain control and to decrease restlessness.

2.27 After establishing IV access, what would be the best for the nurse to document immediately after procedure?

① The type of catheter used and number of venipuncture attempts.

② The type of IV fluid hung and equipment used.

③ The date, time, venipuncture site, type and gauge of catheter, and IV fluid hung.

④ Type, amount, and flow rate of IV fluid, condition of IV site.

2.28 Which would be the most appropriate to assign to the LPN?

① A client who is being discharged and needs new diabetic teaching.

② A client who is a new admission with chest pain.

③ A client who is receiving chemotherapy.

④ A client who has the diagnosis of Myasthenia Gravis.

2.29 While assessing the incision of a 2-day postoperative client, a shiny pink open area is noted with underlying visible bowel. Which action should the nurse take first?

① Cover gaping area with sterile gauze soaked in normal saline.

② Reapply sterile dressing after cleaning with peroxide.

③ Pack opened area with sterile ¾ inch gauze soaked in normal saline.

④ Apply Neosporin ointment and cover with Tegaderm dressing.

2.30 Which intervention indicates the nurse has an understanding of safe medication administration for the pediatric client?

① Validate the order with the chart after the medication has been administered.

② Verify client identify by looking at the arm bracelet prior to administering the medication.

③ Contact the pharmacist for clarification of all the possible adverse reactions which may occur prior to giving any medication.

④ Administer the medication in the child's formula to prevent an increase in anxiety.

2.31 Which nursing implication is important regarding spinal anesthesia?

① The client should be adequately hydrated in order to prevent hypotension after anesthesia is established.

② The client must be NPO at least 12 hours prior to the initiation of the anesthesia to decrease the risk of aspiration.

③ Assess the client for any allergies to Betadine or iodine preparations.

④ Determine the specific gravity of the urine and prepare the client for a central line.

2.32 Which of these clients should be triaged first?
A 74-year-old client:

① who is taking NSAIDs for arthritic pain, experiencing epigastric pain, HR – 90.
② who has a decline in the cranial nerve #1, reporting a problem with presbyscusis and prebyopia.
③ with thin skin, alteration in depth perception, and episodes of incontinence.
④ with fixed, dilated pupils, and is asystole.

2.33 Which symptom would cause a nurse to be concerned about post infusion phlebitis in a client who has been on an IVPB antibiotic mixed in D_5W every 8 hours for four days?

① Tenderness at the IV site.
② Increased swelling at the insertion site.
③ Reddened area or red streaks at the site.
④ Leaking of fluid around the IV catheter.

2.34 After taking the vital signs of a client returning from abdominal exploratory surgery, which action should be taken next?

① Position the client on her left side supported with pillows.
② Check the chart and determine the status of fluid balance from surgery.
③ Check the client's abdominal dressing for any evidence of bleeding.
④ Monitor the incision and pulmonary status for presence of infection.

2.35 To evaluate the adverse reactions from antibiotic therapy in a client with a postoperative infection and receiving ceftriaxone sodium (Rocephin) IVPB every day, the nurse should monitor:

① surface of the tongue.
② hemoglobin and hematocrit.
③ skin surfaces in skin folds.
④ changes in urine characteristics.

2.36 When irrigating a draining wound with a sterile saline solution, which sequence would be most appropriate for the nurse to follow?

① Pour solution, wash hands, and remove soiled dressing.
② Wash hands, prepare sterile field, remove soiled dressing.
③ Prepare sterile field, put on sterile gloves, and remove soiled dressing.
④ Remove soiled dressing, flush wound, wash hands.

2.37 To maintain client safety, which equipment should be readily available when inserting an Ewall tube?

① Suction equipment
② Blood pressure cuff
③ Levine tube
④ Emesis basin

2.38 Which would have the highest priority when caring for a terminally ill client during the final stage of dying?

① Encourage family to discuss legal matters with an attorney.
② Provide privacy for the client and his family to spend time together.
③ Keep client sedate.
④ Encourage family to limit visiting hours so they can rest.

2.39 The charge nurse demonstrates an understanding of appropriate delegation when she makes which client assignment to the LPN?

① A psychotic client
② A client receiving chemotherapy
③ A client in Buck's traction
④ A client receiving a blood transfusion

2.40 Which statement indicates the client has an appropriate understanding of how to adequately use the Albuterol and Vanceril inhalers?

① "I will wait 10 minutes between the 2 medications."
② "It doesn't matter how long I wait or the order in which they are taken."
③ "I will wait 2-3 minutes between taking the Vanceril and the Albuterol inhalers."
④ "I will wait 1-3 minutes between taking the Albuterol and Vanceril inhalers."

2.41 To protect a post heart transplant client from potential sources of infection, the nurse would:

  ① keep client in total isolation.
  ② limit participation in unit activities.
  ③ adhere to and monitor strict hand-washing techniques.
  ④ monitor vital signs, especially temperature, every 2 hours.

2.42 Which instruction is correct regarding the colletion of a specimen from a 4-year-old suspected of having pinworms?

  ① Collect the specimen 30 minutes after the child falls asleep at night.
  ② Save a portion of the child's first stool of the day, and take it to the physician's office immediately.
  ③ Collect the specimen in the early morning with a piece of scotch tape touched to the child's anus.
  ④ Feed the child a high fat meal; then save the first stool following the meal.

2.43 Which nursing action has the highest priority for a teenager admitted with burns to 50% of the body?

  ① Counseling regarding problems of body image.
  ② Maintain respiratory isolation.
  ③ Maintain aseptic technique during procedures.
  ④ Encourage peers to visit on a regular basis.

2.44 Which observation indicates a mother needs further teaching regarding protecting the newborn from infection?

  ① Applies alcohol to the umbilical cord after a diaper change.
  ② Positions the diaper below the umbilicus.
  ③ Does not wash her hands prior to handling the newborn.
  ④ Applies sterile gauze with petroleum jelly to the circumcision.

2.45 To promote safety in the care of a client receiving internal radiation therapy, the nurse would:

  ① restrict visitors who may have an upper respiratoryinfection.
  ② assign only male care givers to the client.
  ③ plan nursing activities to decrease nurse exposure.
  ④ wear a lead lined apron whenever delivering client care.

2.46 To promote safety in the environment of a client with a marked depression of T cells, the nurse would:

  ① keep a linen hamper immediately outside the room.
  ② use sterile linens.
  ③ provide masks for anyone entering the room.
  ④ discard any standing water left in containers or equipment.

2.47 After the nurse receives report, which of these clients should be assessed first?

  ① a client with COPD who is experiencing some shortness of breath with exertion.
  ② a client who had a CVA and has been hospitalized for 1 week.
  ③ a client who had a laminectomy 2 days ago and is complaining of pain.
  ④ a client with diabetes who is diaphoretic, with nausea, and is vomiting.

2.48 Which nursing observation would indicate a major complication in a client who suffered a thermal injury two weeks ago?

  ① Increased heart rate and elevated blood pressure.
  ② Temperature of 100.6°F and decreased respiratory rate.
  ③ Increased heart rate and decreased respiratory rate.
  ④ Increased respiratory rate and decreased blood pressure.

2.49 Which nursing action regarding intubation equipment/ supplies is most appropriate following intubation of a postoperative client who had a respiratory arrest?

  ① Soak the intubation equipment in concentrated Betadine solution.
  ② Place intubation blade in bag and arrange for gas sterilization.
  ③ Soak intubation blade in Cidex solution.
  ④ Wash with soap and water and allow to air dry.

2.50 Which statement concerning the transmission of head lice would be most important for the nurse to teach?

  ① Head lice occur primarily in lower socioeconomic groups.
  ② Transmission is airborne through insect vectors.
  ③ Infestation is reduced in cold weather.
  ④ Transmission is most common where there are crowded living conditions.

2.51 What is the correct procedure for obtaining a throat culture from a client with pharyngitis?

   ① Quickly rub a cotton swab over both tonsillar areas and posterior pharynx.
   ② Obtain a sputum container for the client to use.
   ③ Following irrigation with warm saline, the pharynx is swabbed.
   ④ Hyperextend the client's head and neck for the procedure.

2.52 Which technique is correct when changing a large abdominal dressing on an incision with a Penrose drain?

   ① Remove dressing layers one at a time.
   ② Clean the wound with Betadine solution and hydrogen peroxide.
   ③ Clean drainage area first.
   ④ If the dressing adheres to the wound, pull gently and firmly.

2.53 The nurse comes out of report and has several orders to initiate with a client who has R-28 and is congested, HR-90, and T-102.4. Which of these orders should be implemented first?

   ① Blood cultures.
   ② Evaluate vital signs.
   ③ Start an IV.
   ④ Start Rocephin.

2.54 Which nursing observation would indicate a serious complication of impetigo?

   ① White patches on buccal mucosa.
   ② Hearing loss.
   ③ Respiratory wheezes.
   ④ Periorbital edema.

2.55 Which assignment would be most appropriate to assign to the pregnant nurse?

   ① A client with HIV.
   ② A client with a cervical radium implant.
   ③ A client with syphilis.
   ④ A client with cytomegalovirus (CMV).

2.56 How should the nurse administer the DPT immunization to a 6-month old?

   ① By mouth in three divided doses.
   ② As an IM injection into the gluteus maximus.
   ③ As an injection into the vastus lateralis.
   ④ As a Z track injection into the deltoid.

2.57 After the nurse receives shift report, which of these clients should the nurse assess first?

   ① A 30-year-old female client refusing to take cimetidine (Tagamet) before breakfast.
   ② A 40-year-old male client scheduled for a cholecystectomy and complaining of chills.
   ③ A 50-year-old female client with right-sided weakness, asking to go to the bathroom.
   ④ A 60-year-old male with an NG tube who had a bowel resection 2 days ago.

2.58 Which action is necessary to maintain asepsis during a sterile dressing change?

   ① After scrubbing for the procedure, hold your elbows close to your body.
   ② Unused sterile dressing tray can be used for the next client if used within 15 minutes.
   ③ If you splash a liquid on the sterile field, start over again.
   ④ If you drop a dressing, leave it until you have completed the procedure.

2.59 Which statement made by a parent indicates a correct understanding of poison prevention at home?

   ① "We store gasoline for the lawn mower in the garage."
   ② "All our medications are kept in their original containers."
   ③ "We keep all our cleaning products in the bathroom."
   ④ "I keep most of our medications in my purse."

2.60 Which sequence is correct when providing care for a client immediately prior to surgery?

   ① Administer preoperative medication, client signs operative permit, determine vital signs.
   ② Check operative permit for signature, advise client to remain in bed, administer preoperative medication.
   ③ Remove client's dentures, administer preoperative medication, client empties bladder.
   ④ Verify client has been NPO. Client empties bladder; family leaves room.

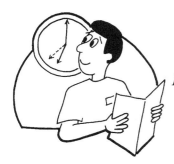

Hey! Why don't you take a break!

Answers & Rationales

2.1 ④ Potassium chloride must be diluted and administered at a rate no faster than 20mEq/hr. Options #1 and #2 are correct after the order has been corrected. Option #3, Lidocaine, should not be added to this IV.

2.2 ② Diarrhea predisposes AIDS clients to decubiti which can lead to significant infection. Therefore, sterile sheets are indicated to reduce risk. Options #1, #3, and #4 do not decrease the risk of infection.

2.3 ② Sterile gloves and dressings are used in the application of dressings to wounds. Option #4 is incorrect because protective isolation is not appropriate for this client. Sterile gloves are not necessary for removing the soiled dressings.

2.4 ③ Inderal is contraindicated in clients with CHF. It is possible the doctor overlooked this in reordering all of the client's previous medications. The oxygen, and digoxin are appropriate. There is no specific order regarding the rate of infusion or any fluids to be infused. Since the client is on po fluids, this is probably a heparin/saline lock. This order should be clarified. However, Option #3 is a priority.

2.5 ④ This option is most appropriate due to a decreased risk of being infected. Option #1 is incorrect because those with a cytomegalovirus positive titer are often immunosuppressed clients who should be protected from other pathogens. Option #2 is incorrect because CMV is fetotoxic, and those who are pregnant should not care for CMV+ clients. Option #3 is incorrect because those with no protective titer are an increased risk for developing the disease if exposed.

2.6 ③ Respiratory precautions call for masks and gloves to be worn to prevent the spread of the causative organism. Options #1, #2, and #4 are not essential in respiratory isolation.

2.7 ④ Option #4 is correct. Rescuing the client is always the priority. "RACE" will assist you in remembering fire safety. R = rescue client; A = activate an alarm; C = confine the fire; and E -= extinguish the fire.

2.8 ② Placing the client on frequent observation status would be the first action to ensure the client's safety. Option #1 is incorrect because it should not be assumed that the client will be able to use the call light appropriately. Option #3 should never be the first option used by a professional nurse. Current standards require not only a physician's order, but a time limit, exact type of restraint to be used, and the specific rationale for restraint. Option #4 may be suggested to the family at a later time.

2.9 ② The hallmark of asepsis is hand-washing. Option #1 is incorrect because the question addresses medical aseptic technique, not sterile procedure. Option #3 is not necessary. Option #4 is incorrect because the client should use only prescribed medications on the wound.

2.10 ① Both clients have lost major protective mechanisms and are at risk for infection. Options #2 and #3 and #4 are incorrect due to the infection risk they pose.

2.11 ① A disoriented client with irregular vital signs represents a grave safety risk. Options #2, #3, and #4 may increase the need for nursing interaction/assessment and are secondary to\ Option #1.

2.12 ② Prior planning for burn wound treatment should include organizing and planning for the mechanics of the procedure as well as the emotional support necessary for the client. Options #1, #3, and #4 may be appropriate but do not take priority over Option #2.

2.13 ④ Option #4 is correct. Maintaining client confidentiality/privacy is most important to this situation. Options #1, #2, and #3 do not address this concern with privacy. These answers focus on the journalist and hospital. The correct answer is the answer that is client-focused.

2.14 ④ Contamination of equipment mandates new equipment be employed. Options #1 and #3 are not adequate—the catheter is still contaminated. Option #2 may be appropriate later, but obtaining a new monitoring device is a priority.

2.15 ③ It is important to prevent venous stasis by increasing the flow of venous return. Options #1 and #2 will increase the risk associated with DVT. Option #4 will not affect the course of deep vein thrombosis.

2.16 ③ Option #3 is correct. Clients who have a hypersensitivity to penicillin may experience the same reaction to Cefaclor (Ceclor). Option #1 is incorrect. Option #2 is important but Option #3 is a priority in this situation. Option #4 is a consideration for this drug, but is not a priority when drug order may be unsafe.

2.17 ① The doctor's orders do not address the seriousness of the client's condition. The doctor should be notified immediately. However, the client should not be left alone. Options #2, #3, and #4 do not address the seriousness of the client's immediate needs.

2.18 ① The sickest client is the pneumonia client, and his needs should be addressed first. This client has an increased temperature, which may indicate his pneumonia is getting worse; and his confusion may be indicative of hypoxia. His status should be evaluated immediately. Premature beats of 4-6 per hour are benign and not unusual for a cardiac client. The elderly lady may be uncomfortable, but the respiratory status of the pneumonia client is priority. A blood sugar of 170 mg% is abnormally high and should be addressed. However, the respiratory status of the pneumonia client is the highest priority.

2.19 ② A decrease in gastric pH could indicate the hypersecretion of hydrogen ions—a predisposing factor to stress ulcer formation. Options #1, #3, and #4 are expected findings in burn wound resolution.

2.20 ④ Option #4 is correct. The priority of care prior to administering nay medication is to verify the identify of the client. A large number of medication errors are a result of administering the medication to the wrong client. The other options are not correct for this question.

2.21 ③ A decrease in physiological shortness of breath and restlessness is a desired outcome criteria of pain management. Options #1, #2, and #4 are undesired responses.

2.22 ① The best way to handle the situation is to begin charting on the next line and have the day nurse make a late entry for the omitted information. Options #2, #3, and #4 would be illegal.

2.23 ② Option #2 is correct. The L&D nurse provides care for clients with pregnancy induced hypertension. These assessments and plans of care would correlate with the nurse's skills. Options #1, #3, and #4 would not be appropriate for this nurse. L&D nurses do not routinely provide care for children. Options #3 and #4 require an understanding of cardiology.

2.24 ③ Any suspected reaction to drugs should be reported to the physician and noted on the list of possible allergies. Option #1 would be noted, but is not as high a priority as Option #3. Options #2 and #4 are inappropriate.

2.25 ④ The information in Option #4 best describes the essential information that should be charted after a dressing change for a wound of this type. Options #1, #2 and #3 contain important information. However, the information in #4 is more important.

2.26 ③ The client may be developing increased intra-cranial pressure and should be monitored closely. Option #4, Demerol, is not given for pain control. It will mask the signs of increased intracranial pressure. Option #2, restraining, is not necessary at this time, and pulling against restraints will increase intracranial pressure. Option #1, continued stimulation, does not provide any benefit for this client.

2.27 ③ Option #3 is the most correct answer. Options #1 and #2 are appropriate but not as inclusive as Option #3. Option #4 should be included in the once-per-shift documentation. This question states "after establishing IV access."

2.28 ④ Option #1 is incorrect because it requires initia teaching. The LPN can reinforce teaching, but it is currently not in the scope of practice to do the initial teaching. Option #2 would require initial assessment. LPNs can do on-going assessment, but it is not in the scope of practice to complete the initial assessment. Option #3 would require IV management and specialized assessment skills so it is not a priority to Option #4.

2.29 ① Evisceration is treated immediately by application of sterile gauze soaked in sterile normal saline followed by notification of the physician. Options #2, #3, and #4 are not correct responses to this complication.

2.30 ② It is imperative to verify the identity prior to implementing any procedure with any client. Medication errors often result from inappropriate identification. Option #1 is incorrect because it should be validated prior to administering it. Option #3 is unnecessary. Nurses must be aware of possible side effects as well as adverse reactions; however, it is not necessary to address with the pharmacist prior to every drug. Option #4 is inappropriate since the child may refuse the bottle. It should be given with a medication syringe or dropper.

2.31 ① It is important that the client be well hydrated to prevent hypotensive problems after the spinal anesthesia is initiated. Option #2 is unnecessary. Option #3 is not necessary as iodine dyes are usually not used. Option #4 is irrelevant to the procedure.

2.32 ① Option #1 is correct. This client is presenting with symptoms of a bleeding ulcer with the history of the NSAIDs and the location of the pain and elevated heart rate. Options #2 and #3 are normal findings and do not need to be triaged. Option #4—the client is dead.

2.33 ③ Postinfusion phlebitis is characterized by inflammation and reddened areas around the site of needle puncture and up the length of the vein. Option #1 is fairly common. Option #2 may be indicative of infiltration. Option #4 is not indicative of phlebitis.

2.34 ③ The dressing should be checked on admission to the room and frequently for several hours. Options #1 and #2 are not priority at this time. Option #4 is inappropriate as it is too soon for infection to occur secondary to surgery.

2.35 ① Long-term use of Rocephin can cause over-growth of organisms such as *Candida albicans*; therefore, monitoring of the tongue and oral cavity is recommended. Options #2, #3, and #4 do not reflect a problem with this medication.

2.36 ② Hand-washing should be done prior to beginning any procedure—especially irrigating a wound. Options #1, #3, and #4 are in the incorrect sequence.

2.37 ① The Ewall tube is a large orogastric tube designed for rapid lavage. Insertion often causes gagging and vomiting such that suction equipment must be immediately available to reduce risky aspiration. Options #2, #3, and #4 are not as high priority.

2.38 ② A priority is to provide privacy. Options #1 and #3 are inappropriate at this time. Option #4 is partially correct about rest, but incorrect regarding the limiting of visiting hours.

2.39 ③ This client is the lowest acuity out of the group and requires the least specialized care. The scope of practice for the LPN would allow her to care for this client. Options #1, #2, and #4 require care from the RN which is out of the LPN's scope of practice.

2.40 ④ The bronchodilator should be taken prior to the steroid inhaler and a period of 1–3 minutes should be between the 2 medications. Options #1, #2, and #3 are incorrect.

2.41 ③ One of the most important nursing strategies with a client who is immunosuppressed is adherence to, and monitoring hand-washing of others to prevent transmission of sources of infection. Option #1 is not necessary although a private room might be helpful. Option #2 would allow the client to further withdraw and limits their opportunities for corrective milieu experiences. Option #4 is more often than necessary unless there is a temperature elevation.

2.42 ③ Pinworms crawl outside the anus early in the morning to lay their eggs. This specimen should be collected early in the morning before the child awakens. Option #1 is not the optimum time for collecting the eggs and may result in a false negative test. Option #2 is incorrect because pinworms are rarely found in the stool. Option #4 is incorrect protocol for this test.

2.43 ③ Safety is a priority for the client who is at high risk for infection. Option #1 may be necessary at some point, but safety issues come first. Option #2 is incorrect because the appropriate isolation technique should be protective—not respiratory—isolation. Option #4 is important for an adolescent but is not a priority over safety.

2.44 ③ Proper hand-washing is a priority in preventing infection. Options #1, #2, and #4 are correct and do not indicate a need for further teaching.

2.45 ③ The principles for radiation safety are time, distance, and shielding. The nurse should decrease the time she spends at close distance to the client. Option #1 is incorrect because all visitors must keep distance from the client. Option #2 is incorrect since radiation is as harmful to males as to females. Option #4 is used when the nurse has to spend any length of time at close distance with the client—not for routine care.

2.46 ④ Water should not be allowed to stand in containers, such as respiratory or suction equipment, because this could act as a culture medium. Option #1 is incorrect because the protocol for handling soiled articles is accomplished within universal precautions guidelines using double biohazard bags. Option #2 is incorrect because sterile linens are used for burn and OR clients. Option #3 is not protocol unless the client or visitor has an active pulmonary infection.

2.47 ④ The diabetic client is presenting with hypoglycemia. This can be dangerous. Option #1 may be expected with COPD. Options #2 and #3 are not priorities to Option #4.

2.48 ④ Increased respiratory rate and decreased blood pressure may indicate burn wound sepsis—a life-threatening complication of thermal injury. Options #1, #2, and #3 should be investigated further but alone do not represent significant compromise.

2.49 ② Sterilization of equipment after exposure to body fluids of a client is protocol. Options #1, #3, and #4 are incorrect because they do not provide sterility.

2.50 ④ Crowded living conditions where there is sharing of clothing and physical closeness increases the likelihood of transmission. Option #1 is incorrect because head lice occur in all socio-economic levels. Option #2 is incorrect because lice are transmitted by close contact. Option #3 is incorrect because weather is not a deterrent although more cases are seen in the winter in some areas due to the sharing of hats.

2.51 ① The tonsilar and pharyngeal areas are quickly swabbed to avoid client discomfort. Option #2 is incorrect because this would not reflect throat bacteria. Option #3 should not be done to obtain an adequate sample for culture. Option #4 is incorrect because the client should hold his head upright—not hyperextended.

2.52 ① To avoid dislodging the drain, remove the dressing layers one at a time. Option #2 is incorrect because the wound should not be cleaned with both a Betadine solution and hydrogen peroxide. Option #3 is incorrect because the wound is cleaned from the center outward to the edges and from top to bottom. Option #4 could tear the skin and dislodge the drain.

2.53 ① The priority is to determine the organism the client is growing in order to determine the correct antibiotic. If the antibiotic, Option #4, is implemented first, then the blood cultures will not be accurate. Option #2 has been reported in the stem of the question and is not necessary to duplicate at this time. Option #3 is not a priority to Option #1.

2.54 ④ Periorbital edema is indicative of post-streptococcal glomerulonephritis, a possible complication of impetigo. Option #1 describes a fungal infection. Options #2 and #3 can be caused by many other factors.

2.55 ① An HIV client would not present a risk to the pregnant woman if she does not come in contact with the body secretions. Options #2, #3, and #4 could result in teratogenic effects to the fetus.

2.56 ③ Because the muscle mass of an infant is small, the intramuscular injection should be given in the lateral aspect of the thigh (vastus lateralis). Option #1 is incorrect since the injection is not administered PO. Option #2 is incorrect because the gluteus does not have enough muscle mass. Option #4 is not necessary, and the deltoid is an incorrect area for this method of administration.

2.57 ② Option #2 is correct. The client is scheduled for surgery and has a sign of infection (chills)! Option #1 does not give any indication of any complications or any specific information about the client to indicate he would be a priority. Option #3 does not require a nurse. This client does need assistance but the RN is not required for this client. Option #4 is high risk for potential complications, but none are indicated at this time. Option #2 has already developed a complication.

2.58 ④ To maintain a sterile field, all items in that field must remain sterile. Leave the contaminated dressing until the procedure is completed. Option #1 is incorrect because elbows are held away from the body. Option #2 is incorrect because sterile materials can be used only for one client; and if unused, must be discarded, or re-sterilized. Option #3 is unnecessary because a liquid can be covered with a sterile towel.

2.59 ② All medications should be kept in their original container and out of reach. Options #1, #3, and #4 are not appropriate safety measures to prevent accidental poisonings.

2.60 ② The operative permit must be signed prior to the client receiving his preoperative medication. The client is considered incapacitated after receiving a narcotic. Options #1 and #3 both administer the medication prior to the permit being signed. Option #4 is important information, but it is unnecessary for the family to leave the room.

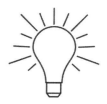

That's right!

Far out in the ocean
On a moonlit night,
A circle of dolphins
Slips out of sight.
They're on a mission
Of the grandest scale,
To spread the word
To every minnow and whale:
That life's an illusion
Just waiting for you—
To believe in your dreams
So that they can come true!
—Michael Dooley

Health Promotion and Maintenance

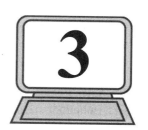

From what we get, we make a living;
what we give, however, makes a life.
—*Arthur Ashe*

✔ **Clarification of this test...**

The minimum standard includes performing and directiong activities that promote and maintain the health of client/family.

Activities in this chapter are not as heavily weighted as many of the activities in pharmacology or fluid-gas. Activities that may be tested in this chapter include:

- ☞ Identify client's allergy and intervene as needed (food, latex and other environmental allergies).
- ☞ Perform a risk assessment (sensory, impairment, potential for falls, level of mobility, skin integrity).
- ☞ Perform comprehensive health assessment (physical, psychosocial and health history).
- ☞ Provide care that meets special needs for the adult client 19–64 years.
- ☞ Provide care that meets special needs for the older client 65–85 years.
- ☞ Provide care that meets special needs for the older client over 85 years.
- ☞ Provide care that meets special needs for the preschool client ages 1 month to 4 years.
- ☞ Provide care that meets special needs for the school age client 7–12 years.
- ☞ Evaluate and monitor the client's height and weight.
- ☞ Provide care that meets special needs for the adolescent client 13–18 years.
- ☞ Provide perinatal education.
- ☞ Provide post-partum care.
- ☞ Assess rediness to learn, learning preferences and barriers to learning.
- ☞ Provide prenatal care.
- ☞ Perform age-specific screening examinations (scoliosis assessment, breast examinations, testicular examinations).
- ☞ Provide information about health maintenance recommendations (physician visits, immunizations).

3.1   What equipment would be necessary to complete an evaluation of cranial nerves 9 and 10 during a physical assessment?

  ① A cotton ball
  ② A pen light
  ③ An opthalmoscope
  ④ A tongue depressor and flashlight

3.2   A client that is involved in a homosexual relationship is scheduled for abdominal surgery. During surgery, the partner requests information regarding her status. What would be the appropriate response from the nurse?

  ① "The physician will be out to inform you after the surgery is complete."
  ② "HIPPA regulations and state laws will provide guidelines to assist with this decision."
  ③ "Let me go back and get an update. I will be right back with a report."
  ④ "She is doing fine; just sit back and relax."

3.3   As the nurse is making midnight rounds, a geriatric client complains that his feet are cold. Which action would the nurse do first?

  ① Examine the feet for presence of pulses and adequacy of circulation.
  ② Elevate the foot of the bed and rub the feet to increase circulation.
  ③ Fill a hot water bottle, wrap it in a case, and place on the feet.
  ④ Bring a warm drink to relax and warm the client.

3.4   Which technique would be best in caring for a client following receiving a diagnosis of a state IV tumor in the brain?

  ① Offering the client pamphlets on support groups for brain cancer.
  ② Asking the client if there is anything he or his family needs.
  ③ Reminding the client that advances in technology are occurring every day.
  ④ Providing accurate information about the disease process and treatment options.

3.5   A 14-year-old is first day postoperative after a Harrington Rod placement. Which sign would be most indicative of positive relief from the pain medication? Client:

  ① verbalizes pain has decreased.
  ② refuses more pain medicine.
  ③ is agitated with visitors in the room.
  ④ cooperates with incentive spirometry exercise.

3.6   A female client is diagnosed with human papilloma virus (HPV). Which client statement illustrates an understanding of the possible sequelae of this illness? "I will:

  ① take all of the antibiotics until they are finished."
  ② use only prescribed douches to avoid a recurrence."
  ③ return for a pap smear in 6 months."
  ④ avoid using tampons for 8 weeks."

3.7   Which of these questions is the highest priority for the nurse when discussing safety for a 4-year-old with the parents?

  ① "Do you have all of your kitchen cabinets locked?"
  ② "Do the parents in your neighborhood feel comfortable reporting strangers?"
  ③ "Are you able to discuss your child's disagreements while playing with his friends to other parents?"
  ④ "Does your child have appropriate safety equipment for the games he plays?"

3.8   A geriatric client, newly diagnosed with diabetes, is being discharged. She is alert, oriented and able to independently maintain her activities of daily living. Treatment will consist of a 1500-caloric diabetic diet, insulin, and regular exercise by walking 30 minutes a day. What is a priority concern at the time the client is discharged?

  ① Does the client have adequate vision and manual dexterity to administer her own insulin?
  ② Does the client understand the impact diabetes will have on her lifestyle?
  ③ Since the client is living alone, does she need Home Health Care to check on her daily?
  ④ Does the client understand how to perform her daily urinary sugar and acetone determinations?

3.9 The family members of an 85-year-old think their father is masturbating. Which response by the nurse would be best?

① "I understand your concern because this is not a normal part of aging."
② "I would not worry about this behavior. He will stop soon."
③ "This is considered a normal behavior."
④ "The best thing you can do is talk to your father about this behavior."

3.10 Which clinical situation indicates the nurse has an accurate understanding of how to complete a physical assessment?

① The nurse uses the diaphragm of the stethoscope to auscultate S3 and S4.
② The nurse uses the Snellen chart to evaluate the first cranial nerve.
③ The nurse uses the bell of the stethoscope to auscultate S1 and S2.
④ The nurse assesses the abdomen by inspecting, auscultating, percussing, and palpating.

3.11 A mother tells you that the 7-year-old sibling of a child with cystic fibrosis is having difficulty in school, fights frequently with playmates and throws his toys. Which response by the nurse would be best?

① "Did he have these behaviors before his sister was diagnosed?"
② "That is typical of 7-year-olds."
③ "Spend time with each child daily, and it will stop."
④ "He is jealous of the attention his sister is receiving."

3.12 During a discussion with the nurse, parents share their feelings of frustration with their 14-year-old who refuses to wear a back brace after surgery for scoliosis. The nurse's best response would be that the teenager is probably concerned with:

① her image.
② being separated from her peers.
③ loss of control.
④ physical discomfort.

3.13 A pelvic exam is planned on a 15-year-old client with sharp bilateral pelvic pain. Which nursing action would be most appropriate?

① Request removal of all clothing.
② Collect a urine and fecal specimen.
③ Give a brief explanation of the procedure.
④ Begin health teaching related to sexually-transmitted diseases.

3.14 A hypertensive client returns to the clinic for re-evaluation of his medication. His blood pressure is 180/100. The nurse questions the client regarding how he is taking his medication. What response by the client indicates that he understands and has been taking the medication as prescribed?

① "I take my medication every morning. If my blood pressure is high, I take another dose in the evening."
② "I take my medication every day at the same time regardless of how I feel. I have not missed any doses."
③ "I take my medication every day and make sure that I drink a large amount of liquid each time I take it."
④ "If I have a headache, I don't take my medication. If I miss the morning dose, then I take two pills in the evening."

3.15 An 8-lb., 6-oz. infant is delivered to a diabetic mother. Which nursing intervention would be implemented when the neonate becomes jittery and lethargic?

① Administer insulin.
② Administer oxygen.
③ Feed the infant glucose water (10%).
④ Place infant in a warmer.

3.16 What question would be most important to ask a male client who is in for a digital rectal examination?

① "Have you noticed a change in the force of the urinary stream?"
② "Have you noticed a change in tolerance of certain foods in your diet?"
③ "Do you notice polyuria in the AM?"
④ "Do you notice any burning with urination or any odor to the urine?"

3.17 A 21-year-old female has just been told by the physician that her biopsy results indicate breast cancer. What would be the most appropriate next action for the nurse to take?

① Ask the client if she has any questions.
② Encourage client to talk about her feelings.
③ Leave client alone for awhile.
④ Call the chaplain for the client.

3.18 A female client reports that for the last 4 months a lump in her right breast has been growing larger. The nurse should recommend the client take which action?

① Notify her physician to schedule a mammogram.
② Begin taking large doses of vitamins.
③ Limit sodium intake.
④ Immediately stop any hormone treatment.

3.19 The nurse is preparing a 40-year-old client for diagnostic tests to determine if she has a malignancy in her reproductive system. The client is having difficulty concentrating, appears tense, and is wringing her hands constantly. Which response should the nurse make?

① "You seem to be anxious about the tests. Tell me what you are thinking about."
② "You need to pay more attention to what I'm saying. You'll be less anxious if you understand these tests."
③ "Why are you so restless? Your physician is very good."
④ "I know you're worried about these tests, but I'm sure everything will be fine."

3.20 The nurse assesses a prolonged late deceleration of the fetal heart rate while the client is receiving oxytocin (Pitocin) IV to stimulate labor. The priority nursing intervention would be to:

① turn off the infusion.
② turn client to left.
③ change the fluids to Ringer's Lactate.
④ increase mainline IV rate.

3.21 Which plan would best promote bonding between the mother and her newborn that is in pediatric intensive care for jaundice?

① Allow the mother to visit and participate in the newborn's care.
② Take the infant to the mother's room for feeding.
③ Place a picture of the infant at the mother's bedside.
④ Provide the newborn with an article that bears the mother's scent.

3.22 A nurse would be concerned with the quality of home care of a toddler if she assesses the toddler:

① Has a bruise on the knee.
② Cries and is fearful when parents leave.
③ Is lacking required immunizations.
④ Throws a temper tantrum during an injection.

3.23 Which assessments would be a priority in documenting the nursing history of a 2-year-old upon admission to the hospital?

① The child's rituals and routines at home.
② The child's understanding of hospitalization.
③ The child's ability to be separated from parents.
④ The parent's methods for dealing with temper tantrums.

3.24 While doing a physical examination with a 2-year-old child, which assessment should be done last?

① Rectal temperature
② Breath sounds
③ Apical heart rate
④ Motor functions

3.25 Which nursing approach would be most appropriate to use while administering an oral medication to a 4-month-old?

① Place medication in 45 cc of formula.
② Place medication in an empty nipple.
③ Place medication in a full bottle of formula.
④ Place in supine position. Administer medication using a plastic syringe.

3.26 Which intervention would be a priority during the care of a 2-month-old after surgery?

① Minimize stimuli for the infant.
② Restrain all extremities.
③ Encourage stroking of the infant.
④ Demonstrate to the mother how she can assist with her infant's care.

3.27 Which statement made by the new mother indicates an understanding of screening for PKU for her newborn son who she is breastfeeding?

① "I will have him tested 24 hours after birth."
② "I will return to the clinic in 48 hours for the screening."
③ "I will return in 1 week to obtain blood samples."
④ "I will return in 1 month for the screening."

3.28 While performing a physical examination on a newborn, which assessment should be reported to the physician?

① Head circumference of 40 cm.
② Chest circumference of 32 cm.
③ Acrocyanosis and edema of the scalp.
④ Heart rate of 160 and respirations of 40.

3.29 To assist the mother in providing appropriate foods for her 2-year-old child, the nurse would identify which priority as being the highest?

① Provide the child with finger foods.
② Allow the child to eat favorite foods.
③ Encourage a diet higher in protein than other nutrients.
④ Limit the number of snacks during the day.

3.30 Which action by the mother of a preschooler would indicate a disturbed family interaction?

① Tells her child that if he does not sit down and shut up she will leave him there.
② Explains that the injection will burn like a bee sting.
③ Tells her child that the injection can be given while he's in her lap.
④ Reassures child that it is acceptable to cry.

3.31 In planning anticipatory guidance for parents of a beginning school-aged child, it is most important for the nurse to include information on:

① teaching the child to read and write.
② teaching the child sex education at home.
③ giving the child responsibility around the house.
④ expecting stormy behavior.

3.32 Which statement by the parent of a toddler indicates a lack of understanding of this child's nutritional needs?

① "I spend a lot of time planning and preparing my family's meals."
② "I realize she eats more at some meals than at others."
③ "She is a picky eater so I give her one of my vitamins every day."
④ "She likes starchy foods so I decorate them with vegetables."

3.33 What is the priority plan for preventing falls in the older adult?

① Recommend removing all the rugs in the home.
② Encourage installation of appropriate lighting in the home.
③ Review the normal aging changes that place one at risk.
④ Complete a comprehensive risk assessment.

3.34 What should the nurse emphasize when guiding parents teaching their children about human sexuality?

① Parents should determine exactly what the child knows and wants to know before answering questions.
② Parents' words will have more influence than their actions.
③ Anatomic terms should be avoided because they are difficult for the child to understand and learn.
④ Children should be allowed to play "physician" as it will satisfy their sexual curiosity.

3.35 What is most important to teach a child's parents about the treatment of pediculosis capitis (head lice) with Kwell shampoo?

① Treatment should be continued every other day for 1 week with a follow-up treatment in 14 days.
② Clothing and personal belongings require only normal cleansing with soap and water.
③ Application of the shampoo may be repeated at a later date to destroy any surviving live lice.
④ Never repeat the shampoo application as it is readily absorbed through the scalp.

3.36 A physician should be notified about which observation of a mother during her third trimester of pregnancy?

① Epigastric pain.
② Shortness of breath.
③ Increase in rectal pressure.
④ A total weight gain of 33 pounds.

3.37 During the nursing history interview, a preschool client's mother reports frequent hospitalizations for gastroenteritis. Which question would reveal the most information regarding the cause of these frequent readmissions?

① "Are there other children in the family?"
② "Does the child attend a day care center?"
③ "Does your child play with neighborhood children?"
④ "Is the child current with his immunizations?"

3.38 Which assessment indicates a need to order a magnesium sulfate blood level?

① Urine output decreased from 70 cc/hour to 30 cc/hour.
② Respiratory rate increased from 14/min. to 18/min.
③ Hypertonic patellar reflexes.
④ Blood pressure 150/90 increased to 170/100.

3.39 Which client would be the most appropriate for the nurse to administer Rh immune globulin (RhoGam)?

① A client with a husband who is Rh positive.
② A client with a positive indirect antiglobulin (indirect Coomb's) test.
③ A client who is sensitized to the Rh antigen.
④ A client who is Rh negative and has an Rh positive infant.

3.40 Which of these schedules would be the most appropriate to recommend to a pre-menopausal woman regarding her self breast exam?

① One week prior to the monthly period
② One week after the menstrual period
③ During every shower
④ The same day monthly

3.41 Which fetal monitor pattern would indicate a problem with a cord compression?

① Early decelerations
② Late decelerations
③ Variable decelerations
④ Loss of variability

3.42 Before administering calcium gluconate 10% 500 mg IVP stat, it is most important that the nurse assess:

① stability of the respiratory system.
② adequacy of urine output.
③ patency of the vein.
④ availability of magnesium sulfate injection.

3.43 After the termination of pre-term labor, what action by a client would indicate her ability to monitor herself at home for fetal well being?

① Count uterine contractions.
② Measure her urine output.
③ Count fetal kicks.
④ Weigh herself daily.

3.44 A 12-year-old child receiving intravenous theophylline (Aminophylline) for respiratory distress, presents signs of tachycardia and irritability. Which plan would be the most appropriate?

① Decrease external stimuli in the child's room.
① Administer an analgesic as ordered.
③ Notify the physician and advise him of child's status.
④ Document the assessments and continue to observe.

3.45 After the anesthesiologist administers an epidural, which nursing action has the highest priority?

① Decrease IV fluid to prevent fluid overload.
② Assess fetal heart monitor for variable decelerations.
③ Place the client on her right side.
④ Evaluate the blood pressure.

3.46 During the fourth state of labor, where would the nurse normally palpate the client's fundus?

① 3 cm below the umbilicus
② At the umbilicus
③ 2 cm above the umbilicus
④ To the right of the umbilicus

3.47 A 28-hour-old newborn begins to exhibit a high pitched cry, irritability, diarrhea, sneezing, and frequent tremors. What is the priority assessment for the nurse to evaluate?

① Cardiac arrhythmias
① History of maternal drug abuse
③ Maternal sepsis
④ Newborn sepsis

3.48   Which nursing interventions would be a priority in preventing complications of a Cesarean birth?

① Turn, cough, deep breathe
② Limit fluid intake.
③ High carbohydrate diet
④ Evaluate skin integrity.

3.49   Which observation indicates the client's family may have misunderstood the purpose of an apnea monitor?

① The parents leave the infant for brief periods.
② The parents sleep by the infant's crib.
③ The monitor is removed during the infant's bath.
④ A family member closely watches the monitor all the time.

3.50   At the peak of a contraction, fluid gushes from a client's vagina. The nurse should immediately:

① evaluate for a prolapsed cord.
② evaluate fetal monitor for early decelerations.
③ perform a pH on the fluid to determine it is amniotic fluid.
④ evaluate fetal monitor for an increase in the variability.

3.51   The mother of a 2-year-old reports that her son is becoming a very picky eater. What would be the best response from the nurse?

① "This is a common behavior since he is becoming more autonomous. Try giving him some finger foods."
② "You may try setting better limits between meals regarding snacks."
③ "Try mixing his food together so there is not so much to select from."
④ "I will report this to the nurse practitioner. He may have a virus."

3.52   Which statement made by a mother who is breast feeding most indicates a need for further teaching about birth control? "I will:

① go to my physician and get fitted for a diaphragm."
② have my husband use a condom."
③ get a prescription from my physician for the pill."
④ practice abstinence during my fertile time."

3.53   Which statement by the parents of a newborn indicates a need for further teaching about newborn care? "We will:

① notify the physician for absence of breathing for 10 seconds."
② notify the physician for more than one episode of projectile vomiting."
③ notify the physician if the infant's temperature is greater than 101°F."
④ rock and cuddle our infant to promote trust."

3.54   Following an abdominal hysterectomy, which action would be a priority in preventing thrombophlebitis?

① Place the knee gatch down.
② Increase the fluid intake.
③ Encourage turning, coughing, and deep breathing every 2 hours.
④ Encourage active leg exercises and ambulation.

3.55   A 3-month-old is placed in Bryant's traction for congenital hip dysplasia. Which toy would be appropriate to offer the infant during hospitalization?

① Rattle
② Stuffed animal
③ Colorful blocks
④ Tape of nursery rhymes

3.56   During the history, which information from a 20-year-old client would indicate a risk for development of testicular cancer?

① Genital Herpes
② Hydrocele
③ Measles
④ Undescended testicle

3.57   While planning care for an elderly client with dementia, which plan would be a priority?

① Encourage dependency with activities of daily living.
② Provide flexibility in schedules due to mental confusion.
③ Limit reminiscing due to poor memory.
④ Speak slowly and in a face-to-face position.

3.58 Which observation would most likely represent care-giver burnout in the daughter of an 80-year-old Alzheimer's client?

    ① Failure of daughter to get parent into wheelchair daily.
    ② Home environment extremely cluttered at each visit.
    ③ Daughter remains involved in family's activities.
    ④ Husband is seen assisting in mother-in-law care.

3.59 During the newborn assessment, the nurse is evaluating the rooting reflex. Locate where the nurse would stroke to elicit this response.

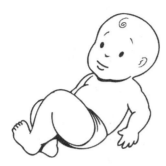

3.60 While assessing cranial nerve 11, which part of the body would the nurse ask the client to move?

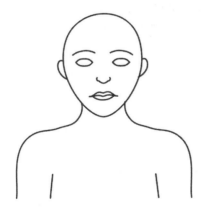

Answers & Rationales

3.1 ④ Cranial nerves 9 and 10 are the glossopharyngeal and vagus nerves. The gag reflex would be evaluated. Options #1, #2, and #3 are inappropriate for these cranial nerves.

3.2 ② Due to the HIPPA regulations and individual state laws, not all partners are recognized as legal partners. Since the NCLEX is a national exam, the answers must represent all states. Option #1 is nurse avoidance. Option #3 violates HIPPA regulations. Option #4 is providing false reassurance and is not therapeutic.

3.3 ① Assessment must be done prior to implementation. The client may have decreased circulation that has increased in severity over the past few hours. Options #2 and #3 are contraindicated. Option #4 is secondary.

3.4 ④ Option #4 is correct. Providing information for the client is the best technique for a new diagnosis. Option #1 is not educating the client and addressing concerns. Option #2 is secondary. Option #3 is not addressing the diagnosis.

3.5 ④ This is the most objective way to quantify the effectiveness of the pain medicine. The nurse can measure breathing. If the client is still in pain, there will be reluctance to take deep breaths. Options #1 and #2 are not measurable. Option #3 is not measurable and may indicate pain is still present.

3.6 ③ Several strains of the human papillomavirus (HPV) are associated with cervical cancer. Option #1 is incorrect because antibiotics are not used for viral infections. Option #2 is incorrect because douches will not prevent recurrence. Option #4 is incorrect because tampons do not contribute to the problem as in toxic shock syndrome.

3.7 ④ Option #4 is a priority due to the developmental stage of the 4-year-old. They are into initiative vs. guilt. The 4-year-old is very active and safety is most important. Option #1 would be priority for the toddler. Options #2 and #3 are important but not a priority.

3.8 ① It is very important that the geriatric client have the visual and manual skills to administer their insulin. Options #2 and #3 are important to determine; but Option #1 is a priority. Urinary tests are not commonly used to monitor diabetics.

3.9 ③ Masturbation is an activity that some elderly engage in. Options #1 and #2 are inappropriate. Option #4 might embarrass the father and may cause feelings of guilt and anxiety.

3.10 ④ Option #4 is correct. The diaphragm of the stethoscope is used to auscultate high pitch sounds such as S_1 and S_2. Option #1 is incorrect. Option #2 is used to evaluate the 2nd cranial nerve. Option #3 should be the diaphragm. The bell is used for S_3 and S_4.

3.11 ① Obtain information about his behavior before the diagnosis to be able to assess a cause for the disruptive behavior. Option #2 is not accurate. Options #3 and #4 may be correct. However, the nurse must assess behavior prior to his sibling's illness.

3.12 ① Adolescents have a concern with their image. Erikson has identified this state as "Identity versus Role Diffusion." Option #2 is a concern of this stage, but is not appropriate for what the question is asking. Option #3 is more appropriate for a school-age child. Option #4 is incorrect for this situation.

3.13 ③ Preparation of client is important for all procedures, especially in this case. A pelvic exam can be extremely embarrassing for a 15-year-old. Options #1, #2, and #4 are appropriate after explanation and client preparation, or after the procedure is completed.

3.14 ② This option best describes how the client should take the medication for hypertension. It is important that he take it every day. However, it may be a problem if he is consuming a large amount of water during the day. If he is taking the medication correctly, he needs to have the medication reevaluated since his blood pressure remains high.

3.15 ③ After birth, the infant of a diabetic mother is often hypoglycemic. Option #1 would maximize the problem. Option #2 would be used if the neonate was hypoxic. Option #4 is a routine nursing action for all newborns.

3.16 ① Option #1 is correct. This change would be most indicative of a potential complication with (BPH) benign prostate hypertrophy. Options #2, #3, and #4 are incorrect. Option #4 would be indicative of an infection.

3.17 ② Encouraging the client to talk about feelings allows the client to cry or express her reaction. Options #1, #3, and #4 do not allow for immediate expression of reaction to this crisis.

3.18 ① A mammogram is an x-ray of the breast. It usually shows the presence of a lesion if one is present. Positive zero radiography (type of mammogram) has the ability to detect carcinomas 1 to 2 years prior to formation of a palpable 1 cm. lesion. Option #2 is incorrect because specific vitamin therapy may be useful in some cases. It is not curative alone. Option #3 is incorrect because sodium has not been associated with breast cancer. Option #4 is incorrect because hormones have not been known to cause breast cancer.

3.19 ① This response acknowledges the client's concerns and allows exploration of her fears. Options #2, #3, and #4 provide false reassurance and do not allow the client an opportunity to express and deal with her feelings.

3.20 ① Stopping the infusion will decrease contractions and possibly remove uterine pressure on the fetus, which is a possible cause of the deceleration. Option #2 may help the deceleration, but it is not priority. Options #3 and #4 will have no influence.

3.21 ① Option #1 is the best intervention to promote contact and feedback needed for bonding between the mother and the newborn. Option #2 is not appropriate. Taking the infant back and forth to the mother's room increases the risk of infection to other infants in the nursery. Option #3 does not replace the benefits of touch and eye contact needed for effective bonding. Option #4 only increases comfort for the infant and does not give feedback to the mother.

3.22 ③ This may indicate a lack of concern for child's well-being and may be a sign of poor quality of home care. Option #1 is a common assessment during the toddler years. Options #2 and #4 are expected behaviors for a toddler.

3.23 ① During a crisis such as hospitalization, children are able to establish a sense of security through a consistency of the rituals and routines from home. Option #2 is inappropriate for this age. Option #3 is incorrect because separation anxiety is a major fear during this age. Option #4 is not as high a priority as Option #1 in decreasing psychological trauma from hospitalization.

3.24 ① This, as any other invasive procedure, should be done last so it doesn't alter the cardiopulmonary assessment of the child. Options #2, #3, and #4 should be done before Option #1.

3.25 ② This is a convenient method for administering medications to an infant. Options #1 and #3 are incorrect. Medication is not usually added to infant's formula feeding. Option #4 is partially correct. However, the infant is never placed in a reclining position during procedure due to potential aspiration.

3.26 ③ Tactile stimulation is imperative for an infant's normal emotional development. After the trauma of surgery, sensory deprivation can cause failure to thrive. Options #1 and #2 are incorrect and would lead to further deprivation. Option #4 is secondary.

3.27 ③ Option #3 is correct since the newborn is only getting colostrum for the first few days. This screening may have a possible false negative result with the initial screening. Options #1, #2, and #4 are inaccurate and would not provide valid information.

3.28 ① Average circumference of the head for a neonate ranges between 32 to 36 cm. An increase in size may indicate hydrocephaly or increased intracranial pressure. Options #2, #3, and #4 are normal newborn assessments.

3.29 ① The child is going through the autonomy versus shame and doubt stage. Finger foods allow the child the necessary independence for this stage. Options #2 and #4 may or may not be correct because the child may eat food without appropriate nutrients. Option #3 does not represent accurate nutritional information.

3.30 ① Threatening a child with abandonment will destroy the child's trust in his family. Option #2 is not necessarily accurate but does not indicate a disturbed family interaction. Option #3 is inappropriate but does not indicate a disturbance in family interaction. Option #4 indicates a healthy interaction.

3.31 ③ Giving children responsibilities allows them to develop feelings of competence and self-esteem through their industry. Option #1 may require some assistance from the parents, but children this age learn at their own rate. Option #2 may be premature. Option #4 usually does not occur until about age 11.

3.32 ③ Children should not be given adult doses of vitamins because a child's need for vitamins is different than adults. Toddlers are picky eaters, and children's daily vitamins are appropriate. Option #1 shows concern about family nutrition. Option #2 is accurate because toddlers usually eat only one or two adequate meals each day. Nutritious snacks are helpful in assuring adequate nutritional intake. Option #4 is true because toddlers do prefer a "white diet" of starchy foods.

3.33 ④ Option #4 is priority in preventing falls. Options #1, #2, and #3 would be a part of doing a complete assessment.

3.34 ① Children often have misinformation about human sexuality; and if not identified, the child will incorporate the misinformation into the parent's answer. To be able to answer a question adequately, it is important to determine what the child wants to know. Option #2 is contra to human behavior. Option #3 is incorrect because most experts believe correct anatomic names are appropriate. Option #4, "oh please…"

3.35 ③ Kwell shampoo should be used as directed as it is an organic solvent and can be toxic as well as absorbed through the skin of the scalp. It may be repeated, but usually at least 5–7 days after the first application. Option #1 is too often for applying the shampoo. Option #2 is incorrect because very hot water and a special detergent (Rid) need to be used for cleansing clothing and personal belongings. Option #4 is incorrect because the shampooing must be repeated after the eggs hatch.

3.36 ① Epigastric pain is usually indicative of an impending seizure. Options #2 and #3 are expected observations. Option #4 is important to address but is not a priority to Option #1.

3.37 ② Environments where there are increased numbers of children, such as day care centers, are more likely to have infections due to close living conditions facilitating the transmission of disease. Options #1 and #4 do not pose a problem or solution regarding gastroenteritis. Option #3 is a possible source of infection but not as likely as a day care center.

3.38 ① Magnesium sulfate is metabolized and excreted by the kidneys. A decrease in the urine output can lead to toxicity. Option #2 indicates an improvement. Options #3 and #4 are incorrect because these assessments indicate a need to start magnesium sulfate.

3.39 ④ RhoGam is administered to this client to prevent sensitization to the Rh antigen. Option #1 is irrelevant because it is the mother and infant's Rh type that the decision is based on. Option #2 may or may not be correct depending on what specific antibody was detected. If the mother has anti-D and did not receive antenatal RhoGam, she is sensitized and not a candidate. Option #3 is incorrect because the client is sensitized and RhoGam is given to prevent sensitization from occurring.

3.40 ② Option #2 is correct because this is when the breasts are least congested. Option #1 is when the breasts are most congested. Option #3 is unnecessary. The recommended frequency is monthly. Option #4 is for post-menopausal women.

3.41 ③ Variable decelerations indicate a problem with cord compression. Option #1 indicates head compression. Option #2 indicates uteroplacental insufficiency. Option #4 could indicate fetal acidosis, fetal neurological immaturity, or maternal medication.

3.42 ③ If injected into the extravascular tissues, calcium gluconate can cause a severe chemical burn. Options #1 and #2 are unnecessary in this situation. Option #4 is irrelevant.

3.43 ③ Being able to count fetal kicks assures the fetus is moving and makes the mother aware of the importance of monitoring fetal movement daily. Option #1 might indicate the onset of premature labor. Options #2 and #4 relate to maternal, more than fetal well-being.

3.44 ③ Tachycardia and irritability are signs of toxicity which need to be reported to the physician. Option #1 may help to cope with current symptoms. Option #2 may mask the signs of toxicity. Option #4 is not taking any action to resolve the problem.

3.45 ④ A side effect of an epidural is hypotension from the vasodilation which occurs. Option #1 is incorrect because the client must be well hydrated before and after the procedure. Option #2 may be done as ongoing management but is not a priority. Option #3 is incorrect because the client would be placed on her left side to promote uterine perfusion.

3.46 ② The uterus is normally contracted and palpable at the umbilicus. Options #1 and #3 are incorrect. It is unusual to palpate the fundus above or below the umbilicus during this stage. Option #4 is incorrect because this may indicate a problem with a distended bladder.

3.47 ② Option #2 is correct. Signs of drug withdrawal are more frequently associated with central nervous system alterations, gastrointestinal disturbances, and tachypnea. Options #1, #3, and #4 are secondary to Option #1.

3.48 ① This response represents preventive care for respiratory congestion resulting from anesthesia and shallow respirations due to abdominal incision. Option #2 contains incorrect information because fluids would be encouraged. Option #3 does not have a specific preventive characteristic. Option #4 is not a usual complication.

3.49 ④ Watching the monitor indicates a feeling that the monitor may not alarm to let them know if their infant quits breathing. Options #1, #2, and #3 are appropriate behaviors.

3.50 ① Option #1 is most important due to safety. Option #2 reflects head compression. Option #3 is not an immediate concern. The fetus is the priority! Option #4 is good; increase in oxygenation is not a problem.

3.51 ① Finger foods will assist the child in establishing his autonomy. Options #2 and #3 are inappropriate. This age of child does not like food mixed together. There are no other concerns stated by the mother to make the nurse even consider a virus.

3.52 ③ The pill (oral contraceptive) will suppress production of breast milk. During breast-feeding, another method of contraception should be used. Options #1, #2, and #4 could be used and do not indicate a need for further teaching.

3.53 ① This is normal for a neonate. Apnea lasting longer than 15 seconds should be reported. Options #2, #3, and #4 do not indicate a need for further teaching.

3.54 ④ Ambulation and active leg exercises will increase the circulation and will decrease the risk of developing thrombophlebitis. Option #1 would increase the risk as blood would pool in the lower extremities. Option #2 is inappropriate. Option #3 is appropriate for minimizing pulmonary complications.

3.55 ① A 3-month-old can grasp a rattle. Options #2 and #4 are correct but not a priority to Option #1. Option #3 is for an older child.

3.56 ④ Option #4—undescended testicles make the client high risk for testicular cancer. Mumps, inguinal hernia in childhood, orchitis, and testicular cancer in the contra lateral testis are other predisposing factors. Options #1, #2, and #3 are not factors that contribute to testicular cancer.

3.57 ④ This is most effective when communicating with an elderly client. Option #1 is incorrect because independence is encouraged. Option #2 is incorrect because schedules need to be routine, reinforced, and repeated. Flexibility leads to confusion. Option #3 is incorrect because reminiscing helps the client resume progression through the grief process associated with disappointing life event and increases self-esteem.

3.58 ② Cluttered environment may represent depression and burnout. Option #1 may be impossible for the daughter to do alone. Options #3 and #4 are very healthy and desirable.

3.59

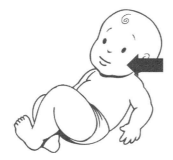

3.60 Cranial nerve 11 is the spinal accessory.

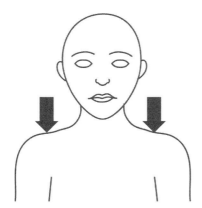

Psycho-Social Integrity

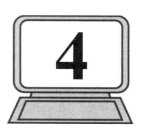

Never believe that a few caring people can't change the world.
For, indeed, that's all that ever have.
—Margaret Mead

✔ **Clarification of this test...**

The minimum standard includes performing and directing activities related to caring for client/family with emotional, mental and social problems including behavioral interventions.

☞ Use therapeutic communication techniques to provide support for the client or family.

☞ Act as a client advocate.

☞ Implement measures to manage/prevent possible complications of client's condition (suicide).

☞ Assess client for drug/alcohol-related dependencies, withdrawal or toxicities.

☞ Assess psychosocial, spiritual, cultural and occupational factors affecting care..

☞ Provide a therapeutic environment for client with emotional/behavioral issues.

☞ Incorporate client's cultural practice and beliefs when planning and providing care.

☞ Assess client risk for abuse/neglect.

☞ Assess and plan interventions that meet the client's emotional and spiritual needs.

☞ Provide support to client and/or family in coping with life changes (loss, new diagnosis, role change, stress).

☞ Maintain continuity of care between/among health care agencies.

☞ Assist client/family to identify/participate in activities fitting his/her age, preference, physical capacity and psychological capacity.

☞ Assess family dynamics (structure, bonding, communication, boundaries, coping mechanisims).

☞ Intervene with a client who has alteration in nutritional intake.

☞ Comply with federal/state/instituional policy regarding the use of client restraints and/or safety devices.

☞ Provide end-of-life care to clients and families.

4.1 A 10-year-old client with AIDS asks if he is going to die. The best response is:

① "Let's talk about getting well instead of dying."
② "What do you think?"
③ "I don't know."
④ "Ask your doctor."

4.2 A 1-year-old is scheduled for open-heart surgery. The mother begins to cry and says, "I'm a terrible mother!" The best response is:

① "Do you want to talk about the surgery?"
② to place a comforting arm around the mother.
③ "Is your family here to be with you?"
④ "You have done everything that you can and the baby is in the best of hands."

4.3 The physician has ordered chlorpromazine (Thorazine) to control an alcoholic client's restlessness, agitation, and irritability following surgery. The nurse would check the order with the physician because:

① the client's symptoms reflect alcohol withdrawal.
② the client may be allergic to this medication.
③ the client is not psychotic.
④ physician's orders are routinely checked.

4.4 A client with a terminal diagnosis asks the nurse what she thinks about complementary medicine for the treatment of cancer. The nurse notices that the client has stopped her 5-FU (fluorouracil) treatments. What is an appropriate response?

① Inquire about the type of complementary therapy the client is using.
② Question the client as to how she felt while taking the 5-FU injections.
③ Explain the importance of taking the 5-FU, as it is the only approved therapy for her type of cancer.
④ Tell the client she is making a big mistake as alternative or complementary medicine is considered "quackery."

4.5 The client throws her lunch tray and yells that nobody cares for her. Which intervention has priority?

① Remove the client from the lunch room.
② Try to gain her trust.
③ Speak strongly and ask her to stop.
④ Administer her PRN medication.

4.6 Your client admitted to the mental health unit experiencing hallucinations is not wearing an identification band. What is your best action before giving your client a scheduled medication?

① Compare the picture and the hospital identification number on the medication administration record (MAR) to the information in the client's chart.
② Ask the client to verify his or her name and the date of birth before giving the medication.
③ Ask another staff member who knows the client to give the medication for you.
④ Use the client's photograph and the hospital identification number on the client's chart and compare this to the client's physical appearance.

4.7 A client with a severe thought disturbance has not been taking medication and appears to be more actively hallucinating. The client claims that the medicine makes him too drowsy during the day. Which action by the nurse is most likely to increase medication compliance?

① Ask the physician to schedule the client's entire dose at bedtime.
② Tell the client he is getting sicker and must take his medicine.
③ Teach the client about the side effects of the medication.
④ Ask the family to talk to the client about this problem.

4.8 A client, admitted for treatment of alcohol dependence, displays the following symptoms: slurred speech, ataxia, uncoordinated movements, and headache. Which nursing action should be taken first?

① Observe the client for 8 hours to collect additional data.
② Perform a complete physical assessment.
③ Collect a urine specimen for a drug screen.
④ Encourage the client to talk about whatever is bothering him.

4.9 When a client has dementia, which stressor would be identified as the most critical for the family?

① Client's unwillingness to eat food with the family.
② Client's inability to recognize and communicate with the family.
③ Lack of knowledge about community resources for day care.
④ Client's loss of continence.

4.10   Before giving medication to a client who identifies himself as Jesus Christ, which action by the nurse is necessary?

① Ask several nursing assistants to be available for safety.
② Ask the priest to come and speak with the client.
③ Check the client's name band to make sure of the client's identify.
④ Make sure the client has eaten a full meal.

4.11   Because of a borderline client's mood swings, limited problem-solving strategies, and self-concept disturbance, the treatment team has determined the client is at high risk for violence, either directed at self or others. The nurse should observe the client for early clues to which behavior?

① Intense but disruptive relationships
② Superficial interactions
③ Persistent sense of boredom and loneliness
④ Self-mutilation or suicidal gestures

4.12   Following the death of a female client who is Muslim, the nurse should plan on providing the family with:

① a private room to gather the family for grieving.
② a muslin wrap, preferably white, for the body.
③ post-mortem care of the body by a female nurse.
④ immediate referral to a crematory.

4.13   An elderly man diagnosed with major depression is demonstrating decreased problem-solving ability, psychomotor retardation, and social isolation. In planning activities for this client during the early phase of hospitalization, which nursing action would be appropriate?

① Prepare and give him a schedule of activities to follow and monitor his participation.
② Encourage him to choose his own activities.
③ Allow him some time to get acclimated to the milieu before scheduling activities.
④ Allow him to rest quietly to restore his energy and fatigue level.

14.14   Which of these psychiatric clients should be evaluated first?

① depressed client sitting on the floor rocking back and forth.
② bipolar client pacing and clenching fist.
③ psychotic client who is having a delusion that she is the Queen of England.
④ schizophrenic client laughing and waving hands up in the air.

4.15   Which plan would be most important to assist a client to cope with sexual problems resulting from a chronic disease?

① Discuss the importance of decreasing sexual activity.
② Recommend counseling for the client's partner.
③ Recommend periods of abstinence after engaging in sexual activity.
④ Discuss alternate forms of sexual expression.

4.16   A client is started on doxepin hydrochloride (Sinequan) 75 mg PO TID. The nurse should recommend a change in the client's therapy in which response occurs? The client:

① refuses to speak and sits quietly in the room.
② becomes excitable and develops tremors.
③ refuses to eat breakfast.
④ sleeps 18 hours a day.

4.17   An elderly man diagnosed as chronically mentally ill due to schizophrenia, is being followed in a partial hospitalization program. He has been on long-term antipsychotic medication and recently has developed some symptoms of tardive dyskinesia. The documentation on this client should include:

① assessment of ADL (self-care) ability.
② Folstein Mini-Mental Status Examination.
③ AIMS (Abnormal Involuntary Movement Scale).
④ MOAS (Modified Overt Aggression Scale).

4.18   The nurse should instruct a client taking Disulfiram (Antabuse) to avoid which medication?

① Over-the-counter cough/cold preparations.
② Cardiac and antihypertensive medications.
③ Aspirin and/or Tylenol.
④ Antacids.

4.19   Which plan is most appropriate for meeting the needs for a Hindu family after the loved one has died?

① Allow the family to wash the body.
② Allow the priest to touch the body.
③ Allow chanting to be done during the "last rites."
④ Do not consult with family about organ donations since it is considered a sin.

4.20   A client was minimally injured in a motor vehicle crash six months ago though his friend was killed. The client comes to Student Health Services with complaints of not being able to study, not sleeping, and thinks "I'm going crazy." The most important information for the nurse to obtain is:

① complete physical and social history.
② complete drug and alcohol history including reports from a drug screen.
③ review of significant events in the last year.
④ coping behaviors concerning the motor vehicle crash and friend's death.

4.21   Which nursing intervention would be an initial approach in symptom reduction for a client with a phobic disorder?

① Referral for psychopharmacologic intervention.
② Group psychotherapy.
③ Systematic desensitization.
④ Biofeedback.

4.22   Which nursing action is of primary importance during the implementation of a behavior modification treatment program?

① Confirm that all staff members understand and comply with the treatment plan.
② Establish mutually-agreed-upon, realistic goals,
③ Ensure that the potent reinforcers (rewards) are important to the client.
④ Establish a fixed interval schedule for reinforcement.

4.23   Which of these statements made by a female client who has been abused by her spouse indicates the counseling has been effective?

① "I know my husband will never hurt me again."
② "I know it is my fault that he hits me."
③ "I promise I will get him to promise that he will not do it again."
④ "I have made arrangements to go to the battered women's shelter the next time he hits me."

4.24   An elderly client is frantically yelling for the nurse. The nurse enters the room as the client states, "See it? It's the devil!" What would be the most therapeutic response?

① "The devil is here?"
② "Show me where the devil appeared to you."
③ "I don't see the devil, but I understand that it is real to you."
④ "The devil is not here. Your mind is playing tricks on you."

4.25   Which of these clinical findings is the first sign of opiod withdrawal?

① abdominal cramping
② diaphoresis
③ fever
④ nausea

4.26   An alcoholic client who occasionally uses marijuana and cocaine is attending his second group therapy meeting. The client comments, "I am having difficulty sitting still. Am I bothering some of the group members? Maybe I should stop coming to these group meetings." Which nursing action is most appropriate?

① Encourage client to share problem with the group.
② Remove client from the group and further assess needs.
③ Recognize that this is manipulative behavior and encourage client to remain in the group.
④ Tell client not to be concerned about the group members and to continue in the group.

4.27   Clients with eating disorders should be instructed to watch for possible problems with:

① aggressive behavior and feeling angry.
② self-identity and self-esteem
③ focusing on reality.
④ family boundary intrusions.

4.28   Which evaluation indicates a disoriented client with poor nutrition has made a positive response to the plan of care?

① Reports relationship of weight loss to change in mental status.
② Identifies basic four food groups.
③ States he needs to drink more water.
④ Feeds self when the nurse stays with and cues him.

4.29 What would be the most important initial goal in caring for a client with a nursing diagnosis of rape trauma syndrome: acute phase?

① Within 3–5 months, the client will state that the memory of the event is less vivid and distressing.

② The client will indicate a willingness to keep a follow-up appointment with a rape crisis counselor.

③ The client will be able to describe the results of the physical examination that was performed in the ER.

④ The client will begin to express her reactions and feelings about the assault before leaving the ER.

4.30 Policemen bring a client to the emergency room after she had been standing barefoot in the rain for more than 2 hours. The policemen report that the woman had to be restrained after she resisted and became agitated. The first action is to:

① do a preliminary physical exam.

② reassure the client that she is safe and maintain safety.

③ ascertain the client's mental status.

④ orient the client to place and time.

4.31 After 2 days in a psychiatric emergency service, a paranoid client refuses to give any information other than name and age. The primary goal of nursing care is to:

① present reality to the client.

② persuade the client to reveal more.

③ try to develop a trusting relationship with the client.

④ introduce the client to other clients in the emergency room.

4.32 An adolescents client is being discharged after an attempted suicide. What would be the priority of care for this client?

① Schedule the follow-up visit for the family and client.

② Review the side effects of the prescribed anti-depressant medication.

③ Obtain the client's signature on the behavior contract.

④ Encourage client to attend group therapy every Wednesday evening.

4.33 Which behavior would be associated with a dysfunctional family process related to impaired communication?

① Acknowledgement of personal needs and role responsibilities.

② Congruence between verbal and nonverbal messages.

③ Appropriate response to other family members' needs.

④ Inability to meet emotional needs of family members.

4.34 A psychiatric client with the diagnosis of schizophrenia tells the nurse that he is the President of the United States. What would be the priority action for the nurse?

① Confront the client regarding this delusion and bring him back to reality.

② Reflect this statement back to the client to encourage therapeutic communication.

③ Respond with an open-ended response to get client to further discuss his thoughts.

④ Verify the identity of the client prior to administering his medications.

4.35 Before undergoing an electroconvulsive therapy (ECT), the client reports being very anxious. Which action by the nurse would be the most therapeutic?

① Allow the client to have a cup of coffee to calm down.

② Encourage the client to sit quietly in her room and listen to a relaxation tape.

③ Administer lorazepan (Ativan) 1 mg IM to the client.

④ Ask if you can remain with client and discuss any fears.

4.36 Which assessment data would indicate a severely paranoid client is likely to need nursing interventions to promote self-care abilities?

① Speaks in a low, monotone voice.

② Has had suicidal ideation on 2 previous admissions.

③ Is very fearful that people are putting poison in his food.

④ Is unable to make eye contact with the nurse.

4.37 A gardener goes to the physician with a complaint of a potential or occupational hazard. What clinical finding would the nurse anticipate to assess?

① Eggs (nits) attached to the hair shaft in the head.
② A painful local reaction of vesicles with an erythematosus louse on the upper lip.
③ Linear patches of vesicles with an erythematosus base.
④ A dark asymmetrical mole with an irregular border on the client's back.

4.38 Which nursing action would be most appropriate in helping an elderly depressed client complete activities of daily living?

① Medicate the client before the activities are begun.
② Develop a written schedule of activities, allowing extra time.
③ Assist the client with grooming activities for her so it doesn't take so long.
④ Provide frequent forceful direction to keep the client focused.

4.39 Which plan would be most likely to help the family of an emotionally disturbed client in managing behavior at home after discharge from inpatient treatment?

① Refer the family to Alliance for the Mentally Ill meetings for educational programs and support groups.
② Provide the family with pamphlets that describe the desired action and side effects of medications the client is taking.
③ Tell the family that it is not their fault that the client behaves inappropriately.
④ Involve the family in the assessment of the client when he is first admitted to the hospital.

4.40 A client with a reactive depression has the greatest chance of success in activities that require psychic and physical energy if the nurse schedules activities in the:

① morning hours
② noontime
③ afternoon
④ evening hours

4.41 Which nursing intervention is most important when caring for a client who has just been placed in physical restraints?

① Prepare PRN dose of psychotropic medication.
② Check that the restraints have been applied correctly.
③ Review hospital policy regarding duration of restraints.
④ Monitor client's needs for hydration and nutrition while restrained.

4.42 The nurse's initial priority when managing a physically assaultive client is to:

① restrict client to room.
② place client on a 1-1 supervision.
③ restore the client's self-control and help prevent further loss of control.
④ clear the immediate area of other clients to prevent harm.

4.43 Which nursing action is most appropriate when a client presents a suicide plan and a request for confidentiality?

① Encourage client to think very carefully before being self-destructive.
② Agree to keep the information strictly confidential.
③ Inform client that confidentiality cannot be kept.
④ Encourage client to express her feelings.

4.44 The nurse recognizes that the client with obsessive-compulsive rituals is attempting to:

① control other people.
② increase self esteem.
③ avoid severe levels of anxiety.
④ express and manage anxiety.

4.45 A client on lithium (Lithane) therapy should be on which dietary plan to receive adequate nutritional requirements?

① Restricted sodium diet with increased fluid intake.
② High calorie diet with sodium and potassium restriction and adequate fluid intake.
③ Regular diet with normal sodium and adequate fluid intake.
④ Reduced calorie diet with a reduced sodium and increased fluid intake.

4.46 In coordinating a community placement for an alcoholic schizophrenic client who has been homeless, the nurse should:

① collaborate with members of the client's family to explore placement options.
② collaborate with health care team and the client to schedule a pre-discharge visit to residential placement facility.
③ visit the placement facility alone to make an independent decision about the facility and report to the client and family.
④ review with the client specific rules of the facility.

4.47 Which behavior indicates a client is beginning to develop a trusting relationship with the nurse?

① The client describes delusions to the nurse.
② The client can describe his feelings to the nurse.
③ The nurse feels more comfortable with the client.
④ The client states feeling less anxious.

4.48 Which post electroconvulsive therapy (ECT) treatment observations would the nurse report to the physician?

① Headache
② Disruption in short and long-term memory
③ Transient confusional state
④ Backache

4.49 Which information would indicate that the therapeutic interaction is in the working stage with a client who has an addiction problem? Select all that apply:

① The client reluctantly discusses the family history of addiction.
② The client addresses how the addiction has resulted in family distress.
③ The client experiences difficulty with identifying personal strengths.
④ The client discusses the financial burden related to the addiction.
⑤ The client is uncomfortable in meeting with the nurse.
⑥ The client discusses the addiction's effects on the children.

4.50 The initial priority of a nurse in dealing with a client who is a victim of interpersonal violence is to:

① encourage the client to verbalize feelings.
② assess for physical trauma.
③ provide privacy for the client during the interview.
④ help the client identify and mobilize resources and support systems.

4.51 An initial positive outcome of treatment with a victim of paternal sexual abuse would be when the client is able to:

① acknowledge willing participation in an incestuous relationship.
② reestablish a trusting relationship with mother.
③ verbalize that she is not responsible for the sexual abuse.
④ describe feelings of anxiety when speaking about father and the sexual abuse.

4.52 A client was recently diagnosed with cancer. Which intervention would be most appropriate to assist the client in dealing with his severe anxiety?

① During periods of stress, distract the client through activities.
② Review the stages of the grieving process.
③ Provide client with written information about chemotherapy.
④ Encourage client to discuss thoughts, feelings, and concerns with nurse.

4.53 Which nursing intervention is the highest priority for a client receiving aripiprazole (Ablify) for a diagnosis of schizophrenia?

① Recommend that the client reduces his alcohol intake to one drink per day.
② Instruct client to take the medication only before meals.
③ Review the importance of taking Ablify at bedtime since it causes sedation.
④ Advise to increase his exercising in order to optimize the drug action.

4.54 The nurse understands that a therapeutic nurse-client relationship is characterized by:

① establishing priorities and goals for the client.
② utilizing the nursing process to establish client goals.
③ collaborating to establish mutually-agreed upon goals and priorities.
④ directing interactions to assist the client to meet needs.

4.55 A client with terminal cancer is nearing the end of life. Which plan would best meet the client's emotional needs?

   ① Provide the client with a room where family can be present.
   ② Make sure that the client has an advanced directive on the chart.
   ③ Consult the hospital chaplain or client's personal spiritual advisor.
   ④ Provide the client with a journal to record final thoughts for family and friends.

4.56 A 17-year-old is beginning chemotherapy for her malignancy. Which statement indicates she has a realistic perception of her health status?

   ① "I will be cured after my therapy is completed."
   ② "I may need to get a wig during my chemotherapy."
   ③ "I will be able to continue my current school schedule."
   ④ "I must have done something to cause this illness."

4.57 Which response is a positive response to fluoxetine HCL (Prozac)?

   ① Hand tremors and leg twitching.
   ② Increased ability to sleep.
   ③ Increased energy level and participation in unit activities.
   ④ Hypervigilance and scanning of the environment.

4.58 Which nursing intervention is most important when working with clients with a diagnosis of dementia?

   ① Reinforce the client's thought patterns.
   ② When speaking with the client, use simple, short sentences.
   ③ Administer anti-anxiety medications.
   ④ Facilitate an exercise program with the client's physical limitations.

4.59 Which assessment should have priority in an initial assessment of an alcoholic client?

   ① Has the client been taking over-the-counter medication?
   ② What has been the client's usual daily intake of alcohol?
   ③ When did the client have his last drink?
   ④ Has the client ever had a withdrawal seizure?

4.60 The priority plan for a client diagnosed with dissociative disorder is to:

   ① assist the client in understanding the relationship between anxiety and dissociation.
   ② assess the client's level and reason for memory loss.
   ③ assist the client to incorporate the dissociated material into conscious memories.
   ④ establish an honest, non-judgmental and safe relationship with the client.

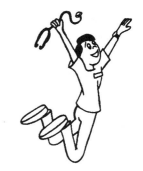

Yes! You're getting the hang of it!

Answers & Rationales

4.1 ② One of the most important concepts is to listen to client concerns. Options #1, #3, and #4 will take away this opportunity.

4.2 ④ Option #4 is the priority answer. It is important to promote a sense of hope. Option #1 would provide for listening to client/family concerns, and Options #2 and #3 may provide comfort.

4.3 ① This medication is contraindicated for the treatment of alcohol withdrawal symptoms. The medication will lower the client's seizure threshold and blood pressure, causing potentially serious medical consequences. Options #2, #3, and #4 are not the best rationale for checking with the physician about this order.

4.4 ① It is important for the nurse to respect a client's wishes for stopping treatment and choosing other forms of care, such as the use of complementary medicine. Offering information and having an open attitude about alternative therapies is part of a holistic approach to nursing management of the client.

4.5 ① Option #1 is the answer. It is important to remove the combative client from a setting where she might harm herself and others. Option #2 is important, but if she is yelling, it would not be the top priority. Option #3 is setting limits and is an appropriate second action. Option #4 would be last if all else fails.

4.6 ④ Option #4 is correct. Using a client photograph for identification is acceptable in behavioral and long-term care areas. Option #1 compares one chart item to another. It does not identify the client. Option #2 is incorrect because a client experiencing hallucinations may not be able to respond reliably. Option #3 is inappropriate.

4.7 ① Medication dose non-compliance is often associated with negative side effects and a multiple dosing daily schedule. When the client has only one daily dose at bedtime, it is easier for him to remember to take the medication. The other advantage is that the sedative effects of the drug peak while the client is sleeping. Options #2 and #4 do not offer concrete solutions and may foster dependent behaviors. Option #3 may help to some degree, but a more concrete solution is possible.

4.8 ② The best way to identify possible physical complications of alcohol dependence is through a complete physical assessment. Option #1 is important but will not provide the data that a physical assessment would. This may be a medical emergency requiring an immediate intervention. Option #3 is also a helpful source of data but can be done after the physical assessment is finished. Option #4 is inaccurate since the symptoms are most likely caused by physical and not psychological stressors.

4.9 ② This confirms a deteriorating condition and increases feelings of loss among family members. Options #1, #3, and #4 are all stressors for those dealing with a family member with dementia but are usually less critical.

4.10 ③ It is always necessary for the nurse to verify the client's identity before administering medications, particularly when the client cannot verbalize his identity. Options #1, #2, and #4 will be unnecessary.

4.11 ④ This is a common form of behavior displayed by the borderline client, which places her at a great risk for violence. Options #1, #2, and #3 are behaviors the client is likely to display, but they are not as clearly related to the high risk for violent behavior.

4.12 ③ The Muslim culture believes that the same sex should provide care after death. Option #1 is incorrect because the Muslim culture grieves at home. Option #2 is secondary to Option #1. Option #4 is incorrect because cremation is not practiced in the Muslim culture.

4.13 ① A regular daily routine of scheduled activities provides structure and decreases the degree of problem-solving. Depressed clients need to have structure provided because of impairment in decision-making and problem-solving. Options #2, #3, and #4 may promote further social isolation and increase the client's impairments. This may further decrease the client's self esteem.

4.14 ② Option #2 needs to be evaluated first due to safety issues. Options #1, #3 and #4 are not going to hurt anyone.

4.15 ④ Option #4 is most important in encouraging client to fulfill an important part of life which is being intimate with his wife. Options #1, #2 and #3 do not support alternative plans.

4.16 ② Doxepin HCL (Sinequan) is an antidepressant. Signs of overdosage include excitability and tremors. Options #1, #3, and #4 are not relevant to this condition.

4.17 ③ While all of these assessment tools are relevant to a thorough assessment of an elderly, chronically, mentally ill client, the AIMS (Abnormal Involuntary Movement Scale) is the most widely accepted examination to test for the presence of tardive dyskinesia. Option #1 is incorrect because it assesses activities of daily living and is not specific for tardive dyskinesia. Option #2 is to measure cognitive function. Option #4 is an assessment tool for determining the nature, severity, and prevalence of aggression.

4.18 ① Clients started on Disulfiram (Antabuse) must avoid any form of alcohol or they will develop a severe reaction. Most over-the-counter cough/cold preparations contain varying levels of alcohol and will produce a strong reaction. A client who ingests even small amounts of alcohol may experience flushed skin, pounding headache, tachycardia, chest pain, shortness of breath, blurred vision, hypotension, and possible confusion. Option #2 needs to be evaluated by the client's physician and should not be discontinued. Options #3 and #4 are over-the-counter medications that do not contain alcohol and will not produce an adverse reaction.

4.19 ① Option #1 is correct for the Hindu family. For an Islam family member death, only relatives or a priest may touch the body. The family washes the body and then turns it to face Mecca. Option #3 is appropriate for a Buddhist family. Option #4 is not true. Donation of organs may be done.

4.20 ④ All of these options are important and relevant to a thorough physiopsychosocial evaluation. However, initially ascertaining focused information about a very traumatic event, is helpful and provides the nurse with an opportunity to understand how this client has coped up to this point with a tragedy that has made him vulnerable.

4.21 ③ Phobic disorders can be attributed to learning theory, that they are learned responses. Therefore, learned responses can be unlearned through certain techniques such as behavioral modification. Systematic desensitization is a form of behavior modification. It is a strategy utilized in conjunction with deep muscle relaxation that is designed to decrease the extreme response to anxiety-producing situations as they are gradually exposed and then exposure is increased. The goal is to eradicate the phobic response while replacing it with the relaxation response. Options #1 and #2 are reasonable treatment options as the nurse is obtaining further information. Option #4 is usually more useful for reducing stress associated with physiologically-based disorders.

4.22 ① To successfully implement a behavior modification plan, all staff members need to be included in the program development and to allow time for discussion of concerns from each nursing staff member. Consistency and follow-through is of utmost importance to prevent or diminish the level of manipulation by the staff or client during the implementation of this program. Options #2, #3, and #4 are important in designing an effective behavior modification program. However, Option #1 is a priority.

4.23 ④ Option #4 is correct. Most abused women eventually leave the situation. Interventions may not produce quick outcomes, but they can begin to facilitate the process of healing. Options #1, #2, and #3 are incorrect. Option #1—the husband will not change without identifying cause of anxiety and altering the manner he deals with it. Options #2 and #3 do not indicate counseling was effective.

4.24 ③ The nurse does not want to reinforce the client's hallucinatory experiences. Option #1 is incorrect because reflection techniques usually do not work in this situation. Option #2 is incorrect because attempts to reason or argue with the client may entrench him more firmly into this distortion. Option #4 is a direct challenge to the client's belief about sensory-perceptual intake and may increase mistrust and conflict between the nurse and client.

4.25 ② Option #2 is correct. Diaphoresis can occur between 6–12 hours. Abdominal cramping, fever and nausea may occur later between 48–72 hours.

4.26 ① The client is probably experiencing some mild level of anxiety related to detoxification as well as his participation in the group process. He needs reinforcement and encouragement to continue attending the group meetings and to share his feelings. Options #2, #3, and #4 would not be therapeutic.

4.27 ② Clients with eating disorders experience difficulty with self identity and self-esteem which inhibits their ability to be a self advocate and act assertively. Some assertiveness techniques that are taught include: giving and receiving criticism, giving and accepting compliments, accepting apologies, being able to say no and set limits on what they can realistically do, rather than just doing what others want them to do. Options #1 and #4 are secondary because these clients may have problems with family boundary intrusion and having difficulty with feelings of anger. Family therapy sessions can be helpful in identifying some of these feelings and difficulties with family boundaries. Option #3 is usually not an issue.

4.28 ④ A disoriented client who is not able to be an independent self-care agent will need cueing from the nurse to accomplish self-feeding. Options #1, #2, and #3 are not usually indicative of a client who is disoriented. They are more characteristic of a client with a higher level of cognitive functioning.

4.29 ④ It is the nurse's initial priority to encourage the client to begin dealing with what happened by verbalizing her feelings and gaining some perspective. Options #1, #2, and #3 are valid goals that would also need to be addressed, but Option #4 is priority.

4.30 ② The major priority of the nurse is to provide and maintain safety for the client who is unable to provide for herself. A safe environment will generate trust and rapport. This will decrease resistance to the next critical steps. Options #1, #3, and #4 are important but cannot be done effectively until Option #2 is accomplished.

4.31 ③ In working with the resistant and paranoid client, the nurse must first try to develop a trusting relationship. Only if a trusting relationship develops can other important goals be accomplished. Options #1, #2, and #4 may be useful but are not the first priority.

4.32 ③ Option #3 is a priority due to safety and placing some accountability with the client. Options #1, #2 and #4 are an important part of the plan but are not a priority to Option #3.

4.33 ④ One of the functions of a family system is to assist the members in getting their physiologic, emotional and safety needs met. When the family is unequipped, unable or unwilling to do this function, this is a behavior consistent with a dysfunctional family process. Options #1, #2, and #3 are all behavioral indications of a functional family unit.

4.34 ④ Option #4 is a priority due to safety. Option #1 is partially correct, but nurses do not confront this client. Options #2 and #3 are part of therapeutic communication and are not answering the question.

4.35 ④ This allows the client some control over how to mutually deal with the anxiety related to ECT. The interpersonal contact provided by remaining with the client and discussing any fears will assist in anxiety reduction. Option #1 is inappropriate because the client must remain NPO before the ECT treatment, and coffee (especially caffeinated) is a CNS stimulant which could escalate her anxiety. Option #2 represents nurse avoidance but could be a beneficial strategy if the exercise had been instructed and practiced with the nurse. Option #3 is incorrect because medicating anxiety does not encourage the development of any additional coping strategies. Only if the level of anxiety were severe would psychopharmacologic intervention be necessary.

4.36 ③ When the client is fearful of being poisoned, he will not eat willingly and may suffer from problems with nutrition. Options #1 and #4 will have little bearing on his self-care abilities. Option #2 warrants further observation for depressive symptoms which might impair self-care, but at this point, there is no evidence to support this.

4.37 ④ Option #4 is correct. This is indicative of a melanoma and may occur to skin exposed to the sun frequently. Melanoma tend to be asymmetrical with border irregularity, color variegation, and a diameter greater than 6 mm.

4.38 ② A written schedule with built-in extra time will allow the client to understand what is expected and will allow her to participate at a slower pace. Options #1, #3, and #4 will not increase the client's independence and may interfere with the client's self-esteem.

4.39 ① This group provides ongoing support and educational information. People who attend have common needs and goals focused on managing the client's behavior at home. Options #2, #3, and #4 may be helpful, but will not have the ongoing impact that Option #1 would have.

4.40 ① Typically a client with reactive depression has the highest level of physical and psychic energy in the morning. Options #2, #3, and #4 are incorrect because energy levels decrease as the day progresses.

4.41 ② While a client is restrained, physiological integrity is important. Monitoring the positioning, tightness and peripheral circulation are essential. The nurse documents the client's response and clinical status after being restrained. Option #1 is inappropriate for the client in restraints. Option #3 is important but secondary to Option #2. Option #4 is important after the client is safely restrained.

4.42 ④ The most important priority in the nursing management of an assaultive client is to maintain safety of the client and others. A quick assessment of the situation, psychological intervention, chemical intervention and possible physical control are important when managing the physically-assaultive client. Option #1 may be a useful strategy before the client becomes assaultive. However, once the client is assaultive, he may continue this behavior in his room without any redirection and support. Option #2 may be unsafe to the other person. Option #3 is helpful but not a priority.

4.43 ③ The nurse must let the client know that this information will be shared with the staff so the client's safety can be preserved. Options #1, #2, and #4 are inaccurate because they do not answer the client's immediate concern while giving accurate information about the nurse's responsibility.

4.44 ③ Obsessive-compulsive rituals are an attempt to avoid or alleviate increasing levels of anxiety. Options #1 and #2 are incorrect because the client is not trying to increase his self-esteem or control others with his ritualistic behaviors. These behaviors, however, do have a significant impact on others. The important element in this disorder is that the person or client does not want to repeat the act but feels compelled to do so. Option #4 is incorrect because the ritual is not a method of expressing anxiety but a strategy to avoid it.

4.45 ③ The client receiving Lithium needs to maintain a regular diet with adequate fluid intake (approximately 2–3 liters per day). Lithium is a salt preparation, and its retention within the body is directly related to the body's sodium and fluid salience. Option #1 is incorrect because a depletion of sodium is to be avoided because Lithium replaces sodium in the cells, therefore precipitating Lithium toxicity. Options #2 and #4 are incorrect because diets that are low in sodium, regardless of caloric intake, do not provide adequate nutritional balance for Lithium regulation.

4.46 ② It is important that the multidisciplinary team discuss and collaborate with the client all discharge placements. The client will need support and assistance in making decisions about discharge and residential living arrangements. Option #1 may not be optimum because of possible co-dependence. Option #3 is incorrect because if the nurse visits independent of the client, that can diminish the sense of self worth and decision-making. Option #4 is incorrect because reviewing rules with the client prematurely can inhibit the opportunity to explore feelings about this decision.

4.47 ② The client who is suspicious and delusional begins to demonstrate trusting behaviors when he/she shares their feelings with the nurse. Option #1 is incorrect because their delusional system is an indication of anxiety and delusions will increase with greater anxiety. Trust with the nurse is not related to an explanation of the client's delusions. Option #3 is incorrect because the nurse's response can be an indication of transference counter-transference issues and is not indicative of the client beginning to enter a trusting relationship. Option #4 may be secondary to Option #2. It is very beneficial that the client's anxiety level is becoming less intense, and this will facilitate the development of a trusting relationship.

4.48 ④ A client undergoing ECT needs to be instructed by the nurse concerning symptoms that could be experienced during and post ECT. A backache is not a usual effect. A thorough description of the pain in relation to severity, duration, location and what makes the pain better, needs to be assessed and reported to the physician. Options #1, #2, and #3 are expected effects of the procedure.

4.49 ② ④ ⑥ Options #2, #4, and #6 are correct. Option #1— the client is reluctant and still not confident with self. Option #3—client is not comfortable enough to be self-aware of positive attributes. Option #5—client is not comfortable with nurse which means there is still not a degree of comfort with interaction.

4.50 ② The victim of interpersonal violence may have physical trauma and concealed injuries. This assessment is of utmost importance so that the client's physiologic integrity is maintained. Options #1, #3, and #4 are done concurrently as the nurse is assessing for physical injury. Privacy and encouraging the client to verbalize feelings are important. Facilitating the client to identify and rally their family or significant others to assist them during the crisis is important in the care of the victim of interpersonal violence.

4.51 ③ A positive outcome of treatment of a sexually-abused client is the verbalization that they are not responsible for the sexual abuse. The victim needs assistance to challenge the "belief of victims" which includes, "I am bad and deserve the abuse." Option #1 continues the myth of badness and that they deserved the abuse and actively consented to it. Option #2 is an outcome that would be positive but usually is not an initial result of treatment. Option #4 is an expected outcome—though not a positive one.

4.52 ④ Option #4 is most therapeutic for reducing anxiety. Option #1 does not encourage personal growth. Option #2 does not deal with the anxiety. Option #3 addresses knowledge but not feelings.

4.53 ③ Option #3 is correct. Aripiprazole is an antipsychotic agent referred to as a dopamine system stabilizer. Since these antipsychotic agents cause sedation, sleeping during the night and decreasing daytime drowsiness can be done by administering the agent at bedtime. Option #1 is incorrect because it should be avoided, not limited. Option #2 is incorrect because Ablify may be administered with or without food since it is well absorbed either way. Option #4 is an incorrect statement.

4.54 ③ The therapeutic nurse-client relationship is a mutual learning and corrective emotional experience. The nurse utilizes self and specified clinical techniques in working with the client to facilitate insight and behavioral change. Options #1, #2, and #4 are incorrect because in a nurse-client relationship, the client's needs are of primary concern.

4.55 ① Option #1 is correct. Providing a room for the client's family would be the best plan to meet the client's emotional needs. Option #2 does not meet the client's emotional needs. Option #3 is secondary. Option #4 is secondary.

4.56 ② This statement reflects the client's understanding of the side effects of chemotherapy. Option #1 may or may not occur. Option #3 is not realistic. It may be possible at times, but the question requests a "realistic perception." Option #4 is inaccurate and may reflect blame and guilt.

4.57 ③ Fluoxetine HCL (Prozac) is an "energizing" antidepressant, and as clients begin to demonstrate a positive response, they have an increased energy level and would be able to become more participative in the milieu. Options #1 and #4 can be side effects of the medication. Option #2 is not indicative of Prozac which can actually inhibit sleep and is useful with clients who experience increasing sleeping and psychomotor retardation and lethargy.

4.58 ② The client with dementia has significant difficulty with communication. Therefore, simple and short sentences can enhance the client's ability to process the information. Option #1 is incorrect because reality orientation, not reinforcement of the client's altered thought process, is an important goal. Option #3 is incorrect because anti-anxiety (anxiolytic) agents are not appropriate in the care of a dementia client and can worsen their confusional state. Option #4 is important but secondary to Option #2.

4.59 ③ It is imperative that the nurse obtain the time of the client's last drink so that anticipation of when the client would most likely experience withdrawal symptoms will be known (usually occurring within 48-72 hours after the last drink). Options #1, #2, and #4 are important to note but do not take priority over Option #3.

4.60 ④ The client who experiences a dissociative disorder is protecting himself from intense levels of anxiety that are stressful and beyond coping abilities. This client needs a safe, non-threatening approach because he typically exhibits difficulty in establishing trusting relationships. Options #1, #2, and #3 are all reasonable nursing goals that must be developed within a multidisciplinary approach in collaboration with the client but are secondary to Option #4.

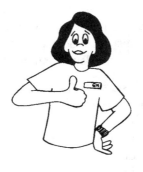

You're doing super!!

Physiological Adaptation: Fluid-Gas

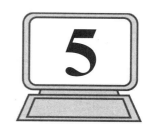

Were there none who were discontented with what they have, the world would never reach anything better.
—Florence Nightingale

✔ **Clarification of this test…**

The minmum standard includes providing direct care for client with acute, chronic or life-threatening conditions.

☞ Evaluate appropriateness/accuracy of order for client.

☞ Assess client's vital signs.

☞ Perform focused assessment or reassessment (cardiac, respiratory).

☞ Perform diagnostic testing (O_2 saturation).

☞ Monitor client's hydration status (I & O, edema, signs and symptoms of dehydration).

☞ Evaluate the results of diagnostic testing.

☞ Initiate, maintain and/or evaluate telemetry monitoring.

☞ Ensure appropriate and safe use of equipment in performing client care procedures and treatments.

☞ Assess client's need for sleep/rest and intervene as needed.

☞ Apply and maintain devices used to promote venous return (anti-embolic stocking, sequential compression device).

☞ Perform nasopharyngeal suctioning.

☞ Provide pulmonary hygiene (chest physiotherapy, spirometry).

☞ Monitor and maintain client on ventilator.

☞ Perform emergency care procedures (cardiopulmonary resuscitation, Heimlich maneuver, respiratory support, automated electronic defibrillator).

☞ Administer oxygen therapy.

5.1 Identify the area where the nurse should place the stethoscope to auscultate the PMI during the physical assessment.

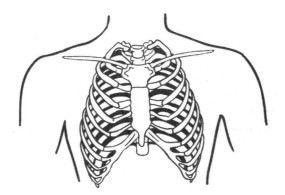

5.2 Your client has returned from having a bowel resection; and as you make rounds at the beginning of your shift, you notice that he is becoming restless. Your first action will be to:

① administer pain medication as ordered.
② order stat labs for electrolytes and blood gasses.
③ ask his family if he has a history of drug or alcohol abuse.
④ assess vital signs and urine output.

5.3 The nurse is caring for a thoracotomy client, one day postoperative, on 40% humidified oxygen. Arterial blood gas (ABG) results are:
- pO_2 90 mmHg
- pCO_2 49 mmHg
- pH 7.30
- HCO_3 26 mEq/1

Based on this information, which nursing action would be best?

① Position in high-Fowler's and encourage coughing and deep breathing. Evaluate airway patency.
② Place in prone position. Request respiratory therapy to perform postural drainage and percussion therapy.
③ Call the physician, and advise him of the arterial blood gas report. Anticipate increase in oxygen percentage.
④ Administer anti-anxiety agent, and assist the client with a rebreathing device to increase oxygen levels.

5.4 The nurse is caring for a client who has a 5-year history of chronic lung disease. The nursing assessment reveals a severely dyspneic client, pulse at 140, respirations labored, and slightly cyanotic. An appropriate nursing action to relieve the client's dyspnea would include:

① administer oxygen at 40% heated mist.
② assist the client to cough and deep breathe.
③ elevate the head of the bed, low flow oxygen.
④ position the client prone and assess breath sounds.

5.5 The pulse oximeter alarms indicating the oxygen saturation is at 86%. What would be the priority action?

① Administering oxygen via mask
② Checking the position of the probe
③ Resetting the pulse oximeter's alarm
④ Completing a cardiovascular assessment

5.6 A client recovering from Streptococcal pneumonia has a chest x-ray which reveals a higher degree of atelectasis in the right lower lobe. Which nursing intervention would be most appropriate?

① Instruct the client to take deep breaths more frequently.
② Reposition client every hour to the right side.
③ Increase frequency of incentive spirometry.
④ Change respiratory treatment to every 2 hours.

5.7 Which nursing assessment would support the complication of right-sided heart failure?

① Increasing respiratory difficulty with exertion.
② Cough productive of a large amount of thick yellow mucus.
③ Peripheral edema and anorexia.
④ Twitching of extremities.

5.8 The nurse is caring for a patient who has a left subclavian Swan Ganz catheter and a right radial arterial line. Which assessment finding requires immediate intervention?

① A dampened arterial line waveform
② Redness at Swan Ganz insertion site
③ Low pulmonary artery pressures
④ A numb, cool right hand

5.9 A 72-year-old client has an order for digoxin (Lanoxin) 0.25 mg PO in the morning. The nurse reviews the following information:
- apical pulse – 68
- respirations – 16
- plasma digoxin level – 2.2 ng/ml

Based on this assessment, which nursing action is appropriate?

① Give the medication on time.
② Withhold the medication; notify the physician.
③ Administer epinephrine 1:1000 stat.
④ Check the client's blood pressure.

5.10 Which instruction would be important for the nurse to include in discharge teaching of a hypertensive client?

① "If you begin to have a headache, double your medication for the next dose."
② "Do not decrease or discontinue your medications, even if your blood pressure feels normal."
③ "If you begin to feel fatigued, decrease your medication for 2 days and call the physician."
④ "Increase your intake of dairy products to replace the calcium you will be losing."

5.11 A client is 3 days postoperative mitral valve replacement. Which recommendation would the nurse include in the nursing care plan to prevent postoperative complications?

① Maintain in supine position to prevent tension on the mediastinal suture line.
② Encourage deep breathing, but discourage coughing because of increased central venous pressure.
③ Decrease fluids to prevent fluid retention and development of congestive heart failure.
④ Encourage early activity to promote ventilation and improve quality of circulation.

5.12 The nurse is caring for a client in ICU. Hemodynamic monitoring is accomplished via a Swan-Ganz catheter. This type of monitoring will provide which piece of information?

① Measures the circulatory volume in the coronary arteries.
② Indirectly measures the pressure in the ventricles.
③ Analyzes the adequacy of pulmonary circulation.
④ Directly measures the adequacy of CO_2 exchange.

5.13 A permanent demand pacemaker set at a rate of 72 is implanted in a client for persistent third degree block. Which nursing assessment would indicate a pacemaker dysfunction?

① Pulse rate of 88 and irregular.
② Apical pulse rate regular at 68.
③ Blood pressure of 110/88, pulse at 78.
④ Tenderness at site of pacemaker implant.

5.14 The nurse is assessing a pregnant client with problems of mitral stenosis and congestive heart failure. What information in the client's history would have a direct correlation with her current problem?

① History of rheumatic fever four years ago.
② Presence of ventricular septal defect as an infant.
③ Heart disease in both the maternal and paternal families.
④ Persistent ear infections and mastoiditis as a child.

5.15 A client is 2 days postoperative aortic aneurysm resection. A complete blood count reveals a decreased red blood cell count. Which symptoms is the nursing assessment most likely to reveal?

① Fatigue, pallor, and exertional dyspnea.
② Nausea, vomiting, and diarrhea.
③ Vertigo, dizziness, and shortness of breath.
④ Malaise, flushing, and tachycardia.

5.16 A client has tested positive for tuberculosis and is started on isoniazid (INH) for 6 months. What information would the nurse plan to include in the client's teaching plan?

① The color of the urine will change.
② Subsequent TB tests will be negative after drug administration.
③ Other medications should be withheld during therapy.
④ Alcohol consumption is contraindicated.

5.17 Which finding would the nurse identify as interfering with the effective functioning of chest tubes?

① 15 cm. water suction on chest tube system.
② An air leak in water seal chamber.
③ Leaking blood around chest tube site.
④ Clots of blood in the chest tube.

5.18 A client is scheduled for a left lower lobe lobectomy. Which nursing observation would most indicate the need for an anti-anxiety agent?

   ① Agitation and decreased level of consciousness.
   ② Lethargy and decreased respiratory rate.
   ③ Restlessness and increased heart rate.
   ④ Hostility and increased blood pressure.

5.19 Organize the following steps to suctioning in chronological order (with 1 being the first step in this procedure).

   ① Put on sterile glove.
   ② Lubricate catheter with normal saline.
   ③ Apply suction for 5–10 seconds.
   ④ Explain procedure to client.
   ⑤ Wash hands thoroughly.

5.20 A client is admitted with dehydration secondary to diarrhea. A nursing history reveals the client has been on daily medications of digoxin (Lanoxin) 0.25 mg and furosemide (Lasix) 40 mg, which are to be continued according to admit orders. Which symptom is most important for the nurse to report to the next shift?

   ① Confusion and reports of yellow lights.
   ② Character and time of daily stools.
   ③ Intake and output for the last 24 hours.
   ④ Irritability toward friends and family.

5.21 You received your client at 1000 from surgery post coronary artery bypass. This is a bedside flow sheet showing your client's chest tube drainage for the shift. What is your best action?

   ① Total the shift amount and enter in the client's chart.
   ② Notify the physician of sudden decrease in output.
   ③ Assess the client for signs of cardiac decompensation.
   ④ Irrigate the client's chest tube.

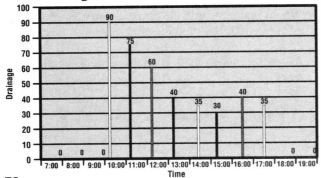

5.22 When changing the tubing on central lines, it is most important for the nurse to instruct the client to:

   ① sit in semi-Fowler's position, and take a deep breath prior to the procedure.
   ② lie down, hold breath, and bear down when the line is opened.
   ③ lie in the left lateral position, and hold breath during the procedure.
   ④ sit in the Fowler's position, and exhale during the procedure.

5.23 Which nursing action would be appropriate for a client with orthopnea, dyspnea, and bibasilar crackles?

   ① Elevate legs to promote venous return.
   ② Decrease the IV fluids, and notify the physician.
   ③ Orient the client to time, place, and situation.
   ④ Prevent complications of immobility.

5.24 A client is 3 hours postoperative thoracotomy. For the past 2 hours, there has been 200 cc per hour of bloody chest drainage. Which action should the nurse take?

   ① Increase the IV fluid rate.
   ② Administer oxygen at 5 liters/min. per face mask.
   ③ Elevate the head of the bed.
   ④ Advise the physician of the amount of drainage.

5.25 The nurse is monitoring a client's ECG strip and notes coupled premature ventricular contractions greater than 10 per min. The nurse should administer which drug?

   ① Atropine sulfate (Atropine) IV.
   ② Isoproterenol (Isuprel) IV.
   ③ Verapamil (Calan) IV.
   ④ Lidocaine hydrochloride (Xylocaine) IV.

5.26 A client awakens during the night with dyspnea, severe anxiety, jugular vein distension (JVD), and frothy pink sputum. After the nurse begins oxygen at 4 liters per nasal cannula, which action should be done next?

   ① Place 2 pillows behind head, and elevate the legs.
   ② Notify physician about change in client's condition.
   ③ Increases IV fluids to liquefy the secretions.
   ④ Dim lights and provide privacy.

5.27 It is 0600 and a client is scheduled for a cardiac catheterization at 0800. Laboratory work completed 5 days ago showed: K 3.0 mEq/L, Na 148 mEq/L, glucose 178 mg/dL. He complains of muscle weakness and cramps. Which nursing action should be implemented at this time?

① Hold 0700 dose of spironolactone (Aldactone).
② Encourage eating bananas for breakfast.
③ Call the physician to suggest a stat K level.
④ Call for a twelve lead ECG.

5.28 A client is being treated for hypovolemia. Which observation would the nurse identify as the desired response to fluid replacement?

① Urine output 160 cc/8 hours.
② Hgb 13 gm, Hct 39%.
③ Arterial pH 7.34.
④ CVP reading of 8 cm. of water pressure.

5.29 The nurse is caring for an intubated, mechanically ventilated patient. The nurse notes a "high pressure alarm" and finds the patient coughing with secretions visible in the endotracheal tube. What are the priority nursing interventions?

① Silence the alarm and sedate the patient for anxiety.
② Ambu the patient and notify respiratory therapy.
③ Suction the patient and monitor pulse oximetry.
④ Disable the alarm and order an arterial blood gas.

5.30 Your client is admitted with arterial blood gasses of 7.57, pCO_2 29, HCO_3 22. In response, the physician orders O_2 nasal cannula at 5L/min. Your priority action is to:

① begin O_2 immediately.
② determine the accuracy of the order.
③ assess for pain.
④ notify the laboratory to repeat the test prior to any action.

5.31 The nurse identifies a nursing diagnosis of disturbed sensory perception related to sleep deprivation in a mechanically ventilated patient in the ICU. What would be the priority nursing intervention for this patient?

① Cluster nursing activities and plan uninterrupted rest periods.
② Administer sedatives and hypnotics at bedtime to promote sleep.
③ Silence the monitor alarms to allow for extended periods of rest.
④ Explain to the patient types of noise and the necessity for the noise.

5.32 A nurse caring for a client with a complete heart block would contact the physician regarding which order?

① Administer Lidocaine (Xylocaine) 50 mg IV push for PVCs in excess of 6 per minute.
② Administer atropine sulfate (Atropine) .05 mg IV for symptomatic bradycardia.
③ Anticipate scheduling client for a temporary pacemaker if pulse continues to decrease.
④ Mix 10 cc of 1:5000 solution of Isoproterenol (Isuprel) in 500 cc D5W for sustained bradycardia below 30.

5.33 A client develops severe crushing chest pain radiating to the left shoulder and arm. Which PRN medication should the nurse administer?

① Diazepam (Valium) PO.
② Meperidine (Demerol) IM
③ Morphine sulfate IV.
④ Nitroglycerine (Nitrostat) SL.

5.34 A client with sudden onset of deep vein thrombosis is started on a Heparin IV drip. Which additional order should the nurse question?

① Cold wet packs to the affected leg.
② Elevate foot of bed 6 inches.
③ Commode privileges without weight bearing.
④ Elastic stockings on unaffected leg.

5.35 A client presents with peripheral venous disease. The nurse will make which assessments with this client?

① Hair loss distal to the occlusion and a cool limb.
② Brawny color of extremity and sudden pain with exercise.
③ Peripheral edema from foot to calf and no pain.
④ Pale extremity when elevated and red when dependent.

5.36 Which assessment data would indicate a client with a chest injury has sustained severe thoracic damage?

① Irregular S_1 and S_2.
② Symmetrical respiratory excursion.
③ Respiratory rate 30.
④ Paradoxical chest movement.

5.37 Which statement made by a client discharged on nitroglycerin sublingual (Nitrostat) would indicate a need for further teaching?

① "I might get a headache when I take it."
② "I should take 4–5 tablets before I call the physician."
③ "I should store them in a dark bottle."
④ "I should purchase a new supply every 6–9 months."

5.38 A client receiving a continuous IV heparin infusion has a partial thromboplastin time (PTT) 1-1/2 times greater than normal. What should the nurse do next?

① Discontinue the heparin infusion.
② Slow down the heparin infusion.
③ Check the prothrombin time (PT) results.
④ Continue to monitor the client.

5.39 A nurse is the first on the scene of a motor vehicle accident. The victim has sucking sounds with respirations at a chest wound site and tracheal deviation toward the uninjured side. Until emergency personnel arrive, the priority nursing action for the nurse is to:

① loosely cover the wound, preferably with a sterile dressing.
② place sand bag over the wound.
③ sit the client up.
④ place a firm, airtight, sterile dressing over the wound.

5.40 The nurse is caring for a client who is immediate postoperative for an abdominal aortic aneurysm repair. Vital signs include: blood pressure 100/70, pulse 120, respirations 24, urine output 75 cc over the past 3 hours. Which nursing action would be a priority for this client?

① Weigh the client to determine postoperative fluid loss.
② Obtain an ECG to evaluate the cause of the tachycardia.
③ Decrease the rate of the IV fluids and start nasal oxygen.
④ Maintain on bed rest; evaluate for decrease in CVP readings.

5.41 Which nursing goal would be appropriate for the client with deep vein thrombosis?

① To decrease inflammatory response in the affected extremity and prevent emboli formation.
② To increase peripheral circulation and oxygenation of affected extremity.
③ To prepare client and family for anticipated vascular surgery on affected extremity.
④ To prevent hypoxia associated with the development of a pulmonary emboli.

5.42 What action should a nurse take if a pleur-evac attached to a chest tube breaks?

① Immediately clamp the chest tube.
② Notify the physician.
③ Place the end of the tube in sterile water.
④ Reposition the client in the Fowler's position.

5.43 The nurse is caring for a client who has been immobilized for 3 days following a perineal prostatectomy. The client begins to experience sudden shortness of breath, chest pain, and coughing with blood-tinged sputum. Immediate nursing actions would include:

① Elevate the head of the bed, begin oxygen, assess respiratory status.
② Assist the client to cough. If unsuccessful, then perform nasotracheal suctioning.
③ Position in supine position with legs elevated. Monitor CVP closely.
④ Administer morphine for chest pain. Obtain a 12 lead ECG to evaluate cardiac status.

5.44 Which client presenting with peripheral edema would be a priority to be evaluated?

    ① A 20-year-old obstetrical client in the third trimester of pregnancy.
    ② A 30-year-old diabetic client who is a hairdresser.
    ③ A 40-year-old male client with hypertension who is taking Verapamil.
    ④ A 50-year-old male client with hypertension who is taking Lasix.

5.45 The nurse would identify which client as being at highest risk for development of a pulmonary emboli?

    ① A 19-year-old four days postpartum with obstetrical history of a placenta previa.
    ② An obese 40-year-old man with multiple pelvic fractures from an auto accident two days ago.
    ③ A 65-year-old woman who is ten days post fractured hip repair and who is in physical therapy daily.
    ④ A 22-year-old leukemic client with a platelet count of 120,000/mm^3 and hemoglobin of 9.0 gm.

5.46 Which clinical finding would be most appropriate for the client who is taking a loop diuretic to report to the nurse practitioner?

    ① Tinnitus
    ② A weight loss of 2 lbs.
    ③ Blood pressure change from 160/98 to 141/90
    ④ An increase in urinary frequency

5.47 Which sign indicates effective CPR?

    ① Adequate capillary refill
    ② Normal skin color
    ③ Symmetrically dilated pupils
    ④ Palpable carotid pulse

5.48 Two hours after a cardiac catheterization, the client begins to bleed from the femoral artery insertion site. Which nursing intervention would be most appropriate?

    ① Assess pedal pulses and apply a sandbag.
    ② Apply manual pressure and notify the physician.
    ③ Place the client in Trendelenburg immediately.
    ④ Elevate the head of the bed 40 degrees and apply an ice pack.

5.49 When obtaining a specimen from a client for sputum culture and sensitivity (C&S), which instruction would be best?

    ① After pursed lip breathing, cough into container.
    ② Upon awakening, cough deeply and expectorate into container.
    ③ Save all sputum for 3 days in covered container.
    ④ After respiratory treatment, expectorate into container.

5.50 Which assessment best indicates proper rehydration in a burn client with an IV order for 200 cc/hr?

    ① 400 cc of po intake over 3 hrs.
    ② Urine output of 100 cc per hr.
    ③ Heart rate of 105 per min.
    ④ Respiratory rate of 32 per min.

5.51 Which method is the most appropriate to assess or measure a client's jugular venous distension?

    ① Inspect the external jugular vein for distention with the client in the supine position.
    ② Observe for pulsations of the jugular vein that fluctuate with client's inspiration/exhalation.
    ③ Place the client in a Trendelenburg position for 5 minutes prior to assessment.
    ④ Recognize that a visible pulse at 2 cm above the sternal angle is recorded as distended.

5.52 Prior to sending a client for a cardiac catheterization, a priority nursing assessment finding to report to the physician would be:

    ① allergy to iodine and/or shell fish.
    ② diminished palpable peripheral pulses.
    ③ cool lower extremities bilaterally.
    ④ anxiety over pending procedure.

5.53 Which nursing action would compromise safety when administering a tube feeding to a client with a tracheostomy?

    ① Place the client in supine position.
    ② Aspirate and return residual stomach contents.
    ③ Determine placement of tube.
    ④ Check bowel sounds.

5.54 Which method is the best for the nurse to evaluate the effectiveness of tracheal suctioning?

① Note subjective data such as, "My breathing is much improved now."
② Note objective findings such as decreased respiratory rate and pulse.
③ Consult with respiratory therapist to determine effectiveness.
④ Auscultate the chest for change or clearing in adventitious breath sounds.

5.55 While the nurse is providing care for a client who is on a volume cycled positive pressure ventilator, the low volume alarm sounds. What assessment would you anticipate the nurse to make?

① Client is biting on the tubing.
② Excessive fluid is in the ventilator tubing.
③ A leak in the client's endotracheal tube cuff
④ Client is lying on the tubing.

5.56 To assess the right middle lobe (RML) of the lung, the nurse would auscultate at which location?

① Posterior and anterior base of right side.
② Right anterior chest between the fourth and sixth intercostals.
③ Left of the sternum, midclavicular at the fifth intercostal.
④ Posterior chest wall, midaxillary right side.

5.57 During a cardiac assessment, the nurse assesses an S_4. What additional assessments indicate an understanding of the implications of this assessment?

① Occipital headache
② Jugular vein distention
③ Weight loss
④ Hepatosplenomegaly

5.58 Your client becomes extubated while being turned. He is cyanotic and has bradycardia and arrhythmias. Which action would be the highest priority while waiting for a physician to arrive?

① Immediately begin CPR.
② Increase the IV fluids.
③ Provide oxygen by ambuing and maintaining the airway.
④ Prepare the medications for resuscitation.

5.59 Following a cardiac catheterization, which nursing assessment would justify calling the physician?

① Serosanguineous drainage on the femoral dressing.
② Discomfort at the site of the femoral catheter insertion.
③ Appearance of redness at the catheter insertion site.
④ Absence of pulse distal to the catheter insertion site.

5.60 What would be the highest priority for providing care for a client with a pulmonary artery catheter?

① Reporting a reddened area at catheter site.
② Reporting a PA reading of 10.
③ Changing dressing daily.
④ Position client in semi-Fowler's position for tubing change.

Answers & Rationales

5.1 Point to the right interspace at the left midclavicular line.

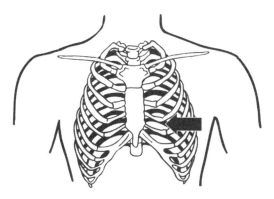

5.2 ④ Post-operative restlessness should create a high degree of suspicion of hypoxemia (for instance—due to bleeding). Vital signs and urine output will give information regarding intravascular volume. Option #1 calls for further assessment to rule out hypoxemia as the cause of the restlessness. Option #2 might be the second priority. Option #3 may indicate an erroneous assumption.

5.3 ① The client is experiencing respiratory acidosis from decreased ventilation. Increasing the quality of ventilation by removing secretions may resolve the problem. Option #2 is used for chronic airway problems. Option #3 is incorrect because the oxygen levels are within the normal range. Action needs to be taken before notifying the physician. Option #4 is for respiratory alkalosis.

5.4 ③ The client is dyspneic, but administering too much oxygen may increase his dyspnea by decreasing his respiratory drive. Position him in high-Fowler's to improve quality of ventilation, and begin oxygen at low liter flow. Option #1 is too high a level of oxygen. Option #2 is not a priority for this client. Option #4 does not address the problem.

5.5 ② Option #2 is correct. The probe may have fallen off. This is the priority action to prevent inappropriate or unnecessary intervention. Options #1, #3, and #4 are incorrect.

5.6 ③ Incentive spirometry is a quantifiable method to assess respiratory effort with deep breathing exercises. Increasing the frequency would be a sound nursing decision in an effort to improve the client's pulmonary status. Option #1 would be effective, however, not as much as Option #3. Option #2 would actually decrease the thoracic expansion of the chest wall on the right side. Option #4 is incorrect because there is no basis to make a judgment about the type of treatment.

5.7 ③ Right-sided heart failure is manifested by a congestion of the venous system resulting in peripheral edema as well as congestion of the gastric veins resulting in anorexia and the eventual development of ascites. Option #1 is a common assessment finding of the chronic lung client. Option #2 is describing a complication of pneumonia. Option #4 is not appropriate to this client.

5.8 ④ Option #4 is correct. A numb, cool hand demonstrates reduced blood flow that can result in limb ischemia. Options #1, #2 and #3 are a concern, but not a priority.

5.9 ② Withhold the medication and notify the physician because the therapeutic plasma level of digoxin is 0.5–2.0 ng/ml. Option #1 is incorrect because the medication should be withheld. Option #3 is not a correct statement. Option #4 is inappropriate because it ignores the blood level of digoxin.

5.10 ② Compliance with medication administration is a serious problem with hypertensive clients. Options #1 and 3 are incorrect because clients must continue their medication, and notify the physician of excessive fatigue or consistent headaches. They should not alter their medication without notifying the physician. Option #4 is incorrect because calcium is not a problem with this client.

5.11 ④ Postoperative open-heart clients should be encouraged to be out of bed and ambulate as soon as possible. Option #1 is incorrect because the client is maintained in semi-Fowler's position. Option #2 is incorrect because coughing and deep breathing should be encouraged. Option #3 is incorrect as fluids are encouraged unless there is evidence of cardiac failure.

5.12 ② The CVP readings measure the pressure of the right ventricle; and the pulmonary artery wedge pressure reading is an indirect pressure of the left ventricle. Options #1, #3, and #4 are not functions of this catheter and do not reflect hemodynamic monitoring.

5.13 ② Anytime the pulse rate drops below the preset rate on the pacemaker, then the pacer is malfunctioning. The pulse should be maintained at a minimal rate set on the pacemaker. Options #1 and #3 do not indicate malfunction of the pacemaker. Option #4 may be an early sign of infection at the site.

5.14 ① By far the most common cause of mitral valve problems is a history of rheumatic fever with subsequent complication of carditis that affect the valve. Options #2, #3, and #4 do not contribute to mitral valve disease.

5.15 ① These "constitutional symptoms" are characteristic of most types of anemia and are predominantly the result of tissue hypoxia secondary to inadequate red blood cells. Options #2, #3, and #4 are not as indicative of the loss of red blood cells.

5.16 ④ Alcohol consumption while on INH therapy has been reported to increase isoniazid-related hepatitis. Therefore, clients should be cautioned to restrict consumption of alcohol. Options #1, #2, and #3 are untrue.

5.17 ② An air leak would not allow negative pressure to be reestablished and would hinder complete resolution of the pneumothorax. Therefore, partial atelectasis could be noted. Option #1 is an appropriate order for chest tubes. Option #3 does not hinder the chest tube functioning. Option #4 would be an expected finding. It would be important for the nurse to ensure tube patency.

5.18 ③ The most indicative observation for anti-anxiety drugs is restlessness and increase in heart rate due to circulating catecholamines (fight or flight syndrome). Options #1 and #2 are more indicative of preoperative complications and should be reported before medications are given. Option #4 may be best treated by ventilating feelings.

5.19 #4 would be done first.
#5 would be done second.
#1 would be done third.
#2 would be done fourth.
#3 would be done last.

5.20 ① This describes characteristic signs and symptoms of digoxin toxicity. Digoxin toxicity is a great concern in the presence of diarrhea or any circumstance that leads to alteration in fluid and electrolyte balance. This is especially true with the young or elderly. Options #2, #3, and #4 are appropriate for this client, but are not as high a priority as Option #1.

5.21 ③ Option #3 is the most appropriate action when chest tube drainage has abruptly decreased or stopped. The change in drainage may indicate a blockage of the tube, cardiac tamponade, or internal bleeding into the mediastinum. Further assessment of cardiac function is indicated. Option #1 is appropriate documentation but does not include an appropriate response to a potentially life-threatening change in client status. Option #2 will be done after further assessment. Option #4 is inappropriate without further reassessment and identification of the cause.

5.22 ② This option is the safest procedure. Since the catheter goes into the thoracic cavity, it is subjected to changes in pressure which increase the risk of air emboli. Options #1, #3, and #4 are unsafe.

5.23 ② Orthopnea, dyspnea, and crackles are signs and symptoms of fluid excess. Decreasing the IV fluids is the priority. Option #1 would worsen the situation. Options #3 and #4 are not of priority to the situation.

5.24 ④ Chest drainage in excess of 100 cc/hr. is not normal and the physician should be notified. Options #1, #2, and #3 may all be appropriate after the physician is notified.

5.25 ④ Lidocaine is the drug of choice for frequent premature ventricular contractions occurring in excess of 6–10 per minute, or if they are coupled, or in a consecutive series which may result in ventricular tachycardia. Options #1, #2, and #3 are not used in treating ventricular irritability.

5.26 ② The next priority is to notify the physician since the signs indicate pulmonary edema. Options #1 and #3 would increase fluids to the lungs. Option #4 is incorrect because the nurse should stay with the client for reassurance.

5.27 ③ The signs and symptoms are indicative of hypokalemia. A stat serum K level is needed to confirm the K level prior to going for cardiac catheterization. Option #1 is incorrect because Aldactone is potassium sparing and is an oral medication. Option #2 is not feasible prior to the cardiac catheterization since the client is NPO. Option #4 is unnecessary.

5.28 ④ The normal range for CVP is 3-8 cm water pressure (or 5-6 mmHg). A reading of 8 cm H_2O would indicate a desired response from fluid replacement. Option #1 indicates a hypovolemic state. Option #2 is inappropriate for this situation. Option #3 is acidosis which can result from various problems.

5.29 ③ Option #3 is correct. A high pressure alarm signals increased pressure in the airways. In the presence of visible secretions in the endotracheal tube, suctioning the patient and monitoring pulse oximetry is priority to reducing airway pressure. Option #1 is never appropriate. Options #2 and #4 are inappropriate actions.

5.30 ① This blood gasses indicates that the client needs oxygen immediately. Option #2: This order is within normal limits and does not need questioning. Option #3: It is always appropriate to asses for pain, but starting the oxygen has priority here. Option #4 would be costly and unnecessary.

5.31 ① Option #1 is correct. Clustering nursing activities promotes sleep-wake cycles. Option #2—sedatives and hypnotics disrupt normal sleep patterns. Option #3—silencing the monitors is a safety violation. Option #4—explaining the necessity for the noise is not therapeutic.

5.32 ① In complete heart block, the AV node blocks all impulses from the SA node so the atria and ventricles beat independently. Because Lidocaine suppresses ventricular irritability, it may diminish the existing ventricular response. All cardiac depressants are contraindicated in presence of complete heart block. Options #2, #3, and #4 are appropriate treatments.

5.33 ③ Morphine sulfate is given to reduce pain, anxiety, and cardiac workload. Option #1 does not reduce this type of pain. Option #2 is less common because it may induce vomiting and initiate a vagal response. Option #4 is incorrect because the nurse would administer it by IV to reduce pain and decrease overload. A client at home may have taken NTG SL.

5.34 ① Warm, moist heat is used to relieve the pain and treat the inflammation. Options #2, #3, and #4 are appropriate therapy.

5.35 ③ Venous disease results from obstruction such as thrombus, thrombophlebitis, or incompetent valves. Signs and symptoms include: little or no pain, brawn (reddish-brown skin color), cyanotic if dependent, stasis dermatitis, limb warm to touch, statis ulcers, and peripheral edema present which may be from foot to calf. Options #1, #2, and #4 would be assessed with arterial insufficiency. While in Option #2 part of it describes venous insufficiency, the sudden pain is a result of arterial complications.

5.36 ④ Paradoxical chest movement occurs with a flail chest. Immediate treatment of flail chest is directed toward improvement of ventilation and oxygenation as well as stabilization of the chest wall. Option #1 describes normal heart sounds. Option #2 is a normal finding. Option #3 occurs with increased anxiety.

5.37 ② The recommended dose is 1 tablet sublingual which can be followed at 5-minute intervals with 2 more doses. After 3 doses without pain relief, medical attention should be sought. Options #1, #3, and #4 are all appropriate statements.

5.38 ④ An expected result of Heparin therapy is prolonged PTT of 1.5–2.5 times the control, without signs of hemorrhage. Options #1 and #2 do not indicate a reason to discontinue or slow infusion since the PTT is appropriately prolonged. Option #3 is incorrect because the prothrombin time (PT) test is useful for assessing warfarin (Coumadin) therapy.

5.39 ① In an open pneumothorax, air enters pleural cavity through an open wound. Placing a sterile dressing loosely over the wound allows air to escape, but not re-enter the pleural space. Options #2 and #4 would prevent air from escaping. Option #3 is inappropriate since a chest tube has not yet been inserted.

5.40 ④ Client is at increased risk for development of hypovolemic shock. The vital signs and urine output correlate with the early signs of shock. CVP needs to be evaluated with previous readings. Option #1 is not a priority. Option #2 is incorrect because an ECG will not determine cause of tachycardia. Option #3 is incorrect because IV fluid will probably be increased.

5.41 ① It is important to prevent the complication of pulmonary emboli in clients at high risk. Option #2 relates to arterial disease. Option #3 is incorrect because surgery is not anticipated for this client. Option #4 is incorrect because preventing the problem is first priority.

5.42 ③ Option #3 is the safest for the client and will allow the nurse time to set up another pleurevac. Option #1 is unsafe and could result in a mediastinal shift. The majority of physicians will request the chest tubes not be clamped. Option #2 is not a priority. Option #4 is incorrect.

5.43 ① Based on the client's history, current immobility, and assessment factors, this client is experiencing a pulmonary emboli. Priority nursing care is to prevent severe hypoxia and maintain ventilation. Option #2 is not appropriate. Option #3 is for hypotension. Option #4 is for a cardiac client.

5.44 ③ An undesirable effect from calcium channel blockers may be peripheral edema. Options #1 and #2 are not priorities. Peripheral edema would be an expected assessment in these 2 clients. Option #4 is receiving Lasix for the peripheral edema.

5.45 ② Obesity, immobility, and pooling of blood in the pelvic cavity contribute to development of pulmonary emboli. Options #1 and #4 are high risk for shock and bleeding complications. Option #3 is incorrect because the client is not immobilized.

5.46 ① A potential adverse reaction is ototoxicity. Tinnitus may result from this problem. Options #2, #3, and #4 are expected outcomes from this medication.

5.47 ④ Palpable carotid pulse is the indicator of effective CPR. Options #1, #2, and #3 are not as objective or definitive.

5.48 ② Option #2 is correct. The client is bleeding and the intervention is to stop it. Option #1 is incorrect. The assessment of the pulses is not going to stop the bleeding. Option #3 is incorrect. Option #4 is not appropriate for this situation.

5.49 ② Specimens should be obtained in the early morning because secretions develop during the night. Option #1 is incorrect because coughing deeply is indicated but not pursed lip breathing. Option #3 is appropriate for Acid-Fast Stain. Option #4 is incorrect because the earliest specimen is most desirable.

5.50 ② This indicates appropriate renal function. Option #1 doesn't evaluate renal sufficiency. Options #3 and #4 are too rapid which indicates a hypovolemic state.

5.51 ② In measuring JVD, pulsations that fluctuate upon respirations are observed. Options #1 and #3 are incorrect because the client is positioned at a 45-degree angle, and the nurse inspects the internal jugular vein. Option #4 is incorrect because 2 cm or less is considered normal.

5.52 ① Allergies to iodine and/or seafood must be reported immediately prior to a cardiac catheterization to avoid anaphylactic shock during the procedure. Options #2, #3, and #4 are not specific for this procedure.

5.53 ① To minimize risk for aspiration, the client should be maintained in semi-Fowler's position. Options #2, #3, and #4 are all appropriate interventions.

5.54 ④ To assess the effectiveness of suctioning, the nurse auscultates the client's chest to determine if the adventitious sounds are cleared and to ensure the airway is clear of secretions. Option #1 is subjective data and not as conclusive. Option #2 is correct but not as specific to suctioning as Option #4. Option #3 is inappropriate.

5.55 ③ Option #3 is correct. When the low alarm sounds, this usually indicates a leak. Options #1, #2, and #4 would result in a high volume alarm.

5.56 ② The RML is found right anterior between the fourth and sixth intercostal spaces. Options #1 and #4 are incorrect because the RML cannot be auscultated from the posterior. Option #3 is the point of maximum impulse or apical pulse.

5.57 ① S_4 is indicative of problems with hypertension. A client may present with an occipital headache upon arising in the morning, blurred vision, and an elevated blood pressure. Options #2 and #4 are related to right-sided heart failure. Option #3 is incorrect.

5.58 ③ Airway is the priority. The client's clinical changes have occurred due to hypoxia. Providing oxygen will maintain the client until the physician can reintubate. Option #1 is inappropriate since the client still has a pulse. Option #2 is incorrect since the hypoxia is not secondary to hypovolemia. Option #4 is not a priority over the client.

5.59 ④ The absence of the femoral pulse is a grave situation as it denotes lack of blood supply to the lower extremity. The physician should be notified immediately. Option #1 is to be expected. The appearance of a hematoma at the insertion site or excessive bleeding would be important information to notify the physician since that would indicate probable arterial bleeding. Options #2 and #3 are to be expected as part of the inflammatory response after the femoral catheter insertion.

5.60 ① Preventing infection is a priority for any client with central line. Option #2 is within the normal range. Option #3 is not necessary. Gauze dressings are changed every 48 hours. Transparent dressings may not be changed for 5–7 days.

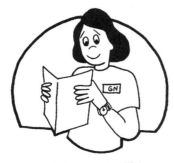

More notes!?!

Reduction of Risk Potential:
Sensory-Perception-Mobility

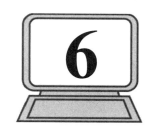

The more you connect with the power within you,
the more you can be free in all areas of your life.
                                        —Louise Hay

✔ **Clarification of this test…**

These questions relate to those activities that will cause increased risk to the client and include: auditory, visual and verbal impairment, increased intracranial pressure, seizure disorders, musculoskeletal and neuromuscular impairment, sleep and rest, —just to name a few.

Examples of these activities include:

☛ Maintain client's skin integrity (skin care, turn, alternation pressure mattress).

☛ Ensure appropriate and safe use of equipment in performing client care procedures and treatments.

☛ Perform a risk assessment (sensory impairment, potential for falls, level of mobility).

☛ Assist client in performance of activities of daily living.

☛ Assess readiness to learn, learning preferences and barriers to learning.

☛ Assess client's need for sleep/rest and intervene as needed.

☛ Use precautions to prevent further injury when moving a client with a musuloskeletal condition (log rolling, abduction pillow).

☛ Provide information for prevention of high risk behaviors.

6.1 For a client with a neurological disorder, which nursing assessment will be most helpful in determining subtle changes in the client's level of consciousness?

① Client posturing
② Glasgow Coma Scale
③ Client thinking pattern
④ Occurrence of hallucinations

6.2 The most important information for the nurse to obtain prior to a computerized axial tomography (CAT) scan concerns:

① problems being in closed spaces.
② allergies to aspirin.
③ intact swallow and gag reflex.
④ full range of motion of all extremities.

6.3 Which client's pain should be assessed initially?

① A client experiencing pain 2 hours after a liver biopsy.
② A client with a long leg cast who was medicated for pain 45 min. earlier.
③ A maternity client who experiences pain during breast feeding.
④ A 4-year-old child who complains of a sore throat after a tonsillectomy.

6.4 Which of these 80-year-old clients should be referred to the physician for further evaluation?

① A client with presbyopia.
② A client with presbycusis.
③ A client with a decreased sensitivity in cranial nerve 1.
④ A client with a depressed cranial nerve 9 and 10.

6.5 At the time of diagnosis, a client with Bell's Palsy is given a supply of eye patches. The client should be cautioned against:

① allowing the cornea of the eye to become dry.
② photosensitivity regarding light on the retina.
③ sudden movement of the head when bending over.
④ contamination from the affected eye to the other eye.

6.6 Which action should the nurse take if a CBC of a client receiving Cephalexin (Keflex) intravenously reflects a significant decrease in red cells and platelets?

① Withhold drug pending notification of physician regarding lab results.
② Administer medication for next 2 scheduled doses and notify physician of CBC changes.
③ Discontinue drug until another CBC can be performed.
④ Proceed with administration of dose without delay.

6.7 While the nurse is irrigating an ear to remove cerumen, the client comments that he is getting dizzy. The nurse would stop the procedure and:

① notify the physician immediately.
② monitor for changes in intracranial pressure.
③ warm the irrigant and resume the procedure.
④ explore the canal with a cotton applicator.

6.8 A client with a recent lumbar spinal cord injury must be repositioned. Nursing actions would include:

① having client raise his leg and turn to opposite side.
② removing the pillow between the client's legs.
③ turning the client smoothly, maintaining straight alignment.
④ moving the client to the middle of the bed.

5.9 A client with a closed head injury begins to vomit. Which assessment is the most important for the nurse to report when calling the physician?

① Increasing lethargy.
② Heart rate 80.
③ Sodium level of 145.
④ Presence of facial symmetry.

6.10 A client returns to the unit after having plastic surgery for left hand reconstruction. The nurse would implement which action to the left hand?

① Apply heat.
② Apply cold packs.
③ Alternate with heat and cold packs.
④ Apply paraffin.

6.11 The nurse is observing a client for complications following a craniotomy. The client begins complaining of thirst and fatigue. Which nursing observation is most important to report to the physician?

① Specific gravity of urine is increased; urine is foul smelling.
② Fluid intake over past 24 hours has been 3000 cc.
③ Urine output in excess of 4000 cc in 24 hours.
④ Presence of diarrhea and excoriation of anal area.

6.12 Before teaching a CVA client about self-care, which plan would be a priority?

① Have the client identify perception of health status.
② Identify the client's strengths and weaknesses.
③ Encourage client to discuss concerns with another CVA client.
④ Provide client with a written plan of therapy.

6.13 Which of these procedures is correct for wrapping a stump after an amputation?

① Make three figure-eight turns to adequately cover the ends of the stump.
② Wrap the ace bandage in a circular motion around the stump.
③ Unroll the bandage upward over the stump and to the front of the leg.
④ Wrap the stump so that it narrows toward the proximal end.

6.14 The client is admitted via the emergency room with a possible cervical spinal cord injury. The most important information for the nurse to obtain is:

① history of accident and type of trauma.
② neurological functioning.
③ respiratory status and tissue perfusion.
④ allergies and pre-existing medical conditions.

6.15 The nurse would identify which ocular response as desirable for the client using Pilocarpine eye drops?

① Pupillary constriction.
② Pupillary dilation.
③ Corneal lubrication.
④ Clearing of injected sclera.

6.16 What would be the highest priority for a client 72 hours after having 2nd-degree burns to 20% of his body in the lower abdominal area, back, and both legs?

① Airway
② Body image
③ Fluid and electrolytes
④ Pain

6.17 Which is the most important postoperative nursing action for the client following a scleral buckling procedure for detached retina?

① Remove reading material to decrease eye strain.
② Closely assess for presence of nausea and prevent vomiting.
③ Assess color of drainage from affected eye.
④ Maintain sterility for q3h saline eye irrigations.

6.18 What would the nurse ask the client to do when evaluating the cranial nerve XI?

① Ask client to smell and identify different odors.
② Ask client to shrug the shoulders.
③ Ask client to read a Snellen chart.
④ Ask client to stick out tongue and move from side to side.

6.19 A client is admitted with a diagnosis of trigeminal neuralgia (Tic Douloureux) involving the maxillary branch of the affected nerve. The nurse would plan nursing care to assist the client with which problem?

① Intermittent blurred vision and tinnitus.
② Intense facial pain on affected side.
③ Attacks of severe dizziness and vertigo.
④ Impaired speech function due to muscle spasm.

6.20 A client with a head injury has an order for hourly neuro checks. During the evaluation, the nurse would anticipate which assessment indicating an early sign of increased intracranial pressure?

① An alteration in the client's ability to answer questions and respond to verbal stimuli.
② Cushing's triad.
③ Decorticate posturing.
④ The presence of Doll's eyes.

6.21 The physician orders a wet-to-dry dressing for your client with a venous stasis ulcer. The correct method of implementing this order is to:

  ① moisten the skin around the ulcer. Then apply a dry gauze dressing.
  ② apply antibacterial ointment to the wound. Then apply a dry gauze dressing.
  ③ apply a wet dressing and allow to dry. Then wet again to remove.
  ④ Apply a wet dressing. Allow to dry; then remove.

6.22 The nurse is caring for an elderly client with bilateral eye patches. Which nursing action would be most beneficial in preventing problems secondary to sensory deprivation?

  ① Maintain client sedation until eye patches are removed.
  ② Isolate client so others will not confuse him.
  ③ Maintain a calm, dark environment conducive to rest.
  ④ Speak to him frequently, and provide frequent touch.

6.23 Which statement made by the parents of a child with hydrocephalus indicates they understand how to care for a child with a ventriculoperitoneal shunt?

  ① "We will position our child on the operative side."
  ② "We will position our child in the semi-Fowler's position after surgery."
  ③ "We will report if our child starts vomiting."
  ④ We will rely on the home health nurse to pump the shunt."

6.24 Which statement by the client best indicates an understanding of and preparedness for a scheduled magnetic resonance imaging (MRI)?

  ① "The dye used in the test will turn my urine green for about 24 hours."
  ② "I will be put to sleep for this procedure. I will return to my room in 2 hours."
  ③ "This procedure will take about 1-1/2 hours to complete. It will be noisy."
  ④ "The wires that will be attached to my head and chest will not cause me any pain."

6.25 When caring for a client with myasthenia gravis, an important nursing consideration would be to:

  ① prevent accidents from falls as a result of vertigo.
  ② maintain fluid and electrolyte replacement.
  ③ control situations that could increase intracranial pressure and cerebral edema.
  ④ assess muscle groups that are affected as they tend to be weaker toward the end of the day.

6.26 The nurse would identify which response as the therapeutic one to mydriatic eye drops?

  ① Pupillary dilation
  ② Decrease in ocular pain
  ③ Resolution of sclera inflammation
  ④ Pinpoint pupils with decreased response

6.27 What is the highest priority following a grand mal seizure?

  ① Remain with client and administer anticonvulsant medication.
  ② Document the events prior to the onset of the seizure.
  ③ Maintain a patent airway by turning client's head to the side and suctioning if necessary.
  ④ Protect client from injuring self by removing constricting clothes.

6.28 In planning the care of a client with an acute episode of Ménière's Syndrome, the nurse would outline teaching to include:

  ① adding salt to food.
  ② avoiding sudden motion of the head.
  ③ restricting fluids to 3–4 glasses daily.
  ④ keeping cotton in affected ear.

6.29 Which instruction would the nurse include in a discharge teaching plan for the client with a diagnosis of glaucoma?

  ① Decrease intake of saturated fats and potassium.
  ② Eye pain and nausea should be reported to the physician.
  ③ Anticipate gradual increase in visual field.
  ④ Eye drops may be discontinued after two weeks.

6.30 Which communication technique would be appropriate for a nurse to implement when caring for a client with a hearing loss?

① Irrigate the ear with warm water to remove any wax obstruction.
② Always touch the client prior to speaking to him.
③ Encourage the client to purchase a hearing aid.
④ Stand in front of him and speak clearly and slowly.

6.31 Which statement made by a client with a left-sided hemi paresis from a CVA indicates an understanding of how to transfer out of the bed?

① "The wheel chair should be on the right side of the bed."
② "The wheel chair should be on the left side of the bed."
③ "I will use a cane."
④ "I will wait for the physical therapist to lift me out of the bed."

6.32 Which client would have the highest potential for skin breakdown?

① A client with functional incontinence.
② A client in Buck's traction.
③ A new postoperative hip replacement.
④ Two-hour postoperative knee replacement.

6.33 A client with a long leg cast on his right leg has a foot that is pale and cool to touch. An analgesic has offered no relief to severe leg pain after 45 minutes. The first action of the nurse should be to:

① apply a heating pad to the right toes.
② repeat the dose of analgesic stat.
③ remove the cast immediately.
④ notify the physician immediately.

6.34 Prior to teaching the client how to appropriately use the cane, which assessment would be a priority? Assessment of:

① gait
② risk
③ emotional status
④ posture

6.35 A client with a closed head injury has a nasogastric tube in place and begins to vomit. What is the highest priority?

① Check the nasogastric tube for appropriate placement.
② Reposition client in bed to the side lying position.
③ Notify physician.
④ Remove the tube immediately.

6.36 Which nursing assessment suggests a complication of a plaster-of-paris cast application on the arm?

① The client states that the wet cast feels "warm."
② The client is able to move his fingers and thumb freely.
③ The client states that his little finger feels "asleep."
④ The wet cast appears gray and smells slightly musty.

6.37 On the second day following a lumbar disc excision, the client complains of mild pain in both legs. The nurse's response is based on which understanding of leg pain in the early postoperative period?

① Should delay early ambulation.
② Can result from swelling which compresses the nerve.
③ Is common for months after surgery.
④ Indicates surgery was unsuccessful.

6.38 An 18-year-old immobilized for trauma to the spinal cord, has periods of diaphoresis, a draining abdominal wound, and diarrhea. An appropriate priority nursing diagnosis is:

① potential constipation related to immobilization.
② impaired skin integrity related to immobilization and secretions.
③ potential for wound infection related to involuntary bowel secretions.
④ potential fluid volume deficit related to secretions.

6.39 The nursing assessment in a client exhibiting symptoms of myxedema should reveal:

① increased pulse rate.
② decreased temperature.
③ fine tremors.
④ increased radioactive iodine uptake level.

6.40 A client with Parkinson's disease has the nursing diagnosis: "potential for injury related to tremors." To promote safety, the nurse would instruct the client about:

① the use of crutches.
② over-filling cup of hot liquids.
③ care of contractures.
④ methods to prevent decubitus formation.

6.41 Which nursing assessment is the most important regarding proper fitting of crutches?

① With the client standing, the top of the crutch should be approximately 2" below the axillary area.
② The bottom of the crutches should be positioned next to the heel of the foot.
③ The arms should be fully extended to the crutch hand grips.
④ The crutches should fit snugly under the arm for weight-bearing.

6.42 Following a left above-the-knee amputation, the nurse is teaching a client regarding positioning. Which response by the client indicates an understanding of the importance of the prone position postoperatively?

① "I need to lie on my stomach to keep from getting a flexion contracture at my left hip."
② "Lying flat keeps my blood flowing and prevents my stump from swelling."
③ "I need to lie on my stomach to prevent a pressure sore on my hips."
④ "I will always elevate my stump when I am in a chair to keep it from swelling."

6.43 A 70-year-old female is diagnosed with a potential cerebral vascular accident (CVA). She presents with left-sided facial paralysis and is unable to move her left side. Her husband attempts to give her a drink of water and she begins choking. What would be the most appropriate nursing action?

① Encourage the husband to use a straw when helping the client drink fluid.
② Explain to the husband that the client is NPO.
③ Reposition client and assist husband to give his wife small sips of fluid.
④ Request him to stop; then assess the client's gag reflex.

6.44 Which nursing measure would be the most appropriate in preventing complications of immobility with an elderly client?

① Consistent use of bedrails
② Physical restraints
③ Encourage isometric muscle contraction.
④ Encourage as much assistance from the caregiver with activities of daily living as needed.

6.45 Which statement made by a client with hypothyroidism started on levothyroxine sodium (Synthroid) indicates a need for further teaching?

① "This medicine might affect my diabetes."
② "I'll take this little pill every day before I have breakfast."
③ "I'll be able to quit taking this pill when I start feeling better."
④ "This medicine will affect the action of my heart pill—Lanoxin."

6.46 To evaluate the desired response of calcium gluconate in treating acute hypoparathyroidism, the nurse would monitor the client most closely for:

① intake and output.
② confusion.
③ tetany.
④ bone deformities.

6.47 In planning discharge teaching for a postoperative client after a lumbar laminectomy, which muscles would the nurse instruct the client to exercise regularly?

① Anal sphincter
② Abdominal
③ Trapezius
④ Rectus femoris

6.48 The nurse would caution the client with hypothyroidism about avoiding:

① warm environmental temperatures.
② narcotic sedatives.
③ increased physical exercise.
④ numbness and tingling of fingers.

6.49 Which nursing measure would be least helpful in maintaining skin integrity?

① Measure lesion size using the two greatest perpendicular diameters and lesion depth or elevation, and document in record.
② Use an air-supported mattress or bed.
③ Educate client regarding how to safely take his iron supplement.
④ Encourage foods high in protein.

6.50 The client with newly diagnosed multiple sclerosis is preparing to go home. The nurse should caution the client about:

① ambulating every day.
② over-exposure to heat or cold.
③ stretching and strengthening exercises.
④ participating in social activities.

6.51 A client who has diabetes mellitus has the following HgB A 1C and fasting blood sugar reports.
7/01 – HgB A1C – High, 7/20 – FBS – normal,
8/01 – FBS - normal, 8/20 – HgB A1C – High.
How would the nurse interpret these results?

① The client is being well managed.
② The client is not being well controlled.
③ The client needs to decrease the daily insulin.
④ The client needs to understand that the HgB A1C evaluates the current management.

6.52 In planning care for the client with hyperthyroidism, the nurse would anticipate the client to require:

① extra blankets for warmth.
② ophthalmic drops on a regular basis.
③ increased sensory stimulation.
④ frequent low calorie snacks.

6.53 Which observation by the nurse would indicate the client is beginning to accept blindness?

① walking in hall without a walking cane
② asking sister to fix her hair
③ surveying her room, touching furniture
④ not listening to TV or radio when alone

6.54 Which nursing intervention is inappropriate in helping a depressed client to sleep more hours per night?

① Teach deep breathing and relaxation techniques.
② Explore what client is thinking and feeling when unable to sleep.
③ Help client express her feelings more clearly.
④ Administer a sedative-hypnotic medication at bedtime.

6.55 Which statement made by the client indicates a correct understanding of steroid therapy for Addison's Disease?

① "I'll take the medicine in the morning because if I take it at night, it might keep me awake."
② "I'll take the same amount from now on."
③ "I'll increase my potassium by eating more bananas."
④ "This medicine probably won't affect my blood pressure."

6.56 Which statement made by the client with Cushing's syndrome indicates a need for further teaching?

① "I realize I'll have to begin an exercise program slowly and gradually."
② "I'm going to have to keep a close eye on my blood pressure."
③ "I'm not really worried about getting pneumonia this winter."
④ "I'll be eating foods low in carbohydrates and salt."

6.57 In planning care for the client with Cushing's syndrome, which nursing action would be highest priority?

① Prevent skin breakdown.
② Prevent infections.
③ Teach client signs and symptoms of hyperglycemia.
④ Prevent fluid overload.

6.58 What is the priority clinical finding that the nurse must monitor for a client who has pheochromocytoma?

① blood pressure
② skin temperature
③ urine for occult blood
④ weight

6.59 Nursing care specific for an adult in Buck's traction would include:

    ① checking site of pins for bleeding or infection.
    ② applying topical or antibiotic ointment as ordered.
    ③ assessing that the elastic bandages are not too loose or too tight.
    ④ removing the bandages daily to lubricate the skin.

6.60 For an elderly client who has just had a prosthetic hip implant, which postoperative position should be maintained?

    ① The affected hip should be internally rotated and flexed.
    ② The affected hip should be adducted when turning the client.
    ③ In the supine position, the knees should be elevated 90 degrees.
    ④ When side-lying, the affected hip should be in a position of abduction.

Answers & Rationales

6.1 ② The Glasgow Coma Coma Scale score best evaluates changes in a client's level of consciousness by evaluating eye opening, motor, and verbal responses. Option #1 indicates increased intracranial pressure. Options #3 and #4 are more appropriate for the psychiatric client.

6.2 ① If the client has claustrophobia, the scan may cause severe anxiety. Option #2 is incorrect because aspirin is not used for the scan. Options #3 and #4 are assessment data related to CVA but not necessary for CT scan.

6.3 ② While it is important to evaluate any client's discomfort, this client could be developing compartmental syndrome and needs immediate attention. It is important to further evaluate the pulse, sensation, movement, color, and temperature. Options #1, #3, and #4 are not a priority to #2. A client will experience discomfort after a liver biopsy. There is a release of oxytocin during breast feeding which will cause some discomfort.

6.4 ④ Option #4 is a concern due to the risk with gagging. The glossopharyngeal (swallowing or gag reflex) and the vagus nerves assist with swallowing. Options #1, #2 and #3 are normal changes.

6.5 ① Paralysis of the eyelid allows the cornea to dry. Patches can be used to keep the eyelid closed to prevent damage. Drops and/or ointments are also used to reduce the chance of corneal damage. Option #2 is incorrect because the problem, properly managed, should not result in a problem with light. Option #3 is for clients with increased intraocular pressure. Option #4 is incorrect because Bell's Palsy is not contagious.

6.6 ① Cephalexin is an antibiotic associated with the development of aplastic anemia. The physician should be notified as soon as the problem is identified. Options #2, #3, and #4 are not appropriate nursing decisions regarding this medication.

6.7 ③ Water that is too cool can elicit dizziness when it comes in contact with the tympanic membrane. Option #1 is not necessary. Option #2 is incorrect because the client is not experiencing increased intraocular pressure. Option #4 could compact the cerumen against the membrane and is never recommended.

6.8 ③ Maintaining straight alignment is necessary to keep the spine straight. Option #1 will increase the twisting of the trunk when the client turns. Option #2 will diminish support to the legs and possibly allow twisting of the hips. Option #4 will not allow the client to be in the center of the bed after the turning.

6.9 ① Changes in level of consciousness, increasing drowsiness or difficulty in arousing (e.g., increasing lethargy), are initial signs of increased intracranial pressure. Options #2, #3, and #4 are normal findings.

6.10 ② Cold packs will cause vasoconstriction which will decrease the edema. Options #1 and #4 are incorrect. Option #3 is used for arthritis.

6.11 ③ In diabetes insipidus, one of the first signs is a significant increase in urine output and pale colored urine. Option #1 is incorrect because the specific gravity is decreased, and foul smelling urine usually indicates infection. Option #2 is incorrect because intake is normal. Option #4 is associated with a client in chemotherapy, but not as often as Option #3.

6.12 ① Before teaching or client learning can occur, the client must identify thoughts about his/her current status including concerns, fears, anxieties, etc. Option #2 is not a priority because the nurse is processing instead of the client. Option #3 is important, but is not a priority over #1. Option #4 will be done at a later time.

6.13 ① Option #1 is correct. Options #2, #3, and #4 are incorrect. Option #3 should be downward over the stump and to the back of the leg. Option #4 should be so that it narrows toward the distal end.

6.14 ③ Respirations are a priority, especially with cervical injuries. Options #1, #2, and #4 are all important but are all secondary to respirations.

6.15 ① Pilocarpine is a miotic which constricts the pupils, allowing the aqueous humor to circulate more freely and reducing the intra-ocular pressure. Options #2, #3, and #4 are not therapeutic responses to Pilocarpine.

6.16 ④ Second-degree burns create a lot of pain for the client. Option #1 would be a priority within the first few hours for upper extremity burns. However, these are on the lower body. Option #2 is a concern, but not a priority to pain. Option #3 is a major concern initially after the burns.

6.17 ② It is important to prevent nausea and vomiting as this would increase the intraocular pressure and could cause damage to the area repaired. Option #1 would not be effective. Option #3 refers to an eye infection. This would be important after the initial operative day. Option #4 is incorrect because eye irrigations are not common following this procedure.

6.18 ② Option #2 is correct for the CNXI (spinal accessory). Option #1 is evaluation of the CNI (olfactory). Option #3 is evaluation of the CNII (optic). Option #4 is evaluation for the CNXII (hypoglossal).

6.19 ② A characteristic of this condition is the intense facial pain experienced along the nerve tract. Nursing care should be directed toward preventing stimuli to the area and decreasing pain. Option #1 does not occur with this condition. Option #3 describes Ménière's disease. Option #4 may occur, but Option #2 is a priority.

6.20 ① Option #1 is an indication in the alteration in the level of consciousness which is the earliest sign of neurological changes. Options #2, #3 and #4 occur later after #1 has occurred. Option #2 includes increased systolic pressure, decreased pulse rate, and irregular respirations. IICP is well-established when this occurs.

6.21 ④ This method aids wound debridement. Option #1 would not be effective. Option #2 will prevent adherence of gauze to wound debris and limit debridement. Option #3 before removal will defeat the purpose of wound debridement.

6.22 ④ The nurse should always speak when entering the room of a client with decreased vision. This makes the client aware of the nurse's presence. Options #1, #2, and #3 are incorrect because the client will become more confused with sensory deprivation.

6.23 ③ The parents need to understand the importance of monitoring and reporting signs of increased intracranial pressure. Vomiting is a sign of IICP. Signs of infection would also be important to report. Options #1 and #2 are incorrect positions. Parents need to understand how to pump the shunt in order to maintain patency.

6.24 ③ This procedure takes approximately 1-1/2 hours, and there is a lot of noise associated with the test. Option #1 is incorrect because there is no dye used for an MRI. Option #2 is incorrect because the client is not anesthetized for this procedure. Option #4 is inappropriate for this situation.

6.25 ④ The client has increased muscle fatigue and needs more assistance towards the end of the day. Option #1 is incorrect because the client does not experience vertigo. Option #2 is incorrect because though fluid and electrolytes are important, they are not a priority over Option #4. Option #3 is incorrect because increased intracranial pressure is not associated with myasthenia gravis.

6.26 ① Mydriatic eye drops are administered to dilate the pupil frequently for ocular surgery. Options #2 and #3 will not occur as a result of the drops. Option #4 is the response of miotic eye drops.

6.27 ③ Option #3 is the priority for safety with airway. Options #1, #2, and #4 are incorrect. While these are correct, they are not a priority to Option #3. Option #2 is incomplete. Documentation should also include during and after the seizure.

6.28 ② Avoiding sudden motion of the head will reduce incidence of vertigo, nausea, and vomiting. Option #1 is incorrect because salt should be restricted. Option #3 is incorrect because fluids should not be restricted. Option #4 is incorrect because cotton will not help the condition.

6.29 ② Eye pain and nausea may be indicative of increased intraocular pressure. Option #1 is for a client with hypertension and atherosclerosis. Option #3 is incorrect because the client may not experience any improvement in vision, but further deterioration may be prevented. Option #4 is incorrect because the eye drops may be continued indefinitely.

6.30 ④ The nurse should always stand in front of the hearing impaired client, and raising the voice is not as effective as clear, slow speech. Option #1 is not necessary. Option #2 is incorrect because it is important that a sensory-impaired client be aware of someone's presence before they are touched. Option #3 may be appropriate at a later time. However, his care needs to be addressed at the present.

6.31 ① When teaching paralyzed clients how to transfer themselves, it is important for them to understand that the strong side leads. Options #2, #3, and #4 are ineffective.

6.32 ① Option #1 would be the highest risk for skin breakdown due to the inability to get to the bathroom. Options #2, #3, and #4 are possibilities but are not priorities to Option #1.

6.33 ④ These are symptoms of compartmental syndrome which must be relieved as soon as possible. The only action within the realm of the nurse is to document observations and secure the physician's intervention immediately. Option #1 is inappropriate response to the symptoms observed. Option #2 is not likely to be ordered q45 min., and it is only palliative. Option #3 is beyond the scope of practice though bivalving is desirable.

6.34 ② Option #2 is a priority due to safety issues. Options #1, #3, and #4 are all important to assess but are not a priority to Option #2.

6.35 ② Option #2 is correct. It is done to decrease risk of aspiration. Options #1, #3, and #4 are incorrect. While the nurse may implement Option #1, it is not a priority to Option #2.

6.36 ③ A wet plaster of Paris cast will generate heat while hardening, appear gray, and smell slightly musty. Loss of sensation may indicate nerve compression. Options #1 and #2 are incorrect because these are normal findings. Option #4 indicates a later sign of complication.

6.37 ② The surgical inflammation can cause some temporary leg pain after disc excision. Option #1 is incorrect because early ambulation should be encouraged and sitting for long times is contraindicated. Option #3 may occur, but a prediction is not made at this time. Option #4 is inaccurate.

6.38 ② Because of the immobility and the bodily secretions, the client's skin is very susceptible to breakdown and needs numerous nursing interventions to prevent this from happening. Options #1, #3, and #4 are not current problems.

6.39 ② With myxedema, there is a slowing of all body functions. Options #1, #3, and #4 are associated with hyperthyroidism.

6.40 ② A full cup of hot liquids may be spilled due to hand tremors, and the client may be burned. Option #1 is inappropriate. Options #3 and #4 are related to the potential for injury but are related to rigidity—not tremors.

6.41 ① The crutches should be positioned about 2" under the axillary area to prevent nerve damage to the brachial plexus area which would result in arm paralysis or numbness. Options #2, #3, and #4 are incorrect positions.

6.42 ① The prone position provides maximum extension of the hip joint and prevents hip flexion contracture. If hip flexion contracture occurs, then it is very difficult to correctly fit or utilize prosthesis. Option #2 contains incorrect information. Option #3 is not a priority. Option #4 can result in contractures.

6.43 ④ Option #4 is the most important nursing action. Options #1 and #3 are similar in that both are giving sips of water. Option #2 may be correct but there is no follow-through assessment.

6.44 ③ This will prevent atrophy of the flexor and extensor muscle groups which will result in optimizing mobility. Options #1 and #2 are inappropriately restraining the client which will result in complications of immobility. Option #4 should say "encourage independence" versus "as much assistance."

6.45 ③ Thyroid hormone replacement is usually continued for life. A sudden discontinuing of the medication may cause a myxedema crisis. Option #1 is a correct statement because thyroid hormones may produce hyperglycemia due to the increased rate of carbohydrate breakdown. Option #2 is a correct statement because taking it before breakfast will prevent insomnia. Option #4 is a correct statement because thyroid hormones enhance toxic effects of digoxin preparations.

6.46 ③ Tetany is the major sign of hypoparathyroidism. Options #1 and #4 are important to monitor but are not top priority. Option #2 is incorrect because bone deformities are most frequently observed with hyperparathyroidism.

6.47 ② Strengthening the abdominal muscles adds support for the muscles supporting the lumbar spine. Options #1 and #4 do not contribute significantly. Option #3 would be secondary.

6.48 ② The client with hypothyroidism is very sensitive to narcotics, barbiturates, and anesthetics. Option #1 is incorrect because the client with hypothyroidism cannot tolerate cold temperatures. Options #3 and #4 do not require caution.

6.49 ① This does not address the question. Options #2, #3, and #4 are very helpful in maintaining skin integrity.

6.50 ② Overexposure to heat or cold may cause damage related to the changes in sensation. Options #1 and #3 are incorrect because the client is encouraged to ambulate as tolerated and participate in an exercise program to include ROM, stretching, and strengthening exercises. Option #4 is inappropriate because a client with multiple sclerosis is encouraged to continue usual activities as much as possible, including social activities.

6.51 ② Option #2 is correct. The HgB A1C are all high which means the blood sugar management is not effective. This value evaluates the previous 3 months of management. Options #1, #3 and #4 are incorrect statements.

6.52 ② Clients with hyperthyroidism frequently exhibit exophthalmos which requires ophthalmic drops on a regular basis. Option #1 is incorrect because the client is usually sensitive to heat. Option #3 is incorrect because the care would include a calm, restful environment with low levels of sensory stimulation. Option #4 is incorrect since these clients need to increase their caloric intake.

6.53 ③ Acceptance of blindness would be exhibited by an exploration of their world. Option #1 demonstrates denial. Option #2 exhibits dependence. Option #4 could be a result of depression.

6.54 ④ Medication which produces dependence should be used only if other nursing measures and antidepressant medications have not worked, and the client is exhausted. Options #1, #2, and #3 are therapeutic interventions to help the client learn how to create an environment conducive to sleep.

6.55 ① If steroids are taken at night, they may cause sleeplessness. Option #2 is incorrect because the dosage has to be regulated according to stress. Option #3 is incorrect because the client with Addison's disease has hyperkalemia. Option #4 is incorrect because steroids cause fluid retention which can increase the blood pressure.

6.56 ③ This statement does not indicate the client realizes that there is an increased susceptibility to infections. Option #1 is a correct statement. Option #2 is a correct statement because these clients may develop hypertension related to sodium and water retention. Option #4 is a correct statement since the diet should be low carbohydrate, low sodium, and high protein.

6.57 ④ Respirations are the first priority. Clients with Cushing's syndrome are prone to fluid overload and CHF due to sodium and water retention. Options #1 and #2 are incorrect because these clients are susceptible to skin breakdown and infections. Option #3 is incorrect because the hyperglycemia due to the impaired glucose tolerance is not the top priority.

6.58 ① Hypertension is a major symptom associated with pheochromocytoma. Diaphoresis, glycosuria, and weight loss are also systems, but an elevation in the blood pressure is the major symptom. Option #3 is not necessary since hematuria is not associated with this medical condition. Options #2 and #4 are incorrect.

6.59 ③ Assessment is needed to make sure circulation is not being compromised. Option #1 is incorrect because Buck's traction is a type of skin traction. Therefore, there are no pins. Option #2 is incorrect because skin traction has no need for topical ointment. Option #4 is incorrect because the skin is not lubricated under the bandages.

6.60 ④ A position of abduction should be maintained. Flexion beyond 60 degrees and internal rotation should be avoided in the early postoperative period. Options #1, #2, and #3 are incorrect.

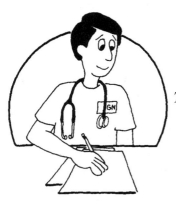

This page is for your notes!

Basic Care and Comfort— Elimination

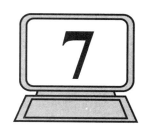

Can't get it? Don't sweat it. Let it come to you!
If it's right, and you hold tight, your dreams will come true!
—Tut

✔ **Clarification of this test...**

The minimum standard includes providing and directing basic care and comfort measures.

☞ Assess and intervene with the client who has an alteration in elimination.

☞ Perform focused assessment or reassessment (GI, renal).

☞ Perform diagnostic testing (occult blood, gastric pH, urine specific gravity).

☞ Provide wound care.

☞ Perform dressing change (wound).

☞ Obtain specimens for diagnostic testing (blood, urine, PKU testing, wound cultures, stool specimens).

☞ Provide pre- and post-operative care.

☞ Educate client/family/staff on infection control measures.

☞ Monitor and maintain devices and equipment used for drainage (surgical wound drains, chest tube suction).

7.1 What would be the priority of care for a client who presents with nausea, diarrhea, muscle weakness, and an abnormal ECG and is taking aldactone, zestril, and glucotrol?

① Evaluate the potassium level.
② Evaluate the sodium level.
③ Review the importance of eating bananas.
④ Assess for signs and symptoms of dehydration.

7.2 An order has been received to obtain a consent for an intravenous pyelogram (IVP). The most important information for the nurse to obtain is:

① color of urine.
② renal history.
③ last bowel movement.
④ iodine sensitivity.

7.3 Which assessment would be most appropriate for monitoring a client's state of hydration?

① Daily weight.
② I & O.
③ Skin turgor.
④ Characteristic of lips and mucous membranes.

7.4 Upon auscultation of a client's bowel sounds, the nurse notes soft gurgling sounds occurring every 5–20 seconds. This indicates:

① excessive intestinal motility.
② reduced intestinal peristalsis.
③ normal sounds.
④ rapid gastric emptying.

7.5 The nurse is assessing a child with a tentative diagnosis of appendicitis. This diagnosis is most often manifested by:

① sharp pain with extreme gastric distention.
② rebound tenderness in the right lower abdominal quadrant, with decreased bowel sounds.
③ growing pain, radiating to the lower back.
④ pain on light palpation in epigastric area with diarrhea.

7.6 Which nursing observation would relate to a post operative complication in the client with postoperative ileostomy?

① The ileostomy does not require daily irrigations to maintain function.
② The stoma appears tight and there is a decreased amount of stool.
③ An impaction appears to be forming in the distal anal area.
④ A weight gain of 5 pounds related to increased fluid retention.

7.7 A client with a permanent colostomy on the transverse colon questions the nurse as to whether or not he will ever be able to establish bowel control. The nursing response would be based on which concept?

① There is little chance that the client will gain an equate control with this colostomy.
② Control may be achieved with colostomy irrigations twice a day.
③ Daily colostomy irrigations and diet are frequently used to main colostomy control.
④ A high residue diet that provides bulk to the stool may be used to maintain bowel control.

7.8. A client on chemotherapy has a WBC count of 1,200/mm. Based on this data, which nursing action should be taken first?

① Check temperature q 4h.
② Monitor urine output.
③ Assess for bleeding gums.
④ Obtain an order for blood cultures.

7.9 Which of the following statements, if made by a client with oliguric renal failure, would indicate a need for further teaching?

① "I will only eat processed foods in moderation."
② "I must limit the amount of salt I eat."
③ "I won't eat pickles and green olives anymore."
④ "I will use a salt substitute instead of table salt."

7.10 Which statement is most appropriate for the nurse to include in the discharge instructions for a client who has a prescription for naproxen (Naprosyn)?

① "Make sure you take the medication with food or meals."
② "Limit your intake of foods containing potassium, such as citrus, bananas, meats, etc."
③ "Limit your intake of sodium to prevent edema."
④ "Limit your intake of fluids while taking this medication."

7.11 A 77-year-old client with iron deficiency anemia has been started on ferrous sulfate tablets. However, they make the client vomit. The best instruction to assist in minimizing this side effect would be to take the medication:

① before meals.
② in the early morning.
③ after meals.
④ bedtime.

7.12 A client with lung cancer and bone metastasis is grimacing and states, "I am a little uncomfortable. May I have something for pain?" Which nursing action should be taken first before administering his pain medication?

① Check the chart to determine last medication.
② Encourage client to refocus on something pleasant.
③ Notify physician that medication is not working.
④ Assess the severity and location of pain.

7.13 Which of these documentations indicate the nurse understands how to accurately evaluate the client's stool for occult blood?

① Collect stool placed in a clean container to examine for pathological organisms.
② Remained on regular diet prior to test being done.
③ Stool sample obtained from one area of the stool.
④ Guaiac testing—positive for occult blood. Paper turned blue.

7.14 Which nursing observations would relate to the complication of intestinal obstruction following an exploratory laparotomy?

① Protruding soft abdomen with frequent diarrhea.
② Distended abdomen with ascites.
③ Minimal bowel sounds in all four quadrants.
④ Distended abdomen with complaints of pain.

7.15 A client with prostatic cancer is admitted to the hospital with neutropenia. Which signs and symptoms are most important for the nurse to report to the next shift?

① Arthralgia and stiffness
② Vertigo and headache
③ General malaise and anxiety
④ Temperature elevation and lethargy

7.16 A client with chronic cancer pain has been receiving Meperidine HC1 (Demerol) 100 mg PO q4h PRN for pain, without much relief. Which change in narcotic pain management would be the most valid suggestion to make to the physician?

① Decrease to twice a day.
② Decrease to every 6 hours PRN.
③ Give every 4 hours around the clock.
④ Give every 2 hours PRN.

7.17 Which priority is first when inserting an indwelling urinary catheter?

① Aseptic technique
② Taping the catheter to the leg
③ Instilling water into the balloon
④ Inserting the catheter to the point where the urine flows

7.18 Based on the assessment findings of oliguria, hyperkalemia, and increased BUN on a client in chronic renal failure, an appropriate nursing diagnosis would be:

① fluid volume excess and electrolyte imbalance related to decreased urinary output.
② altered nutrition less than body requirements related to anorexia and dietary restrictions.
③ knowledge deficit regarding condition and treatment regimen.
④ fluid volume deficit related to fluid restrictions.

7.19 A client is four days postoperative abdominal perineal resection. Which sign is most important for the nurse to report to the physician?

① Moderate amount of serosanguineous drainage on abdominal dressing.
② Nausea, vomiting, and increased abdominal distention.
③ Moderate amount of yellow-green nasogastric drainage and decreased urine output.
④ Urinary output via Foley catheter 160 cc over a 4-hour period.

7.20 In a 7-month-old infant, which is the best way to detect fluid retention?

① Weigh the child daily.
② Test the urine for hematuria.
③ Measure abdominal girth weekly.
④ Count the number of wet diapers.

7.21 What would be a priority in establishing a bladder retraining program?

① Provide a flexible schedule for the client to decrease anxiety.
② Schedule toileting on a planned time schedule.
③ Teach client intermittent self-catheterization.
④ Perform the Crede maneuver tid.

7.22 Which medication order should be questioned for a client who has the diagnosis of diabetes, hypertension, peptic ulcer, and renal failure?

① Carafate
② Inderal
③ Insulin
④ Zestril

7.23 While checking patency of a Salem sump tube, stomach contents are found draining from the air vent. Which nursing action is most appropriate?

① Insert water through air vent.
② Pull sump tube back 2-3 inches.
③ Insert 30 cc air through air vent.
④ Insert new nasogastric tube.

7.24 A client is admitted with frequent, loose stools. Prior to implementing orders to insert a Foley catheter, the nurse would first:

① apply fecal incontinence bag.
② perform perineal care.
③ administer an antidiarrheal agent.
④ insert a rectal tube.

7.25 A client is admitted with renal calculi, and is experiencing severe pain. Meperidine (Demerol) 75 mg IM is given prior to change of shift. Which symptom is most important for the nurse to report to the next shift?

① Nausea with small amount of emesis.
② Pain is 5 on a scale of 1–10.
③ Change in location and character of pain.
④ No known drug allergies.

7.26 A client with renal cancer will be discharged home with a central venous catheter in place. Which of the following statements made by the client indicates a correct understanding of aseptic technique?

① "I should not take showers."
② "I must wash my hands after changing the dressing."
③ "I can reuse my equipment from the day before."
④ "I must wash my hands before changing the dressing."

7.27 During report, the nurse indicates that the client's NG tube quit draining over the last hour. Prior to that, it was draining 100 cc of fluid q 2 hr. Which plan would best assist this client?

① Anchor a new NG tube.
② Reposition the tube to promote drainage.
③ Order a chest X-ray to determine placement.
④ Force 50 cc of normal saline down the tube.

7.28 A client with a Tenchkoff catheter is being discharged home on continuous ambulatory peritoneal dialysis (CAPD). He has not successfully returned the demonstration to verify his understanding of the procedure. Based on this assessment, an appropriately-stated nursing diagnosis is:

① health maintenance alteration due to lack of knowledge.
② knowledge deficit related to CAPD self care.
③ alteration in compliance related to lack of interest.
④ self-care deficit: toileting.

7.29 During peritoneal dialysis, the nurse notes that the outflow is less than the inflow. Which nursing action is most appropriate?

① Reposition the dialysis catheter.
② Irrigate the catheter with 30 cc of normal saline.
③ Change the client's position.
④ Notify the physician immediately.

7.30 A client has a bovine graft inserted into the left arm for hemodialysis. During the immediate postoperative period, the nurse would prevent complications by which action?

① Restart the IV above the level of the graft.
② Take blood pressures only on the right arm.
③ Elevate the left arm above the level of the heart.
④ Check the radial pulse on the left arm q4h.

7.31 A client is experiencing gastric upset after taking his phenazopyridine hydrochloride (Pyridium). Which nursing action is most appropriate?

① Tell client to seek treatment for probable pyelonephritis.
② Notify physician if urine turns red.
③ Discontinue medication if urine becomes cloudy.
④ Instruct client to take the drug with food.

7.32 A fluid challenge of 250 cc of normal saline infused over 15 min. is ordered on a client with possible acute renal failure. The nurse understands that the fluid challenge is given to:

① rule out dehydration as the cause of oliguria.
② increase cardiac output and fluid volume.
③ promote the transfer of intravascular fluid to the intracellular space.
④ dilute the level of waste products in the intravascular fluid.

7.33 A client has been transferred from a nursing home to the hospital with an indwelling urinary catheter. The urine is cloudy and foul smelling. Which nursing measure would be most appropriate?

① Clean the urinary meatus every other day.
② Encourage the client to increase fluid intake.
③ Empty the drainage bag every 2–4 hours.
④ Irrigate the Foley catheter every 8 hours to maintain patency.

7.34 A client has a three-way Foley catheter following a transurethral resection. When would the nurse anticipate running irrigating solution in rapidly?

① The urinary output is increased.
② Bright red drainage or clots are present.
③ Dark brown drainage is present.
④ The client complains of pain.

7.35 A child weighing 80 pounds is sent home in a hip spica cast. Which instruction would be most important to include in the teaching plan designed to promote bowel functioning?

① Give a soap suds enema every day.
② Perform range of motion exercises to the upper extremities four times a day.
③ Give at least six to eight 8-ounce glasses of fluid a day.
④ Give a strong laxative every day.

7.36 Which instruction should be included in the teaching plan of a client taking sulfasalazine (Azulfidine)?

① Restrict fluids to 1500 cc per day.
② Explain to client that the stool may turn to a clay color.
③ The medication should be continued even after symptoms subside.
④ If diarrhea occurs, the client should discontinue the medication.

7.37 What is the priority of care after the urinary catheter is removed?

① Encourage client to eliminate fluid intake.
② Document size of catheter and client's tolerance of procedure.
③ Evaluate client for normal voiding.
④ Documentation of client teaching.

7.38 The nurse is caring for a client with a perforated bowel secondary to a bowel obstruction. At the time the diagnosis is made, which nursing priority would be most important in the care plan?

① Maintain the client in a supine position.
② Notify the client's next of kin.
③ Prepare the client for emergency surgery.
④ Remove the nasogastric tube.

7.39 A client returns to his room following a uretero-lithotomy with a left ureteral catheter in place. Which instruction concerning the catheter would be included in the nursing care plan?

① The catheter may be clamped for short periods of time.
② Teach the client that the urine from this catheter should be clear.
③ Gently advance catheter if there is no drainage for 2 hours.
④ The catheter should be irrigated every 2 hours to maintain patency.

7.40 A client with a diagnosis of ulcerative colitis is receiving sulfasalazine (Azulfidine). What is the desired response to the medication?

① A decrease in the anemia
② Relief of the diarrhea
③ Exacerbation of anorexia
④ Diminish the retention of fluids.

7.41 A client with a peptic ulcer had a partial gastrectomy and vagotomy (Billroth I). In planning the discharge teaching, which instruction to the client should be included?

① Sit up for at least 30 minutes after eating to reduce peristalsis.
② Avoid fluids between meals to promote the transit of food from the stomach to the jejunum.
③ Increase the intake of high carbohydrate foods to prevent dumping syndrome.
④ Avoid eating large meals that are high in simple sugars and liquids.

7.42 Which of these clients would be most appropriate for the RN to assign to the LPN/LVN?

① A 33-year-old client who has kidney stones and has an order for lithotripsy.
② A 43-year-old client with cystitis and is taking po antibiotics.
③ A 53-year-old client with pyelonephritis presenting with acute pain.
④ A 63-year-old client with urinary incontinence starting bladder training.

7.43 Which statement made by a client scheduled to have a TURP would indicate a need for further teaching?

① "If I have this surgery, I will become impotent."
② "I will call the nurse if my bladder feels like it is full."
③ "A catheter will be in place to drain my bladder."
④ "At first my urine may be somewhat bloody."

7.44 An elderly client is admitted to a medical surgical unit with suspected sepsis. Which assessment finding would indicate the need for urinalysis?

① An indwelling catheter
② A small amount dark amber urine
③ An elevated temperature
④ A urine with whitish sediment

7.45 Which instruction is a priority in the nursing care plan of a client experiencing severe pain from renal calculi?

① Administer pain medication as often as ordered.
② Encourage fluid intake to help flush the stone through.
③ Assist the client to ambulate to promote draining the bladder.
④ Irrigate the bladder to maintain urinary patency.

7.46 The nurse would anticipate which assessment findings in a client who has developed a lower intestinal obstruction?

① Nausea, vomiting, abdominal distention
② Explosive, irritating diarrhea
③ Abdominal tenderness with rectal bleeding
④ Mid-epigastric discomfort, tarry stool

7.47 To determine the client's tolerance of total parenteral nutrition (TPN), what would the nurse observe?

① A significant increase in pulse rate
② Decrease in diastolic blood pressure
③ Temperature in excess of 98.6°F.
④ Urine output of at least 30 cc per hour

7.48 Your client is beginning peritoneal dialysis. During the first infusion of dialysate, the client experiences mild abdominal discomfort. You should take which of these actions:

① Stop the infusion.
② Decrease the total infusion volume.
③ Inform the client that the discomfort will subside after a few exchanges.
④ Notify the physician.

7.49 Which of these laboratory findings would be a priority concern for a client with the diagnosis of cystitis?

① Serum hematocrit 36%.
② Serum WBC 6000/mm3.
③ Urine bacteria 105,000 colonies/ml.
④ Urinalysis with 2–3 WBCs present.

7.50 Which clinical finding should be reported prior to administering gentamycin IV piggyback?

① Temperature –101.2 degrees F.
② I+O = 65 cc in one hour.
③ BUN – 29, creatinine – 2.1 mg/dl.
④ WBC – 12,000/mm3.

7.51 Which method would be the best to assess a client's understanding of colostomy care prior to discharge?

① Review teaching materials.
② Have client explain irrigation procedure.
③ Have client demonstrate colostomy care.
④ Observe colostomy film.

7.52 Which action should the nurse instruct the client to do first when assisting to establish a normal urinary pattern?

① Advise him to urinate every 2 hours.
② Explain to him to record when he urinates in the toilet.
③ Have him keep a record of his daily fluid intake.
④ Stress the importance of staying near a bathroom.

7.53 Which nursing diagnosis would be appropriate for a client experiencing chronic renal failure?

① Potential for infection related to retention of urine
② Alteration in nutrition: more than body requirements related to glucose intolerance
③ Altered comfort related to hyperthermia and malaise secondary to uremia
④ Impairment of skin integrity related to pruritus and urea crystallization on skin.

7.54 Which assessment finding would be most indicative of an obstructed urinary catheter?

① Bladder distention
② Increased urge to void
③ Concentrated urine
④ Complaint of burning

7.55 What is the desired response to intestinal antibiotics such as neomycin sulfate?

① Decrease gas formation by anaerobic bacteria.
② Work as an adjunct to systemic antibiotics therapy.
③ Decrease postoperative wound infection by decreasing incidence of peritonitis.
④ Prevent ulcerative colitis in young adults.

7.56 Which statement indicates the nurse needs more information regarding how to provide care for a client with a shunt for hemodialysis?

① "I will feel the shunt for a thrill."
② "I will record blood pressures on the same extremity as the shunt."
③ "I will auscultate a bruit."
④ "I will report any swelling at the shunt site."

7.57 What information would the nurse need to know before administering ioperamide (Imodium) to a client?

① Time of last bowel movement.
② Time of last solid food intake.
③ Total oral intake over the last 8 hours.
④ Character and frequency of stool.

7.58 Twenty-four (24) hours after abdominal surgery, which plan would be priority to prevent complications of flatulence?

① Encourage the client to drink carbonated beverages daily.
② Instruct the client to turn from side to side.
③ Encourage the client to do leg exercises in bed.
④ Assist the client to walk in the hall every 2 hours.

7.59 The first postoperative day after a cholecystectomy, the client drains 375 cc of dark serosanguineous fluid from the gastric tube. The nurse should:

① notify the physician immediately.
② prepare for a blood transfusion.
③ document information in notes.
④ replace fluid to prevent dehydration.

7.60 Nursing management prior to an IVP would include which protocol?

① Having client eat a fat-free meal the evening prior to the examination and radiopaque tablets at bedtime
② Placing a retention urinary catheter to facilitate dilation of the bladder sphincter
③ Using cleansing enemas the evening before to provide for adequate visualization of urinary tract
④ Explaining the importance of following directions regarding voiding during the test

Answers & Rationales

7.1 ① Aldactone is a potassium-sparing diuretic, and when given with Zestril, there is a potential problem with hyperkalemia. Option #2 is inaccurate. Option #3 is high in potassium and could contribute to the complication of hyperkalemia. While Option #4 is appropriate, it is not a priority to Option #1. Since the client has already developed an abnormal ECG, it is apparent there is alteration in the fluid and electrolytes.

7.2 ④ The fluoroscopic exam of the urinary track is visualized after an injection of a radiopaque dye. People who have iodine sensitivity may have an allergic reaction. Although Options #1, #2, and #3 are important in the overall assessment, they do not specifically address iodine sensitivity.

7.3 ① Daily weight is the most appropriate evaluation out of these options. It is the most measurable. While Options #2, #3 and #4 are correct, they are not a priority to Option #1.

7.4 ③ Option #3 is the correct description of bowel sounds. Options #1, #2, and #4 all reflect abnormal bowel sounds related to hypo or hypermotility of the GI tract.

7.5 ② Option #2 is correct. Rebound pain is manifested by pressing firmly over the area known as McBurney's point. The rebound pain, decreased bowel sounds, tender abdomen, and fever, are all characteristic of appendicitis. Options #1, #3, and #4 are incorrect.

7.6 ② If there is a decrease in flow of stool in an ileostomy, along with changes in the appearance of the stoma, it would be important to report these findings to the physician as they might indicate an obstruction or stoma stricture. Option #1 is incorrect because ileostomies are not irrigated. Option #3 is incorrect because the anal area is not functional. Option #4 is related to cardiac or renal problems.

7.7 ③ Diet and irrigations are the common methods used for colostomy control. Option #1 is incorrect because clients gradually are able to "control" and adapt to their individual bowel evacuation routines. Option #2 is incorrect because irrigation of the colostomy is usually needed only once a day. Option #4 is incorrect because diet may assist in control but cannot be used alone and irrigations are more successful.

7.8 ① It is important to monitor for infection which would be evidenced by an elevated temperature in a client who has such a low WBC count. Option #2 is important to monitor because of problems of increased uric acid excretion from chemo-therapeutic drugs but is not applicable to this situation. Option #3 would be associated with a low platelet count. Option #4 would be secondary to Option #1.

7.9 ④ Option #4 is correct. Many salt substitutes contain potassium and could lead to hyperkalemia in clients with renal failure. This must be clarified with the client. Options #1, #2, and #3 indicate an understanding by the client of the need to limit sodium intake.

7.10 ① Option #1 is important to prevent the development of gastric ulcers. This medication is very irritating to the stomach. Options #2, #3, and #4 are not correct in answering this question.

7.11 ③ While the preferred method for taking ferrous sulfate is on an empty stomach, to reduce the side effect of vomiting, it may be administered after meals. If the client does not experience any side effects, the ideal time is 1 hour before, or 2 hours after, meals. Option #1 is incorrect since the client can develop gastrointestinal problems and may experience anorexia as a result. Options #2 and #4 are incorrect since it may cause nausea.

7.12 ④ The first step is to assess the client's pain and determine its severity. Option #1 is incorrect because assessment is done prior to checking the chart for information. Option #2 is incorrect because the pain of metastatic cancer does not usually lend itself to nonmedical measures. Option #3 may be secondary. Further pain management includes intervention before pain becomes intense.

7.13 ④ Option #4 is correct. Options #1, #2, and #3 are incorrect. Option #1 should be in a sterile container. Option #2—client may be on a specific type of diet prior to test being done to minimize false results. Option #3 should be collected from various areas of stool.

7.14 ④ If an obstruction is present, the abdomen will become distended and painful. Options #1 and #2 do not support intestinal obstruction. Option #3 is incorrect because immediately postoperative abdominal surgery, a client's bowel sounds are absent or decreased.

7.15 ④ With a low WBC (neutropenia), the client is at risk for the development of infection. Options #1 and #2 could be experienced but are not most important. Option #3 is more closely associated with anemia.

7.16 ③ Research shows that around-the-clock (ATC) administration of analgesics is more effective in maintaining blood levels to alleviate the pain associated with cancer. Options #1 and #2 actually decrease the amount of pain medication. Option #4 might be too frequent an interval.

7.17 ① Prevention of infection is a priority. Whenever a foreign tube is being introduced into the body, there is always a chance for infection to occur. Option #2 is incorrect. Option #3 is incorrect because it should be sterile water, and even then, it is not a priority. Option #4 contains incorrect information as the catheter is usually inserted 2-3 inches beyond the flow of urine.

7.18 ① In renal failure, oliguria is accompanied by an increased BUN, increased serum potassium, and decreased renal blood flow. Option #2 is incorrect because it addresses other information not in the question. Option #3 does not have "related to" as part of the diagnosis. Option #4 is incorrect because oliguria is decreased urinary output, not increased urinary output.

7.19 ② Abdominal distention, along with the nausea and vomiting, indicate potential development of an ileus, or decreased peristalsis, and should be brought to the attention of the physician as soon as possible. Options #1, #3, and #4 might also be reported as additional data, but are normal findings.

7.20 ① Option #1 is correct. Fluid retention is best detected by weighing daily and noting a gaining trend. Options #2 and #3 are incorrect and will not provide information regarding fluid retention. Option #4 can provide an estimation of the amount of urine output, but not about fluid retention.

7.21 ② This is a priority when establishing a program. Option #1 is incorrect. Option #3 may not always be necessary in all programs. Option #4 would only be appropriate for a client with overflow incontinence.

7.22 ④ Option #4 is correct. Ace inhibitors are contraindicated in clients with renal failure. Options #1, #2, and #3 are incorrect. Option #1 is an ulcer-adherent complex that protects the ulcer against acid, pepsin, and bile salts, thereby promoting ulcer healing. Option #2, While Inderal may decrease the sensitivity to hypoglycemia, which could be a potential problem for the diabetes, it would be beneficial for the hypertension and would not create increased complication with the renal failure. The action is on the beta receptors vs. the kidney, which is the site for the therapeutic action of zestril. Option #3 is necessary for managing the diabetes.

7.23 ③ Clearing the air vent with air will reestablish proper suction in the Salem sump tube. Option #1 is incorrect because it is important not to put fluids through the air vent. Options #2 and #4 are unnecessary at this time.

7.24 ② Careful perineal care should be performed prior to beginning the catheterization procedure to give added cleanliness to the area, especially when diarrhea is present. Option #1 is not necessary. Options #3 and #4 require a physician's order and are not appropriate.

7.25 ③ The location of the pain depends on the location of the renal stone. The character of the pain changes depending on the location or movement of stone. Option #1 often accompanies pain but is not what the question is asking. Options #2 and #4 are important, but not a high priority.

7.26 ④ The foundation of aseptic technique is meticulous hand-washing prior to a procedure. Options #1 and #3 are inappropriate. Option #2 is incomplete.

7.27 ② This will be the best plan to minimize trauma and be effective. Option #1 is not necessary in this situation. Option #3 is inappropriate. Option #4 is incorrect since fluid should never be forced down any tube.

7.28 ② With such an important procedure as CAPD, return demonstration is the most valid way of evaluating health teaching. In this situation the client has a knowledge deficit regarding his care. Options #1, #3, and #4 are not stated appropriately.

7.29 ③ The outflow should always be greater than the inflow. After the dwell time, the dialysate should be diffusing out the extra fluid and waste products. By changing a client's position, you can affect the drainage. Options #1 and #2 are incorrect because peritoneal catheters are surgically placed and are usually not irrigated. Option #4 is done after Option #1 if there is not an increased amount of drainage. Sometimes problems with outflow are related to a full colon.

7.30 ② Blood pressures should always be taken on the arm opposite the one used for hemodialysis. Option #1 is incorrect because IVs should not be started in the grafted arm. Option #3 is not necessary after surgery. Option #4 would not necessarily prevent complications which is what the question is asking.

7.31 ④ Pyridium should be taken with food to minimize gastric distress. Option #1 is not a typical symptom of pyelonephritis. Option #2 is incorrect because this drug normally turns the urine red. Option #3 is incorrect because this drug does not make urine cloudy.

7.32 ① The expected response after a fluid challenge on normal functioning kidneys is an increase in urine output. This will occur if the client's low urine output is due to dehydration. However, if it is due to acute renal failure, the oliguria will continue. Options #2, #3, and #4 contain incorrect information.

7.33 ② Increasing fluids is an appropriate independent nursing action that facilitates the removal of concentrated urine. Options #1 and #3 are incorrect because they do not address the problem of the client's urine. Option #4 is incorrect and cannot be performed without a physician's order.

7.34 ② The three-way Foley catheter should be irrigated rapidly when bright red drainage or clots are present. It should be decreased to about 40 gtts/min when the drainage clears. Options #1, #3, and #4 contain incorrect information.

7.35 ③ Adequate fluids will help maintain regular bowel function. Options #1 and #4 are unnecessary. Option #2, while beneficial, will not promote bowel function.

7.36 ③ Sulfonamides need to be given with lots of fluids to prevent crystallization in the kidney tubules. The client should continue on the medication even after the symptoms subside. They may turn the urine an orange-red color temporarily. If the client has ulcerative colitis, medication would be continued even with diarrhea. Options #1, #2 and #4 contain incorrect information.

7.37 ③ Option #3 is a priority. Within 24 hours client should be voiding normally. Options #1, #2, and #4 are incorrect. Option #1 should be increased. Option #2 is not totally correct. The size of the catheter should have been documented when it is placed. Option #4 is important but is not a priority for this question.

7.38 ③ When the bowel perforates as a result of increased intraluminal pressure within the gut, intestinal juices are released into the peritoneum leading to peritonitis. Option #1 is incorrect because the client is kept in semi-Fowler's position. Option #2 is correct but is not a priority action. Option #4 is incorrect because it would be unwise to remove the nasogastric tube.

7.39 ② After surgery, a small amount of blood-tinged urine is normal. However, the client is taught that the urine should be clear. Options #1, #3, and #4 are incorrect because ureteral catheters are not to be clamped, advanced, or irrigated due to the small size of the ureter and the potential for trauma.

7.40 ② Azulfidine is used to decrease diarrhea. Option #1 is incorrect because one of the side effects of prolonged use of this drug is anemia. Option #3 is incorrect because nausea and vomiting are common reactions. Option #4 is incorrect because this drug has no effect on fluid retention.

7.41 ④ The basic guidelines to teach a post-gastrectomy client are measures to prevent dumping syndrome. Option #1 is incorrect because the client is taught to lie down for 30 minutes after meals. Options #2 and #3 are incorrect because the client is taught to limit the intake of fluids, avoid highly spiced foods, and avoid high carbohydrate foods during meals.

7.42 ② Option #2 is most stable with expected outcomes. Option #1 has a new order. Option #3—the acute pain needs immediate assessment. Option #4 requires new teaching.

7.43 ① Following TURP, the client will not have physiological impotency. Option #2 is correct because this could be an early indication of urinary retention. Options #3 and #4 are correct and indicate the client understands his postoperative management.

7.44 ④ Urine with cloudy sediment most often suggests the presence of infection. Options #1, #2, and #3 are less indicative of urinary tract infection and the need for urinalysis.

7.45 ① Relief of the severe pain associated with renal colic is priority. Option #2 may help the client pass the stone but will not alleviate pain. Option #3 is incorrect because the client will probably not feel like ambulating if they are experiencing renal colic. Option #4 may cause spasm and additional pain.

7.46 ① There is distention above the level of obstruction and initially hyperactive bowel sounds. Options #2, #3, and #4 are incorrect because there would be no stool as motility distal or below the obstruction would cease. Therefore, no diarrhea, rectal bleeding, or a tarry stool would be present.

7.47 ④ If the client is being properly hydrated with a hypertonic IV such as TPN, then the urine output needs to be at least 30 cc/hr. Other nursing actions include the assessment of blood glucose levels. Option #1 might indicate fluid overload. Option #2 might indicate shock or lack of blood volume. Option #3 is incorrect because the temperature should remain normal.

7.48 ③ Option #3 is correct. Mild discomfort is expected with the first few exchanges until the peritoneal space has expanded to accommodate fluid. This will subside after several exchanges. Option #1 is unnecessary unless the client experiences acute pain. Option #2 is incorrect. This will interfere with the effectiveness of the dialysis. Option #4 is not necessary at this time.

7.49 ③ Option #3 is a priority due to count indicating infection. Option #1 is slightly low but is not a priority concern. Option #2—WBC—is within normal limits. Option #4 is not a priority.

7.50 ③ Option #3 is important to report since gentamycin can be nephrotoxic. Options #1 and #4 are indications of an infection which is the reason for administering the antibiotic. Option #2 is a normal clinical finding.

7.51 ③ A return demonstration is the most reliable method to evaluate the effectiveness of teaching. Options #1 and #4 are effective as initial presentation methods when teaching. Option #2 is not as effective as Option #3.

7.52 ③ The client needs to know how much and when they ingest fluid. Option #1 is incorrect because the client is advised to start every 2 hours and gradually progress to 3-4 hours. Option #2 is secondary to Option #3. Option #4 is appropriate but is not a priority in instruction.

7.53 ④ Uremic frost (urea crystallization on skin) leads to itching and potential skin breakdown. Option #1 would be correct if the potential for infection was related to suppressed immune system and/or malnutrition. Option #2 is incorrect because CRF clients have problems with anorexia, vomiting, and diarrhea which would lead to a less-than-body requirement nursing diagnosis. Option #3 is incorrect because altered comfort may be related to the uremic frost, edematous areas, but not elevated temperature.

7.54 ① Bladder distention is one of the earliest signs of obstructed drainage tubing. Options #2, #3, and #4 are indicative of other genitourinary complications.

7.55 ③ Neomycin sulfate is a bowel sterilizer and is used to prevent wound and abdominal infection in the postoperative intestinal surgery client. Options #1, #2, and #4 are incorrect.

7.56 ② It is inappropriate to take blood pressures or draw blood on the extremity that has the shunt. Options #1, #3, and #4 indicate an understanding of how to provide care safely for this client.

7.57 ④ This represents the most important assessment data needed to determine when to administer an "as needed" antidiarrheal. Options #1, #2, and #3 are not necessary in making this decision.

7.58 ④ Having the client ambulate will increase peristalsis, thus decreasing the development of flatus. Option #1 is incorrect because increasing carbonated beverages will increase flatus. Options #2 and #3 are incorrect as they do not address flatulence.

7.59 ③ The amount of drainage for the first postoperative day is approximately 300 to 500 ml. It is important to keep accurate records of the output. Options #1, #2, and #4 are incorrect.

7.60 ③ Because of the need to visualize the abdominal area, cleansing enemas the evening before an IVP are usually ordered. Option #1 is associated with a gall bladder series. Option #2 may be in place but not for the purpose of dilating the bladder sphincter. Option #4 is incorrect because voiding during the test is not a required part of the procedure.

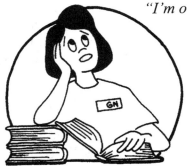

"I'm over half-way through!"

Physiological Adaption: Nutrition

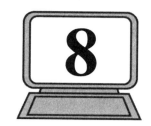

To predict the future, you have to create it.
—Thomas Peters

Thoughts become things.
—Michael Dooley

✔ **Clarification of this test…**

The minimum standard includes performing and directing activities that manage client care such as:

☛ Monitor client's hydration status.

☛ Perform focused assessment.

☛ Plan safe, cost-effective care for the client.

☛ Perform diagnostic testing (glucose monitoring).

☛ Provide client nutrition through continuous or intermittent tube feedings.

☛ Assess and intervene with the client who has an alteration in nutritional intake (adjust diet, change delivery to include method, time and food preferences).

☛ Assess client's food allergies.

☛ Insert/remove nasogastric, urethral catheter or other tubes.

☛ Assess and intervene in client's performance of instrumental activities of daily living (preparing meals).

☛ Perform emergency care procedures (Heimlich maneuver).

8.1 For a client receiving total parenteral nutrition (TPN), the nurse reviews the following lab values:

Glucose = 72 mg/dL
Chloride = 98 mEq/L
Sodium = 138 mEq/L
Potassium = 3.0 mEq/L

Based on this assessment, which nursing action is appropriate?

① Discontinue TPN administration.
② Notify physician and obtain order for potassium supplement.
③ Administer IV glucose immediately.
④ Check client vital signs immediately.

8.2 Which nursing action is most appropriate for a 2-month-old infant with reflux?

① Hold the next feeding.
② Teach the mother CPR.
③ Maintain normal feeding schedule.
④ Elevate the head of the bed.

8.3 A client is taking metoclopramide hydrochloride (Reglan) orally for nausea secondary to chemotherapy. In reference to the timing of the medication, when would the nurse instruct the client to take the medication?

① With each meal
② Thirty minutes before meals
③ One hour after each meal
④ At the same time each day

8.4 Which dietary modifications are important to include in a teaching plan for a client with cirrhosis of the liver?

① Decrease in calories and increase in protein.
② Decrease in carbohydrates and vitamin B.
③ Increase in carbohydrates and calories.
④ Increase in protein and fats.

8.5 A 3-month-old infant is scheduled for a barium swallow in the morning. Prior to the procedure, the most appropriate nursing action would be to:

① offer the infant only clear liquids.
② make the infant NPO for 3 hours.
③ feed the infant regular formula.
④ maintain NPO for 6 hours.

8.6 Which nursing action is most appropriate for a client receiving a tube feeding around the clock?

① Rinse the bag and change the formula every 4 hours.
② Rinse the bag and change the formula every shift.
③ Change the bag and formula every shift.
④ Rinse the bag and change the formula every 2 hours.

8.7 A nurse is obtaining a health history from a mother of a child with failure to thrive. Which assessment would provide the most pertinent data?

① Weight and height
② Urine output
③ Type of feedings
④ Mother-child interactions

8.8 What instructions would a nurse give a diabetic client who has been vomiting for 24 hours and is concerned about blood glucose levels?

① Take only half of the regular insulin dose.
② Attempt to maintain a regular diabetic diet.
③ Limit intake of sweets and sugar.
④ Drink liquids as often as possible.

8.9 What type of foods would be best for an 8-year-old receiving chemotherapy?

① A diet high in nutrients
② Hot and spicy foods
③ Small and frequent meals
④ Foods on a regular schedule to promote a routine

8.10 Which of the following would be the best plan for prevention of constipation during the first trimester of pregnancy?

① Take mineral oil every morning.
② Increase bulk and fiber in the diet.
③ Take a mild laxative as needed.
④ Decrease fluid intake.

8.11 Which of these interventions indicate the nurse needs more information regarding how to safely ensure proper tube placement?

① When confirming tube placement, place the tube's end in a container of water.
② Use a tongue blade and penlight to examine mouth and throat for signs of a coiled section of tubing.
③ Stop advancing tube when tape mark reaches the client's nostril.
④ Inject 10cc of air into tube. At same time, auscultate for air sounds with stethoscope placed over the epigastric region.

8.12 While managing a client's nutritional status during the weaning from total parenteral nutrition (TPN), which nursing intervention should be most appropriate?

① Evaluate weight daily.
② Monitor I&O.
③ Encourage client to eat a variety of foods.
④ Maintain a calorie count.

8.13 Which dietary requirements must be considered for an 8-year-old client with cystic fibrosis?

① High protein, high fat, and high calories
② High protein, low fat, and high calories
③ Low protein, low fat, and low carbohydrates
④ High protein, high fat, and low carbohydrates

8.14 A diabetic client, controlled with oral antihyperglcemic agents, questions the need for postoperative subcutaneous insulin injections. What is the most accurate explanation the nurse would give the client for the injections?

① Tissue injury after surgery decreases blood sugar.
② Anesthesia acts to increase glycogen stores.
③ Being NPO inhibits normal blood sugar control.
④ Surgery often leads to insulin dependency.

8.15 One hour after receiving 7 units of regular insulin, the client presents with diaphoresis, pallor, and tachycardia. The priority nursing action would be:

① notify the physician.
② call the lab for a blood glucose level.
③ offer the client milk and crackers.
④ administer glucagon.

8.16 After a month of taking iron supplements, a client complains of constipation. Based on client tastes, the nurse adapts a diet plan to include:

① oatmeal, green beans, celery.
② strawberries, rice, mushrooms.
③ grits, orange juice, cheddar cheese.
④ pasta, buttermilk, banana.

8.17 Which foods would the nurse discourage the client from eating prior to a parathyroidectomy?

① Milk products
② Green vegetables
③ Seafood
④ Poultry products

8.18 A school-aged child is being treated for Hepatitis A which was diagnosed two weeks ago. He plans to return to school this week with a physician's permit. The school nurse should plan for his return by:

① isolating him from the other children.
② talking with the physician about the reason for his return so soon.
③ no specific health requirements are necessary.
④ not allowing his participation in any sports.

8.19 The nurse is preparing a teaching plan for feeding an infant postoperative repair of a cleft lip. In order to prevent complications, the nurse would teach the mother to:

① feed the infant with a newborn nipple while holding him in the recumbent position.
② clean the suture site with a cotton dipped swab soaked in Betadine.
③ place the infant in prone position after feeding.
④ feed the infant with a rubber-tipped syringe and bubble frequently..

8.20 Which assessment indicative of hypoglycemia would be most important to report to the next shift for a client who received 6 units of regular insulin 3 hours ago?

① Kussmaul's respirations and diaphoresis
② Anorexia and lethargic
③ Diaphoresis and trembling
④ Headache and polyuria

8.21 A teenager with newly diagnosed diabetes is being discharged. Which client statement indicates an understanding of insulin?

① "The peak action for Humulin N insulin is 5–10 hours."
② "The peak action for Semilente insulin is 2–3 hours."
③ "Ultra Lente insulin is effective for 8–12 hours."
④ "The onset action for Humulin R insulin is 1-1-1/2 hours."

8.22 Which statement made by a client with portal hypertension and esophageal varices indicate an understanding of appropriate home management for these medical conditions?

① "I will eat a diet high in protein and fat."
② "I will have periodical blood samples drawn to evaluate my pT."
③ "I will use a stool softener."
④ "I will drink a minimum of 6 glasses of water per day."

8.23 A geriatric client is admitted with a left-sided paralysis. Which data would offer the nurse the most useful information regarding dietary intake? The client's:

① favorite foods.
② ability to chew and swallow.
③ normal bowel schedule.
④ routine meal times before admission.

8.24 A 3-year-old is admitted with nausea and vomiting. The nurse would offer which foods for initial PO intake?

① Ice cream
② Apple juice
③ Orange juice
④ Pudding

8.25 The client with peptic ulcer disease wants to know why he is taking ranitidine (Zantac) at bedtime. Which response is best?

① "When the physician ordered this medication, he said to give it at bedtime."
② "Taking Zantac at bedtime suppresses acid production through the night."
③ "The foods taken during the day may interfere with the effectiveness of the medication."
④ "Antacids interfere with the absorption of other drugs. Therefore, the medication is adminitered at bedtime."

8.26 Organize these steps in chronological order with #1 being the first step for a client who is having a nasogastric tube removed.

① Assist client into semi-Fowler's position.
② Ask client to hold her breath.
③ Assess bowel function by auscultation for peristalsis.
④ Flush tube with 10 ml of normal saline.
⑤ Withdraw the tube gently and steadily.
⑥ Monitor client for nausea, vomiting.

8.27 What is the priority nursing action prior to administering medications through a nasogastric tube?

① Consult a drug book regarding the recommendations for crushing each medication.
② Verify placement of the nasogastric tube in the abdomen through auscultation of air.
③ Calculate the amount of water needed to dissolve each medication.
④ Clean out the pill crushers to get rid of any residue.

8.28 At a health screening clinic, an adult male client's total plasma cholesterol level is reported to be 200 mg/dL. Based on this assessment, which nursing action is most appropriate?

① Refer the client to a physician for appropriate medication.
② Ask the client to lie down immediately.
③ Encourage the client to follow a low-fat diet.
④ Recheck the cholesterol level in two years.

8.29 An 82-year-old client is diagnosed with a vitamin K deficiency due to dietary malabsorption. Which nursing intervention is most appropriate for this client?

① Encourage the client to remain in bed to decrease bleeding potential.
② Carefully check the client's arm after taking blood pressure.
③ Increase client's dietary intake of fruits and fiber.
④ Observe client carefully for signs of angina or cardiac dysrhythmia.

8.30 A client is scheduled for a cholangiogram. Prior to the administration of meglumine diatrizoate (Gastrografin), the nurse should:

① identify the client before administering the medication.
② administer the medication 2 hours before the upper GI.
③ administer an enema after giving the medication.
④ instruct the client to take medication slowly with water.

8.31 A client with a colostomy wants to know if other people will be able to smell him. The best response by the nurse would be:

① "Keep your bag clean to reduce this possibility."
② "You can eat onions, beans and cucumbers."
③ "You could eat oranges, yogurt and drink buttermilk."
④ "You can take a nonprescription medicine that controls smell."

8.32 A client is placed on cephalexin monohydrate (Keflex) prophylactically after surgery. Which foods would the nurse encourage?

① Bran cereals and fruits
② Egg white and lean meats
③ Yogurt and acidophilus milk
④ Fish and poultry meats

8.33 In planning dietary instructions for the client with diverticular disease without symptoms of diverticulitis, the nurse would caution the client to avoid which foods?

① Fresh tomatoes
② Fresh carrots
③ Fresh lettuce
④ Whole-wheat bread

8.34 Which instructions should be given to an adult client in preparation for a plasma cholesterol screening?

① Eat a vegetarian diet for one week before the test.
② Limit alcohol intake to two glasses of wine the day before the test.
③ Abstain from dairy products for 48 hours before the test.
④ Only sips of water should be taken for 12 hours before the test.

8.35 What would be the priority of care for a client who has a blood sugar of 200 at 7:00 AM?

① Increase the PM dose of NPH insulin.
② Increase the AM dose of regular insulin.
③ Wake the client up at 3:00 AM and evaluate the blood sugar.
④ Decrease the PM dose of NPH insulin.

8.36 Which clinical findings indicate a complication from diabetes insipidus?

① Urine specific gravity – 1.001
② Serum sodium - 135
③ Urine output greater than 200 cc/hr.
④ Weight loss of 2 lbs.

8.37 In teaching a newly diagnosed diabetic client how to give insulin injections, the nurse would:

① demonstrate how to give an insulin injection on herself.
② provide the client with a pamphlet on how to give injections.
③ provide the client with a doll to practice her injection technique.
④ let the client practice giving the injection to the nurse.

8.38 Which statement made by the family indicates a correct understanding of the appropriate diet for a child with celiac disease?

① "My child's diet should include raw vegetables, fruits, and crackers."
② "My child's diet should include high carbohydrates, high calories, and high proteins."
③ "The only restriction in my child's diet should be breads and cereals."
④ "My child's diet should include high calories, high protein, and restrict foods containing rye, oats, wheat and barley."

8.39 During the first 24 hours after total parenteral nutrition (TPN) therapy is started, the nurse should:

① monitor vital signs every two hours.
② determine urinalysis results.
③ evaluate blood glucose levels.
④ compare weight with previous weight record.

8.40 To evaluate the progress of the client trying to lose weight, which information would the nurse use?

① Listing of food preferences
② History of weight gain/loss
③ Familial history of obesity
④ Weekly log of weight gain/loss

8.41 Which food would the nurse encourage a low income client to eat to satisfy essential protein needs?

① Legumes
② Red meat
③ Seafood
④ Cheese

8.42 Which assessment would be indicative of hypocalcemia?

① Constipation
② Depressed reflexes
③ Decreased muscle strength
④ Positive Trousseau's sign

8.43 Which of the following dietary modification should the nurse suggest to a client receiving peritoneal dialysis?

① Limit the amount of protein in the diet.
② Eat high fiber foods to help prevent constipation.
③ Encourage dairy products to increase phosphorus.
④ Recommend beans and cheese to assist indigestion.

8.44 Which foods would the nurse include in the diet for a client who has high cholesterol and triglyceride levels?

① Avocados, processed meats
② Red meat, eggs
③ Whole grain cereals, pasta
④ Olives, shell fish, whole milk

8.45 In working with an overweight adolescent with hypertension, the most helpful suggestion the nurse could make regarding long-term health promotion and maintenance would be to:

① avoid participating in organized sports.
② join an adolescent weight reduction support group.
③ limit socialization with non-overweight friends.
④ adhere to a 1000 calorie, low-fat diet.

8.46 Which statement made by a mother of a child with celiac disease indicates an understanding of the appropriate diet?

① "I will need to provide low protein and low fat meals to increase food absorption."
② "My child will need an increase in high fiber foods to prevent problems of constipation."
③ "I understand that wheat and oats are not included in a gluten-free diet."
④ "A high protein diet with easily digested carbohydrates will increase nutrition."

8.47 Which comment would indicate that a pregnant woman understands the recommended dietary caloric increase for pregnancy?

① "I will need to double my calorie intake since I am now eating for two of us."
② "I can add an additional 500 calories by drinking milk shakes."
③ "I need to add 300 calories by increasing intake of basic four food groups."
④ "I really need to watch my calorie intake so I will not gain too much weight."

8.48 To prevent the spread of Hepatitis A, the most effective measure the nurse should teach the client and close associates would be to:

① wash their hands every time they go to the bathroom.
② wash all dishes in a dishwasher.
③ teach drug addicts never to share their used needles.
④ always use condoms during sexual intercourse.

8.49 The nurse may suggest the client take prenatal vitamins daily with:

① orange juice at bedtime.
② breakfast.
③ milk at lunch.
④ water at dinner.

8.50 When teaching a newly diagnosed diabetic about regulating her diabetes at home, the nurse would include which instructions?

① Limit vigorous exercise.
② Eliminate sugar from the diet.
③ Test blood sugar at regular intervals.
④ Limit carbohydrates in the diet.

8.51 A client has a nasogastric tube in place after extensive abdominal surgery. He complains of nausea. His abdomen is distended, and there are no bowel sounds. The first nursing action would be to:

① administer the PRN pain medication and antiemetic.
② irrigate the nasogastric tube with normal saline.
③ re-anchor a new nasogastric tube.
④ check the placement and patency.

8.52 A good menu selection for a client with a gallbladder disturbance would include:

① skimmed milk, banana, broiled fish, lettuce salad.
② skimmed milk, bran cereal, apple, fried eggs.
③ tea, carrots, bran muffins, and pork chops.
④ tea, broccoli, broiled fish, and pie.

8.53 Which foods would reflect appropriate selection for a client on a low residue diet?

① Milk, green beans, whole wheat bread
② Creamed chicken soup, broccoli, pudding
③ Baked chicken, buttered rice, plain gelatin
④ Cabbage salad, fried chicken, applesauce

8.54 Which information should the nurse recognize as being the most pertinent to the diagnosis of cholecystitis?

① Flatulence
② Nausea and vomiting
③ Right upper abdominal pain
④ Dyspepsia

8.55 Which statement made by the client indicates a correct understanding of cholecystectomy?

① "After this surgery, I'll be able to eat anything."
② "I'll be able to drink coffee and colas again."
③ "If I start having a fever, I need to call my physician."
④ "I won't have indigestion or heartburn anymore."

8.56 The nurse should plan on administering levothyroxine (Synthroid) by mouth at which time of day?

① prior to breakfast
② with lunch
③ at bedtime
④ two hours after eating the main meal of the day

8.57 Which outcome best evaluates the effectiveness of health promotion regarding a self-care deficit in relation to feeding?

① The client eats at least one half of all meals and drinks a minimum of 2000 ml/day.
② The client's dentures have been replaced, and he is able to chew.
③ The client will eat without verbalizing suspicions when one particular nurse sits with him.
④ The client appears to have increased energy to complete grooming activities.

8.58 When would the nurse anticipate the client with a gastric ulcer to have pain?

① Two to three hours after a meal
② At night
③ Relieved by ingestion of food
④ One half to one hour after a meal

8.59   Which nursing observations would indicate the
client has developed complications of cholecystitis?

   ① Nausea
   ② Indigestion and frequent belching
   ③ Jaundice
   ④ Right upper abdominal pain

8.60   How would the nurse evaluate if a client is getting
enough Vitamin K in diet?

   ① Client is able to fight an infection.
   ② Client has normal night vision.
   ③ Client has normal clotting of blood.
   ④ Client doesn't break bones when he falls.

Answers & Rationales

8.1 ② The normal plasma potassium level is 3.5—5.5 mEq/L. This client's potassium is low and needs replacement. Options #1, #3, and #4 do not address the problems.

8.2 ④ An infant with reflux should be maintained in an upright position. The head of the bed should be raised at a 30-degree angle. Option #1 may not be necessary, if positioning is effective. Option #2 is an action for the mother versus the infant. Option #3 is incorrect because the client's feedings should be changed to small volume, frequent feedings.

8.3 ② Since metaclopramide facilitates gastric emptying, it must be taken before meals. Options #1 and #3 do not promote optimum effects of the medication. Option #4 is incorrect because the time of administration should be changed to give with the client's meals.

8.4 ③ Option #3 is an appropriate diet for a client with cirrhosis of the liver. Options #1, #2, and #4 are inappropriate for this disorder.

8.5 ② An infant should be NPO 3 hours prior to the procedure. Options #1 and #3 are inappropriate. Option #4 is incorrect because it is not necessary for an infant to be NPO for 6 hours.

8.6 ① Research indicates there is an increased growth of organisms after four hours. Options #2 and #3 are inappropriate due to increased organism growth. Option #4 is not a necessary action to maintain asepsis.

8.7 ① This provides the most pertinent data in assessing actual growth. Option #2 is inappropriate for this situation. Options #3 and #4 are important assessments but are not a priority to Option #1.

8.8 ④ Diabetic ketoacidosis is frequently associated with dehydration. Fluids should be encouraged. Option #1 is incorrect because a diabetic should alter the dose according to serial glucose checks. Option #2 is incorrect because the client is not tolerating PO foods. Option #3 is incorrect because sweets can be used as calories in this situation.

8.9 ③ Offering small and frequent meals will help prevent nausea and enable the client to eat adequate amounts. Option #1 is important but is not a priority to Option #3. Option #2 may promote vomiting. Option #4 does not provide adjustments for the client's illness.

8.10 ② This will assist in preventing constipation. Options #1 and #3 are incorrect for the pregnant woman. Option #4 will lead to more constipation.

8.11 ① Option #1 is the correct answer. This practice is unsafe. If the tube should be mispositioned in trachea, the client may aspirate water. Options #2, #3, and #4 are correct procedures and do not answer the question.

8.12 ④ This is the best method of determining the client's nutritional status. Option #1 and #2 only indicate the client's hydration. Option #3 does not guarantee that this food will be eaten.

8.13 ② The impaired intestinal absorption of cystic fibrosis necessitates a diet higher in protein and calories. Fat is decreased because it may interfere with absorption of other nutrients. Options #1 and #4 contain high fat. Option #3 is not adequate for this child.

8.14 ③ The inability to control diabetes mellitus by diet and oral agents, coupled with surgically-induced metabolic changes, being NPO both prior to and after surgery, necessitates temporary control by insulin. Options #1, #2, and #4 are not true statements.

8.15 ③ The onset of action for regular insulin is 30–60 minutes. The assessment indicates a problem with hypoglycemia. Foods such as milk and crackers should be given if the blood sugar level is around 40 to 60 mg/dL. If orange juice or simple sugar is given, it should be followed with a meal or protein intake. Option #1 is incorrect because action should be taken prior to notifying the physician. Option #2 delays the response to the problem. Option #4 is inappropriate for this client.

8.16 ① This option contains foods highest in fiber to assist in counteracting constipation (green vegetables and grains). Options #2, #3, and #4 do not have as high a fiber content.

8.17 ① A low calcium diet is recommended preoperatively. Options #2, #3, and #4 would not be discouraged.

8.18 ③ Type A Hepatitis is not infectious within a week or so after the onset of jaundice, and the child can return to school. Options #1 and #2 are not necessary. Option #4 depends on the child's energy level.

8.19 ④ The rubber tip can be placed in from the side of the mouth to avoid the operative area and to prevent sucking on the tubing. Infants with cleft lip swallow excessive amounts of air so they require frequent bubbling. Option #1 is unsafe due to aspiration. Option #2 is incorrect. Option #3 is incorrect because the site is cleansed with saline or hydrogen peroxide.

8.20 ③ Regular insulin peaks in 2–4 hours. These are signs of hypoglycemia which may occur. Option #1 is incorrect because Kussmaul's respirations are signs of hyperglycemia. Options #2 and #4 are not indicative of hypoglycemia.

8.21 ① Humulin N, an intermediate acting insulin, has a peak action of 5–12 hours. Option #2 is incorrect because Semilente, a rapid acting insulin, peaks between 8-10 hours. Option #3 is incorrect because Ultra Lente, a long-acting insulin, is effective for 36+ hours. Option #4 is incorrect because the onset of action for regular insulin is between 1/2 to 1 hour.

8.22 ③ Option #3 is appropriate for preventing bleeding from the esophageal varices. Options #1, #2 and #4 do not address the concern with the varices.

8.23 ② The ability of the client to chew and swallow will be the basis of planning. Options #1 and #4 won't make any difference if he cannot chew. Option #3 would be important in avoiding constipation.

8.24 ② Clear liquids should be offered first. As child tolerates these fluids, then full liquids may be offered. Options #1, #3, and #4 are all part of a full liquid diet.

8.25 ② Bedtime administration suppresses nocturnal acid production. Option #1 may be correct, but Option #2 is a more complete answer. Option #3 is incorrect. Although foods sometimes interfere with the effectiveness of some medications, this is not the rationale for giving Zantac at bedtime. Option #4 is incorrect because Zantac is an H_2 antagonist—not an antacid.

8.26 ③ #3 is the first step. #1 is the second step.
③ #4 is the third step. Flushing will ensure
① that the tube doesn't contain stomach
④ contents that could irritate tissues during
② tube removal. #2 is the fourth step. This is
⑤ to close epiglottis. #5 is the fifth step. #6
⑥ is the sixth step. For 48 hours, monitor client for GI dysfunction including nausea, vomiting, abdominal distention, and food intolerance.

8.27 ② The verification of tube placement prevents the instillation of medication into the lungs, which will fill the lungs with fluid and medications leading to aspiratory pneumonia. Option #1 is incorrect because the priority with a nasogastric tube is to verify placement prior to any medication administration. With Option #3, the amount of water needed to administer the medications is not priority. Option #4 is incorrect because cleaning the pill crusher of any residue is important to prevent cross contamination, but is not priority.

8.28 ③ The total cholesterol level for an adult male should be under 200 mg/dL. Higher levels require a low-fat diet. Levels higher than 250 mg/dL may require medication, if diet therapy is not effective. Option #1 is not necessary prior to working on diet. Option #2. Option #4 is incorrect because blood levels should be checked sooner than 2 years.

8.29 ② Due to the potential for bleeding, the client's arm should be observed for bruising after taking a blood pressure reading. Option #1 is incorrect because remaining in bed does not decrease the potential for bleeding. Option #3 does not affect absorption of vitamin K. Option #4 is not appropriate for vitamin K deficiency.

8.30 ① Appropriate identification of client is the first nursing priority after the order is verified (5 Rights of medication administration). Options #2, #3, and #4 are incorrect.

8.31 ① Cleanliness is known to control odor. Option #2 causes gas production. Option #3 is ineffective. Option #4 is incorrect because the client should check with his physician before taking any over-the-counter drugs.

8.32 ③ These foods will help maintain normal intestinal flora. Options #1, #2, and #4 are not necessary to encourage.

8.33 ① Fresh tomatoes should be avoided because they contain indigestible roughage and seeds that may block the neck of a diverticulum. Options #2 and #3 are incorrect because fresh carrots and lettuce are encouraged for a high-fiber content to add bulk to stools. Option #4 is incorrect because the client with diverticulosis is encouraged to eat a diet high in cellulose and hemicellulose types of fiber found in wheat bran and whole-wheat bread.

8.34 ④ Only sips of water are permitted for 12 hours before plasma cholesterol screening for accurate results. Options #1 and #3 are incorrect because a normal diet should be eaten the week before the test. Option #2 is incorrect because alcohol intake will interfere with test results.

8.35 ③ It is important to know what the 3:00 AM blood sugar is to determine if the hyperglycemia is from the somoygi effect. Options #1 and #4 will be adjusted after knowing if the AM blood sugar is the accurate reading or a rebound response to a low blood sugar at 3:00 AM. Option #2 is incorrect.

8.36 ④ Option #4 is correct. Clinical manifestations from diabetes may result in severe dehydration. These manifestations may include: dry skin and mucous membranes; weight loss; decrease in blood pressure; decrease in central venous pressure; weakness; confusion; or speech difficulty in elderly. Options #1 and #3 are clinical manifestations of diabetes insipidus but not complications. Option #2 is normal range.

8.37 ③ A client should be given a doll to practice injection technique. Options #1 and #2 may be appropriate, but Option #3 provides the best teaching method. Option #4 is not recommended.

8.38 ④ Celiac disease is characterized by an intolerance of gluten. Therefore, foods containing rye, oats, wheat, and barley should be restricted from the client's diet. Options #1, #2, and #3 do not reflect appropriate dietary needs for this client.

8.39 ③ Total parenteral nutrition (TPN), or hyper-alimentation, has a high glucose content. Therefore, it is important to monitor glucose levels. Options #1 and #2 are inappropriate. Option #4 is appropriate, but not a priority.

8.40 ④ The weekly log of weight gain/loss would indicate progress of client in losing weight. Options #1, #2, and #3 are important for history taking and planning.

8.41 ① Legumes are an economical source rich in protein. Options #2, #3, and #4 are high in protein but more expensive to purchase.

8.42 ④ A positive Trousseau's sign is indicative of neuromuscular hyperreflexia associated with hypocalcemia. Options #1, #2, and #3 are symptoms associated with hypercalcemia.

8.43 ② Option #2 is correct. Constipation should be avoided with peritoneal dialysis as it will contribute to fullness and discomfort with exchanges. Option #1 is incorrect as protein is lost with peritoneal dialysis and needs to be replaced in the diet. (This is untrue with hemodialysis.) Option #3 is not needed with these clients. Option #4 is incorrect as these foods can lead to gas and constipation which would increase discomfort with exchanges.

8.44 ③ Whole grain cereals have little or no fat content. Options #1, #2, and #4 have high fat content.

8.45 ② This is an excellent means of obtaining information and support while helping the client. Option #1 is incorrect because properly supervised physical activity is desirable, not to be avoided. Option #3 is incorrect because peer relationships are important, not to be avoided. Option #4 is not enough calories for an adolescent, and a diet too low in calories is hard to comply with and may set the adolescent up for failure.

8.46 ③ Celiac Disease is an inborn error in metabolism of rye, wheat, and oat products. Primary dietary management is a gluten-free diet. Options #1, #2, and #4 are not correct statements regarding a gluten-free diet.

8.47 ③ It is recommended to increase intake of a healthy diet by 300 calories. This is for fetal growth, maternal tissues, and the placenta. Option #1 is a common misconception. Option #2 is incorrect because 500 calories are too many calories, and a milkshake is not a good food source because of fat content. Option #4 is not safe for the pregnant client.

8.48 ① Type A Hepatitis is spread by oral-fecal route so it is important to teach effective hand-washing every time the client uses the bathroom, or has genital-rectal contact. Options #2, #3, and #4 are not true for Hepatitis A.

8.49 ① Taking the vitamin with something acid increases the absorption of iron, and taking them with food and at bedtime decreases the possibility of nausea as the client will be asleep. Option #2 is not a priority to Option #1. Options #3 and #4 are incorrect because milk and water are less effective fluids.

8.50 ③ Testing blood sugar levels several times each day gives the client information about the regulation of insulin and blood sugar. This information would be important in assessing the control of this disease process. Option #1 is incorrect because regular exercise should be encouraged. Option #2 is correct for a diabetic. However, Option #3 is a higher priority. Option #4 is not correct for the diabetic diet.

8.51 ④ The first assessment in determining problems with nasogastric tubes is to determine tube placement and patency. Option #1 may be implemented after the placement and patency of the tube are determined. Option #2 would be completed only after Option #4 was completed. Option #3 is inappropriate without further assessment.

8.52 ① The diet would be low in fat, spices, condiments, and coffee. Options #2, #3, and #4 are incorrect because cooked vegetables, raw vegetables (except lettuce), and eggs are usually not tolerated. All fried foods and pastries should be avoided.

8.53 ③ A low residue diet will leave a relatively small amount of residue or indigestible material in the colon. All meats, fish and poultry must be broiled or baked. Options #1, #2, and #4 contain a high residue food.

8.54 ③ The most pertinent to the diagnosis of cholecystitis is the pain in the right upper abdominal quadrant. Options #1, #2, and #4 may indicate other gastrointestinal problems

8.55 ③ A fever may indicate an infection and should be reported to the physician. Options #1, #2, and #4 are incorrect because the client may continue to have trouble with certain foods. Indigestion and heartburn may occur for an indefinite period of time after surgery.

8.56 ① Option #1 is correct since administering levothyroixine (Synthroid) prior to breakfast will reduce the possibility of insomnia, and the body avoids the need to fight the digestion of food with the digestion of the medication due to the 50-80% absorption rate associated with oral forms of this drug. Option #2 is contraindicated because the body will digest the food slowing the absorption rate of the medication. Option #3 is incorrect because insomnia is associated with this drug. Consequently, administration at bedtime will heighten the chances of sleep disruption. Option #4 is incorrect because the main meal of the day is subjective to the client.

8.57 ① This is a concrete measure of the client's eating patterns which indicates adequate intake of a well-balanced diet. Option #2 may not present a well-balanced diet. Option #3 indicates that the client is still experiencing distorted thinking about the foods to eat. Option #4 may not be an accurate measure of adequate nutrition.

8.58 ④ Pain related to a gastric ulcer occurs about 1/2 to 1 hour after a meal, rarely at night, and is not helped by ingestion of food. Options #1, #2, and #3 are features of a duodenal ulcer.

8.59 ③ Jaundice indicates possible stone in the bile duct causing obstruction. Options #1, #2, and #4 are signs and symptoms of cholecystitis and do not necessarily indicate a complication.

8.60 ③ Option #3 is correct. Vitamin K is necessary for clotting. Option #1 may be Vitamin B6 (pyridoxine) which stimulates hemo production for red cells, necessary for antibody formation. Option #2 is Vitamin A retinol. Option #4 is calcium.

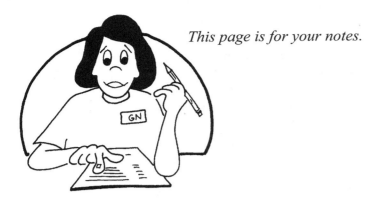

This page is for your notes.

Pharmacology and Parenteral Therapies

Many of lifes failures are people who did not realize how close they were to success when they gave up.

—Unknown

✔ **Clarification of this test…**

The minimum standards include performing and directing activities necessary for safe administration of medications and intravenous therapies.

☛ Prepare medication for administration.

☛ Administer and document meds given by common routes (oral, topical).

☛ Evaluate appropriateness/accuracy of medication order for client.

☛ Review pertinent data prior to medication administration (vital signs, lab results, allergies, potential interactions).

☛ Evaluate and document client's response to medication.

☛ Administer and document meds given by parenteral routes (IV, IM, SQ).

☛ Monitor and maintain infusion sites and rates.

☛ Comply with regulations governing controlled substances (counting/wasting narcotics).

☛ Perform calculations needed for medication administration (educate client/family about medications).

☛ Insert/remove a peripheral intravenous line.

☛ Assess implanted venous access devices.

☛ Administer blood products and evaluate client's response.

9.1   A client in ICU is given procainamide HCl (Pronestyl) slow IV push. The nurse should withhold the next dose for which indication?

① Presence of premature ventricular contractions
② Occurrence of severe hypotension
③ Recurring paroxysmal atrial tachycardia
④ A sedimentation rate of 10

9.2   An anxious adult client has been ordered the following preoperative medications IM:
   • Meperidine HCl (Demerol)
   • promethazine (Phenergan)
   • diazepam (Valium)
Which technique should be used in the administration of these medications?

① The diazepam (Valium) should be placed in a separate syringe.
② All the medications should be placed in one syringe to avoid the discomfort of several injections.
③ Each medication should be placed in a separate syringe for safety.
④ The physician should be notified because these drugs are incompatible.

9.3   Which instruction should be given to a client taking tetracycline HCL?

① Take with a full stomach or a glass of milk.
② Avoid exposure to direct sunlight.
③ Continue taking the medication until client feels better.
④ Avoid the use of soaps or detergents for two weeks.

9.4   A client has taken levothyroxine sodium (Synthroid) 0.4 mg daily for 4 days. Which symptoms suggest that the nurse should recommend a change in the client's medication?

① Nervousness and difficulty sleeping
② Tired with no energy
③ Coarse hair and skin
④ Persistent weight gain

9.5   Which medication would be a priority for the diabetic client to avoid if possible?

① Steroids
② Narcotics
③ Major tranquilizers
④ NSAIDs

9.6   What action should a nurse take for an adult client taking lithium carbonate (Lithane) who has a serum lithium level of 2.0 mEq/L?

① Administer the next dose on time.
② Increase the client's fluid intake.
③ Notify the physician.
④ Encourage the client to rest..

9.7   During the administration of amphotericin B, what would be the priority of nursing care?

① Observe for signs of hyperkalemia.
② Monitor serum glucose.
③ Encourage a diet low in calories and protein.
④ Evaluate the IV site for phlebitis.

9.8   Your COPD client's order reads theophylline (Aminophylline) 300 mg in 100 cc D5W at 36 mg/hr. To deliver the correct dose, the nurse sets the infusion control device at:

① 12 cc/hr.
② 25 cc/hr.
③ 36 cc/hr.
④ 100 cc/hr.

9.9   A client presents in respiratory acidosis and pulmonary edema. What would be the desired outcome after administering furosemide (Lasix) for this client?

① Blood pressure change from 160/92 to 148/88.
② Respiratory rate change from 52 to 48
③ Urine output 100 cc/hr.
④ Breath sounds present with less rales and rhonchi.

9.10 A male nurse is 5'8" tall and weighs 175 pounds. The nurse has selected the gluteus medius muscle for an intramuscular injection. Which size needle should be used?

① 20 gauge, 3-inch needle
② 22 gauge, 1 to 1-1/2 inch needle
③ 25 gauge, 3-inch needle
④ 25 gauge, 5/8 inch needle

9.11 Which medication has an adverse reaction on extrapyramidal effects?

① Lithium (Lithane)
② Haloperidol (Haldol)
③ Chlordiazepoxide (Librium)
④ Nortriptyline (Aventyl)

9.12 A client is given morphine 6 mg IV push for post-operative pain. Following administration of this drug, the nurse observes:
  • P-68
  • R-8
  • BP-100/68
  • Client sleeping quietly
Which nursing action is most appropriate?

① Allow the client to sleep undisturbed.
② Administer oxygen via face mask or nasal prongs.
③ Administer naloxone (Narcan).
④ Keep epinephrine 1:1000 at the bedside.

9.13 During administration of oral medications to an elderly confused client, the client states, "These pills look funny. They belong to the lady down the hall." How should the nurse respond to the client?

① "Your physician has ordered new medications for you. They will help you get well."
② "Remember yesterday when I brought your medications? They look the same."
③ "I'll explain the purpose of medications."
④ "I'll be back after I check your medications again."

9.14 What would be the priority care before pushing a medication via a heparin lock?

① Change the angiocath every 48 hours.
② Change the dressing every 24 hours.
③ Check for a flashback prior to administering the medication.
④ Flush the heparin lock with 25 cc fluid prior to administering the medication.

9.15 Which observation of a client receiving theophylline (Aminophylline) IVPB for an acute respiratory problem would alert the nurse to withhold the medication and notify the physician?

① Hypertension
② Unresponsiveness
③ Polyuria
④ Tachycardia

9.16 Which action would be appropriate for a client receiving a continuous infusion of heparin with a PTT greater than 150 seconds?

① Slow the heparin drip.
② Stop the heparin and notify the physician.
③ Maintain the heparin at the current infusion rate.
④ Increase the infusion rate and notify the physician.

9.17 Which medication should the nurse question?

① Carvedilol (Coreg) for a client with COPD
② Enalapril (Vasotec) for a client being discharged post MI
③ Hydrochlorothiazide (HCTZ) for a client with stage 1 hypertension
④ Digoxin for an adult patient with a heart rate of 64

9.18 A client discharged with sublingual nitroglycerin (Nitrostat) should be taught to:

① take the medication 5 minutes after the pain has started.
② stop taking the medication if a burning sensation is present.
③ take the medication on an empty stomach.
④ avoid abrupt changes in posture.

9.19 While monitoring a client receiving pain relief from client-controlled analgesia (PCA), what would be the priority care for this client?

① Set the pump's hourly infusion rate to equal total cc/hour needed to control pain.
② Evaluate the client for orthostatic hypotension.
③ Monitor the respiratory rate for tachypnea.
④ Inform the client that he can control all of his pain by simply pushing a button.

9.20 Which statement made by the client indicates an understanding of the health promotion teaching regarding lithium (Lithane)? "I will:

    ① increase my fluid intake."
    ② decrease my fluid intake."
    ③ increase my salt intake."
    ④ decrease my salt intake."

9.21 After administering Dimetane-DC cough syrup to a child, the nurse notes that the child becomes excitable and restless. The most appropriate action for the nurse to take is:

    ① report the child's behavior to the physician.
    ② decrease the dose by half in the future.
    ③ have the child drink a glass of warm milk to dilute the medication.
    ④ chart the client's response to the medication and alert the next shift.

9.22 An elderly client experiencing diarrhea for 4 days has been taking Kaopectate at home. Which nursing assessment would indicate a complication of kaolin and pectin mixtures?

    ① Itching
    ② Fecal impaction
    ③ Nausea
    ④ Dysrhythmia

9.23 In the elderly client, which assessment finding would indicate side effects of Meperidine (Demerol) and hydroxyzine hydrochloride (Vistaril)?

    ① Tachypnea
    ② Lethargy
    ③ Hypertension
    ④ Disorientation

9.24 Which side effect needs to be discussed in the teaching session for a client taking an ace inhibitor?

    ① Peripheral edema
    ② Rash with pruritus
    ③ Increase in weight
    ④ Polycythemia

9.25 The nurse is preparing to start a blood transfusion of 250 cc packed cells to her client. Which would be most important for the nurse to consider during this process?

    ① Hang D_5W for flushing blood tubing.
    ② Start transfusion at 60 cc per hour.
    ③ Warm the blood in the microwave.
    ④ Start transfusion with a 19-gauge needle.

9.26 Which parameter should the nurse check before administering oral Verapamil (Calan)?

    ① Electrolytes
    ② Urine output
    ③ Weight
    ④ Heart rate

9.27 In addition to the digitalis levels, it would also be necessary for the nurse to periodically evaluate which lab values on

    ① Creatinine levels
    ② Serum potassium
    ③ Urine potassium and sodium
    ④ Blood urea nitrogen and glucose

9.28 Which observation indicates the most common side effect of Trimethoprim-sulfamethoxazole (Bactrim)?

    ① Hypotonia
    ② Loss of hearing
    ③ Hypotension
    ④ Urticaria

9.29 A client with arterial fibrillation and a pulse of 120, BP 110/60 has received diltiazem (Cardizem) IV. What would be the expected outcome within 15 minutes after administration?

    ① Pulse 90, BP 96/50, atrial fibrillation on cardiac monitor.
    ② Pulse 150, BP 140/90, atrial fibrillation on cardiac monitor.
    ③ Pulse 90, BP 140/90, sinus rhythm on the cardiac monitor.
    ④ Urine output 50 ml/hr, pulse 60, BP 140/80.

9.30 Which fluid should a client taking methenamine mandelate (Mandelamine) for a recurrent urinary tract infection be caused to limit?

① Milk
② Juices
③ Water
④ Tea

9.31 A client has total parenteral nutrition (TPN) infusing at 50 cc per hour. The nurse runs out of fluid prior to a new bag coming to the unit. What would be most important for the nurse to assess with this client?

① Hyperglycemia
② Hyponatremia
③ Hypoglycemia
④ Infection

9.32 Before beginning a dopamine (Intropin) infusion on a client, the nurse should assess:

① urine output.
② weight.
③ patency of IV.
④ pulmonary artery pressures.

9.33 Before administering penicillin to a client, the nurse should check:

① other medications the client is taking.
② client allergy to penicillin.
③ oral temperature.
④ white blood count.

9.34 The nurse's priority action, before administering terbutaline (Brethine) to a client in labor whose pulse is 144, should be to:

① withhold the medication.
② decrease the dose in half.
③ administer the medication.
④ wait 15 minutes; recheck the pulse rate.

9.35 Which measure should the nurse take on a postoperative client who develops a red rash and starts vomiting 20 minutes into a nafcillin (Nafcil) infusion?

① Stop the infusion and notify the physician.
② Stop the infusion, administer nausea medications, and continue the infusion.
③ Complete the infusion and then administer nausea medication.
④ Complete the infusion, monitor and report the rash to the next shift.

9.36 The nurse should administer phenytoin (Dilantin) intravenously in which fluid?

① 5% dextrose
② Ringers lactate
③ 10% dextrose
④ Normal saline

9.37 The physician orders an intramuscular injection of neostigmine (Prostigmin) on a client with a history of asthma. The most appropriate nursing action would be:

① administer the medication.
② check blood pressure and pulse.
③ notify the physician so the medication can be changed.
④ ask the pharmacy if the medication can be given by mouth.

9.38 A client has been taking perphenazine (Trilafon) by mouth for two days and now displays the following:
   • head turned to the side and arched at an angle
   • stiffness, and
   • muscle spasms in neck.
Which PRN medication would the nurse give?

① Promazine (Sparine)
② Biperiden (Akineton)
③ Theothixene (Navane)
④ Haloperidol (Haldol)

9.39 When a client is taking Tetracycline with St. John's Wort, what would be the priority care?

① Recommend that client avoids beer.
② Report a change in the client's mood.
③ Advise client to stay out of the sun.
④ Review the importance of monitoring serum glucose.

9.40 Which statement by a client reflects a correct understanding of alprazolam (Xanax)?

① "I can take it whenever I feel upset."
② "I should not take this with anything but water."
③ "I need to quit drinking white wine."
④ "This medication will help me forget and go on."

9.41 The nurse administers Meperidine (Demerol) 50 mg IM for pain as per physician's orders. Three hours later, the client again complains of pain, and the nurse administers a second injection of Demerol. Which statement describes the nurse's liability?

① She administered the medication appropriately; there is no liability.
② The nurse violated the narcotic law in not having an order to administer the Demerol a second time.
③ The client was not injured. Therefore, the nurse is not liable.
④ The nurse should have waited at least 4 hours then there would be no liability.

9.42 Which instruction should be given to a client with drug-induced Cushing's Syndrome?

① Increase calcium-rich foods to help prevent compression fractures.
② Increase bed rest to decrease stress.
③ Decrease drug dosage gradually.
④ Increase dietary fat intake.

9.43 Which response should the nurse recognize as the desired one to levodopa (L-Dopa) in the treatment of Parkinson's Disease?

① Dyskinesia
② Complete remission of symptoms
③ Less rigidity
④ Decrease in fine motor tremors

9.44 What should be the priority action for a client who is receiving vancomycin (Vancocin) 500 mg IV and develops a flushed neck and face?

① Decrease the rate of the vancomycin (Vancocin).
② Discontinue the infusion.
③ Evaluate the client's temperature and vital signs.
④ Notify provider of care for an order for an antihistamine.

9.45 The best administration schedule for an adult taking a psychostimulant, such as methylphenidate (Ritalin) is:

① breakfast and bedtime.
② early morning, late afternoon.
③ breakfast time—not after 2:00 PM.
④ late afternoon, dinnertime.

9.46 The most appropriate nursing action before administration of Captopril (Capoten) would be to check the client's:

① apical pulse for 60 seconds.
② blood pressure.
③ urine output.
④ temperature.

9.47 A psychiatric client with the diagnosis of schizophrenia tells the nurse that he is the President of the United States. What would be the priority action for the nurse?

① Confront the client regarding this delusion and bring him back to reality.
② Reflect this statement back to the client to encourage therapeutic communication.
③ Respond with an open-ended response to get client to further discuss his thoughts.
④ Verify identify of the client prior to administering his medication.

9.48 What would be most important to monitor on a client who is taking Lisinopril (Zestril)?

① Serum potassium
② Serum pH
③ Serum calcium
④ Heart rate

9.49 A client who weighs 75 kilograms has an order for heparin, 5000 units, subcutaneously (SC) every 12 hours. The vial contains 5000 units/mL and your medication administration record (MAR) indicates that the client should receive 2 milliliters (2 mL). The priority nursing intervention is to:

① question the order.
② administer the 2 milliliters as ordered.
③ perform a stool hemocult on the client prior to administration.
④ check the lab values prior to administration.

9.50 A client presents to your unit in atrial fibrillation. What medication protocol would be most important to implement?

① Inderal
② Isuprel
③ Lidocaine
④ Verapamil

9.51 The physician orders heparin 7,000 U S.C. g8h for a client with deep vein thrombosis. The heparin available is 20,000 units per 1 ml. How many milliliters of heparin should the nurse administer?

① 0.2 ml
② 0.3 ml
③ 0.35 ml
④ 3.5 ml

9.52 Which observations indicate the client is experiencing a side effect(s) of prednisone (Deltasone)?

① Decreased sodium levels and increased urinary output
② Vomiting small amounts of bile-stained fluid
③ Bleeding gums with a decrease in clotting time
④ Ecchymosis and an increase in the retention of fluids

9.53 A client is brought to the ER by his family after severe, extensive burn injury. Which of the following physician orders would you question?

① Begin Lactated Ringers infusion stat.
② Give furosemide 80 mg IV push stat.
③ Give morphine sulfate 2 mg IV push stat.
④ Insert Foley catheter.

9.54 Which instruction would be included in a teaching plan for the client receiving a peripheral vasodilator?

① Take hot showers to promote the vasodilation effect.
② Small amounts of alcohol will enhance the medication.
③ Increase the sodium intake due to excessive loss.
④ Change body positions slowly to reduce dizziness.

9.55 Which of the following nursing actions would be important in the safe administration of oxytocin (Pitocin)?

① Assess respirations and urine output.
② Administer parenterally as the primary IV.
③ Have calcium gluconate available as an antidote.
④ Palpate uterus frequently.

9.56 Prior to the administration of hydralazine (Apresoline), the nurse would evaluate for which symptom?

① A decrease in the pulse pressure
② Pulse rate in excess of 110
③ A significant decrease in blood pressure
④ Presence of confusion and disorientation

9.57 Which response is the desired client response to hydroxyzine (Vistaril)?

① Decrease in anxiety, and control of nausea and vomiting
② Control of diarrhea by direct action on intestinal nerve endings
③ Edema is decreased due to the increased excretion of water.
④ Inflammation in joint is decreased; pain is reduced.

9.58 What nursing action is most appropriate when inserting a vaginal suppository?

① Remove the suppository from the wrapper and lubricate it with Vaseline.
② Instruct client to place in tampon after inserting the vaginal medication.
③ With an applicator on the forefinger of your free hand, insert the suppository about 2" (5 cm) into the vagina.
④ Direct the applicator up initially and then down and forward.

9.59 A provider has ordered timolol (Timoptic) 1 gtt OU bid. Point to the location of the eye where the medication will be placed.

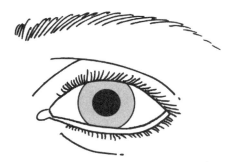

9.60 Which observation is a sign of impending toxicity from an aminoglycoside antibiotic such as gentamycin sulfate (Garamycin)?

① Decrease in blood pressure
② Pulse rate drops from 140 to 90.
③ Decrease in agitation
④ Hearing loss

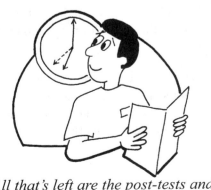

*All that's left are the post-tests and
the simulated exam!!*

Answers & Rationales

9.1 ②   Severe hypotension or bradycardias are signs of adverse reaction with this medication. Options #1 and #3 are not ordinarily side effects of this drug. Option #4 is within normal limits.

9.2 ①   Diazepam (Valium) is not compatible with most other medications and should be administered separately. Option #2 is incorrect because the two drugs are incompatible. Option #3 is unnecessary. Option #4 is inappropriate as the nurse should be knowledgeable about drug interactions and compatibility.

9.3 ②   Photosensitivity occurs with the use of this medication. Option #1 is incorrect because this medication should be taken on an empty stomach. Option #3 is incorrect because the full prescription should be taken. Option #4 is irrelevant.

9.4 ①   Nervousness and insomnia suggest an overdose of thyroid hormone replacement therapy. Options #2, #3, and #4 are symptoms of hypothyroidism—the reason for giving this medication.

9.5 ①   Steroids increase the blood glucose requiring an increase in the insulin intake. Options #2, #3, and #4 are usually safe for diabetic clients.

9.6 ③   The therapeutic level of lithium is 0.5–1.2 mEq/L. Toxic manifestations may occur at levels about 1.5 mEq/L so the physician should be notified. Option #1 will not occur since the client's level is out of the therapeutic range. Options #2 and #4 will not decrease the lithium level.

9.7 ④   This anti-fungal is very irritating to the vein. The IV site must be evaluated frequently for phlebitis. Option #1 is incorrect since the problem that can occur is hypokalemia. Option #2 is incorrect. Option #3 should be a diet high in calories and protein.

9.8 ① $\dfrac{300 \text{ mg}}{100 \text{ cc}} = \dfrac{36 \text{ mg}}{x}$

$300x = 3600 \quad x = 12$

9.9 ④   Lasix is administered to diurese the extra fluid. As the fluid decreases, the breath sounds will have less rales and rhonchi. Option #1 is not specific for this client. It would be an outcome, but not specific for pulmonary edema. Option #2 is insignificant. Option #3 is expected, but the priority is to improve the breath sounds.

9.10 ②   An intramuscular injection at the gluteus medius calls for a needle length of 1 to 1-1/2 inches, and gauge #20 to #22. Option #1 is incorrect because the needle is too long. Option #4 is incorrect because the needle gauge is too small and the needle is too short.

9.11 ②   This medication produces extrapyramidal reactions. Options #1, #3, and #4 do not include extrapyramidal reactions as a possible adverse reaction.

9.12 ③   IV naloxone (Narcan) should be given to reverse respiratory depression. Option #1 is incorrect because the respiratory rate of 8 is too low and necessitates a nursing action. Option #2 is secondary and may not be needed. Option #4 is irrelevant to the situation.

9.13 ④   Even the confused client should have medications rechecked when there is any possibility of an error. Always observe the five Rs of medication administration. Options #1, #2, and #3 are incorrect.

9.14 ③   Checking for a flashback is a priority before administering any medication via a heparin lock. Another alternative would be to flush the lock, but 25 cc is too much fluid. Options #1 and #2 are inappropriate.

9.15 ④ Option #4 is a side effect of Aminophylline. Levels about 20 ug/l are considered toxic. Clients with long-term use of this drug may tolerate higher blood concentration levels. Other side effects which can develop are hypotension, nausea, vomiting, and headache. These must be monitored to minimize the potential problems associated with seizures. Options #1, #2, and #3 are not due to an Aminophylline overdose.

9.16 ② The client is excessively anticoagulated. The heparin should be stopped immediately and the physician notified for further action. Option #1 is incorrect because the client is still receiving the drug, and it should be stopped. Options #3 and #4 are inappropriate actions.

9.17 ① Option #1 is correct. Carvedilol is a non-selective beta blocker medication. It will affect the beta fibers in the lungs causing bronchoconstriction. Option #2—Enalapril is an ACE inhibitor—appropriate post MI. HCTZ—Option #3—is often a first-line treatment for HTN. Option #4—Digoxin should be held if pulse <60.

9.18 ④ Nitroglycerin can cause hypotension. The client should avoid changing positions quickly to decrease the chances of falling. Option #1 is incorrect because the client should be taught to take medication with the onset of pain. Option #2 is incorrect because a burning or stinging sensation indicates the medication is working. Option #3 is incorrect because the client should be taught to place the medication under the tongue and let it melt, not swallow it.

9.19 ② Orthostatic hypotension and respiratory depression may occur from the PCA. Option #1 should read mg/hour. Option #3 is incorrect, and Option #4 may not relieve all the pain.

9.20 ① Increasing fluids is required to maintain a therapeutic lithium (Lithane) level. Option #2 can result in retention resulting in toxicity. Option #3 can lead to lithium excretion and reduce the drug effect. Option #4 can also result in retention resulting in toxicity. A 6-10 G salt intake is required to keep serum level in the therapeutic range.

9.21 ① While this type response to antihistamines is not uncommon in young children, it is undesirable and must be reported to the physician so a change in drug therapy can be initiated. Option #2 is not within the realm of the nurse's scope of practice. The physician, nurse practitioner, or physician's assistant must order dose changes. Option #3 will not affect the medication. Option #4 is incorrect because the physician must be alerted so a preventive action can be taken.

9.22 ② Kaolin and pectin may cause constipation which, although transient, may lead to fecal impaction, especially in the elderly. Options #1, #3, and #4 are not complications of Kaopectate.

9.23 ④ The elderly are prone to paradoxical reactions and can become agitated and disoriented. Options #1 and #3 are inappropriate. Option #2 is an expected finding.

9.24 ② Common side effects of ace inhibitors include angioedema of the face, rash with pruritus, anorexia, hypotension, and decrease or loss of taste perception with weight loss. Option #1 is a side effect of calcium channel blockers. Option #3 is incorrect because these drugs may cause a weight loss. Option #4 is incorrect because this doesn't routinely occur with this category of medication.

9.25 ④ This is necessary to prevent hemolysis of the cells. Option #1 should read normal saline. Option #2 is too fast at the beginning. Option #3 should NEVER be done.

9.26 ④ Verapamil is indicated for the treatment of supraventricular tachycardias so the client's heart rate should be checked prior to administration. Options #1 and #2 are inappropriate actions. Option #3 is not a priority to Option #4.

9.27 ② The serum potassium is very important to monitor while a client is undergoing digitalization (short period of increased doses of digitalis) because low levels can potentiate the effect of the digitalis. Options #1 and #3 assess renal function. Option #4 is incorrect because BUN assesses renal function while the glucose measurement is used in the monitoring of diabetes and other disorders of the pancreas, pituitary, or adrenal glands.

9.28 ④ Mild to moderate rashes are the most common side effects of Bactrim. Options #1, #2, and #3 are not side effects of Bactrim.

9.29 ① Cardizem is given to control the rate of rhythm—not to convert it—even though there are situations when the AV conduction is slowed down enough after Cardizem administration to allow the sinus node to resume as the primary pacemaker. A side effect of Cardizem is hypotension.

9.30 ① Limit intake of alkaline foods and fluids such as milk. Option #2 could be increased to acidify urine. Options #3 and #4 do not need to be restricted.

9.31 ③ Hypoglycemia is a major concern if the bag runs dry and another concentration of dextrose is hung. Option #1 is a concern during the transfusion. Options #2 and #4 are not correct.

9.32 ③ A serious side effect of Dopamine, if extravasation occurs, is sloughing of the surrounding skin and tissue. A patent IV is essential to prevent serious side effects. Option #2 contains correct information but is not a priority over Option #3. Options #1 and #4 are not critical assessments at this time.

9.33 ② Prior to administering any antimicrobial agent, the nurse should determine if the client has any drug sensitivities. Option #1 is true for medications in general, not specifically penicillin, and is secondary in priority. Options #3 and #4 are inappropriate actions.

9.34 ① Maternal tachycardia is a side effect of Brethine. Other side effects include nervousness, tremors, headache, and possible pulmonary edema. Fetal side effects include tachycardia and hypoglycemia. Brethine is usually preferred over ritodrine (Yutopar) because of minimal effects on the blood pressure. Options #2 and #3 could be harmful. Option #4 is incorrect because the pulse is unlikely to decrease enough to give Brethine.

9.35 ① This should be recognized as a drug reaction. The infusion should be stopped, and the physician should be notified. Options #2, #3, and #4 can be harmful.

9.36 ④ Phenytoin may precipitate in any fluid containing dextrose. Options #1, #2, and #3 are inappropriate.

9.37 ③ Cholinergics such as neostigmine can cause bronchoconstriction in asthmatic clients which may precipitate an acute asthmatic attack. Thy physician will need to order an appropriate medication. Option #1 is unsafe due to adverse effects of bronchoconstriction. Option #2 is secondary to Option #3. Option #4 does not address the question.

9.38 ② This medication is an anti-parkinsonian agent used to counteract the extrapyramidal side effect the client is experiencing. Options #1, #3 and #4 are antipsychotic medications which would not relieve the adverse effects.

9.39 ③ Both of these medications can cause photosensitivity. Options #1, #2, and #4 are incorrect.

9.40 ③ Sedative-type drugs should not be taken with alcoholic beverages. Option #1 is unsafe because maximum dose is 4 mg/day. Option #2 is incorrect because GI upset can be reduced if the medication is taken with food. Option #4 is an untrue statement. This drug is given for anxiety disorders or panic attacks.

9.41 ② The order does not state PRN. Therefore, the nurse only had an order for the first injection and not the second one. Options #1, #3, and #4 do not address the fact there was no order for the Demerol to be repeated.

9.42 ③ This is first priority because if steroids are withdrawn suddenly, the client may die of acute adrenal insufficiency. Options #1 and #2 are problems associated with Cushing's Syndrome but are not first priority. Option #4 is incorrect because the cholesterol is already elevated.

9.43 ③ The drugs of choice to treat rigidity are the dopaminergics which include levodopa (L-Dopa). Option #1 is inaccurate and is an adverse side effect of L-Dopa. Option #2 is inaccurate. Option #4 is incorrect because anticholinergic drugs, such as benztropine mesylate (Cogentin) are beneficial for a client whose primary symptom is tremors.

9.44 ① Option #1 is correct. "Red Man Syndrome" occurs when the vancomycin is infused too quickly. Vancomycin should be infused in, over at least 60 minutes. Option #2 is incorrect. Option #3 is not the appropriate action for this clinical situation. Option #4 may help decrease the flushing, but Option #1 is the priority.

9.45 ③ The psychostimulant, methylphenidate (Ritalin) generates increased vigilance and attention in the medically ill, depressed client. However, with this comes hyperalertness, insomnia and tremors. Restricting the hours of scheduled administration can help to diminish the medication's side effects related to insomnia. Administering the last dose at least 6–8 hours before bedtime is preferred.

9.46 ② Captopril is an antihypertensive which necessitates blood pressure assessment prior to administration. Options #1 and #3 are important but not a priority. Option #4 is not necessary to assess prior to the medication administration.

9.47 ④ Option #4 is priority since he is having delusions. It is imperative for the client's identity to be confirmed prior to administering medications for the client's safety. Option #1 is true, however, it is not a priority to Option #4. Options #2 and #3 are incorrect for the client who is delusional. These options would be effective for therapeutic communication.

9.48 ① Option #1 is priority. This medication may cause retention of potassium. Options #2, #3, and #4 are incorrect.

9.49 ① Option #1 is correct. If 2 milliliters are given, the client will receive 10,000 units of Heparin. The order reads for 5,000 units to be administered. This would be an overdose. Questioning the order is the safe action to take. Option #2 would be an unsafe dose. Options #3 and #4 should have been performed prior to removing the medication for administration.

9.50 ④ Verapamil controls rapid ventricular rate in atril flutter or atrial fibrillation by inhibiting the transmembrane calcium flow resulting in the depression of impulse formation in specialized cardiac pacemaker cells. This action results in the slowing of the velocity of conduction of the cardiac impulse. Options #1, #2, and #3 are incorrect for this arrhythmia. Option #1 is effective in treating supraventricular tachycardia, and ventricular tachycardias induced by digitalis or catecholamines. Option #2 is effective in treating AV heart block. Option #3 is effective in treating ventricular arrhythmias.

9.51 ③ Option #3 is correct.

$$\frac{20,000 \text{ U}}{1 \text{ ml}} = \frac{7,000 \text{ U}}{X}$$

$$20,000 \text{ U}/x = 7,000 \text{ U}/ml$$

$$X = \frac{7,000 \text{ ml}}{20,000}$$

$$X = .35 \text{ ml}$$

9.52 ④ Steroids such as prednisone have many side effects such as ecchymosis (large, bruised areas of the skin) and edema. Option #1 is incorrect because the sodium levels would be increased and the urine output decreased. Option #2 would indicate a problem with the gall bladder or liver. Option #3 is incorrect though bleeding gums may occur due to thrombocytopenia. The drugs will not cause a decreased clotting time.

9.53 ② Furosemide is a loop diuretic and would contribute to intravascular fluid volume deficit after burn injury. Option #1 is correct—fluid resuscitation is a priority as severe burns cause fluid shift from the intravascular to the interstitial space. Option #3 is correct as IV morphine is the preferred drug and route for pain management after severe burn. Option #4 is correct as a way to monitor renal function and the effectiveness of fluid resuscitation.

9.54 ④ Vasodilators can cause postural hypotension which can lead to dizziness when changing positions. Option #1 would not be encouraged because a rapid drop in blood pressure could lead to a severe hypotensive episode. Option #2 can potentiate the effects of CNS depressants. Option #3 is incorrect because sodium levels are not affected by vasodilators.

9.55 ④ Oxytocin stimulates the uterus to contract which necessitates the nurse to frequently assess the uterus. A prolonged tetanic contraction can lead to a ruptured uterus. Options #1 and #3 are pertinent to the care of a client receiving magnesium sulfate for pre-eclampsia. Option #2 is incorrect because oxytocin should be given via an infusion pump and never allowed to be the primary IV.

9.56 ③ Prior to administering an antihypertensive medication, it is important to assess the client for a decreased blood pressure. Option #1 is expected in a medication that has vasodilating effects like Apresoline. Option #2 would be consistent with a diagnosis of hypertension. Option #4 would indicate a decrease in oxygenation to the brain.

9.57 ① Vistaril is an antihistamine with CNS depressant, anticholinergic, and antispasmodic activities. Option #2 might refer to a medication like Imodium. Option #3 is often associated with the action of diuretics. Option #4 refers to an anti-inflammatory medication.

9.58 ③ Option #3 is correct. Option #1 is incorrect. It should be lubricated with a water-soluble lubricant. Option #2 should not be done because the tampon would absorb the medication and decrease its effectiveness. Option #4 should read to direct the applicator down initially (toward the spine), and then up and back (toward) the cervix.

9.59 The proper placement of eye drops is the lower conjunctival sac.

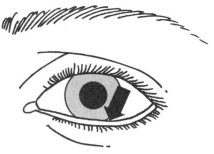

9.60 ④ Ototoxity (hearing loss) is a major adverse reaction from this drug. Other reactions include rash, urticaria, nephrotoxicity, nausea. and vomiting. Options #1, #2, and #3 are incorrect.

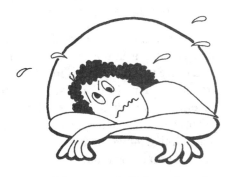

*Way to go! Take a break
before taking the post-tests.*

Post-test #1

The river where you set your foot just now is gone—those waters gave way to this, now this.
— *Heraclitus*

10

✔ **Clarification of this test...**

The two Post-tests are comprehensive, integrated exams and are comparable to the Pretest. We suggest you complete the other chapters prior to taking the post-tests and simulated exam.

10.1 Which measure should be explained to the staff to maintain safety while using the defibrillator?

① Remain clear of the bed when using the defibrillator.
② Check the defibrillator every 24 hours.
③ Ask staff not to leave the defibrillator plugged in.
④ Do not defibrillate over the electrodes.

10.2 What would be the priority plan of care for an elderly client with diabetes, hypertension, BUN– 23, creatinine 2.1, who is scheduled for a CAT Scan with and without contrast?

① Hydrate well prior to the procedure.
② Monitor BP before and after procedure.
③ Make client NPO six hours prior to procedure.
④ Recommend to provider that the scan is only done without contrast.

10.3 Which assessment finding should a nurse report to the physician in a 3-month-old experiencing increased intracranial pressure?

① Pinpoint pupils
② High-pitched cry
③ Decrease in blood pressure
④ Absence of reflexes

10.4 Which approach should be included in the nursing care plan for a client who displays the following: restless and tense behavior, complaints of feeling empty, history of several threats of self-mutilation?

① Monitor weight and dietary intake.
② Medicate with chlordiazepoxide (Librium) for tremors.
③ Provide foods in client's own containers to decrease suspiciousness.
④ Take inventory of unit and remove hazardous or sharp objects.

10.5 When the nurse manager gives information which is pertinent to maintaining the budget of the unit, the nurse manager may:

① share this information with everyone on the unit.
② share this information only with those needing to know for planning.
③ post the information on the bulletin board only.
④ share this information only with other nurses on the unit.

10.6 After a client has a positive Chlamydia trachomatis culture, she and her husband return for counseling. Which question should the nurse ask during the assessment?

① "Do you have contacts to identify?"
② "What is your understanding regarding how Chlamydia is transmitted?"
③ "Do you have questions about the culture and its validity?"
④ "Do you have allergies to the medications?"

10.7 A preschooler is being same day discharged following a tonsillectomy. Which instruction is a priority to include in teaching the mother?

① Observe the child for frequent swallowing.
② Place the child in prone position.
③ Increase the child's fluid intake.
④ Notify the physician if white patches develop on the throat.

10.8 Which assignment would be most appropriate to assign to the CNA? Assist in:

① ambulating a client who had a CVA two weeks ago.
② bathing a client with COPD who is in acute distress.
③ changing a central line dressing.
④ bathing a client with diabetes who is on the ventilator.

10.9 Before administering an IM injection of Meperidine (Demerol) to a client who has received thrombolytic therapy, the nurse should:

① make certain all lab work has been completed.
② verify the order with the physician.
③ check the client's PTT.
④ ascertain that all of the thrombolytic agent has infused.

10.10 The client with cardiomyopathy asks how he will know if he is "over-doing it" when he gets home. The best response is to tell him that:

① fatigue is a good guide.
② the doctor will advise him on specific do's and don'ts.
③ if he begins coughing up increased amounts of sputum, he has overdone it.
④ it is best to let others do as much as possible for him.

10.11 Which comment made by a client who is hospitalized for treatment of uncontrollable aggressive impulses would be most important to record to establish a baseline of data before beginning a behavior modification plan?

① Client tells each nurse that she is his favorite.
② Client has been flirtatious with female members of the staff.
③ Client threatened to hit two clients within a 2-hour time span.
④ Client appears to be insincere and superficial in his interactions.

10.12 A physician orders an analgesic to be administered to a woman in labor who is 9 cm dilated and having contractions every 3 minutes lasting for 50 seconds. Which nursing action would be most important?

① Identify client prior to administering medication.
② Calculate the amount of medicine to be administered.
③ Hold the medication and document in nursing notes.
④ Notify the physician regarding the status of the contractions.

10.13 A mother is admitted to the labor and delivery unit in a sickle cell crisis. Which nursing action is a priority?

① Administer oxygen.
② Turn to right side.
③ Provide adequate hydration.
④ Start antibiotics.

10.14 Which statement made by a 70-year-old client indicates more health promotion regarding safely taking NSAIDs is needed? "I will:

① take the NSAIDs on an empty stomach."
② inform my dentist prior to surgery that I am taking NSAIDs."
③ report tinnitus to my physician."
④ inform my physician if my stool becomes dark and tarry."

10.15 In order to prevent infection with streptococcus viridians in the client with an artificial heart valve, you will teach the client to:

① wash his hands carefully before eating.
② sterilize eating utensils after each use.
③ wear a mask when around children.
④ avoid the use of a Water-Pic.

10.16 An elderly client has an order for phenytoin (Dilantin) IV push. In planning to administer this drug, the nurse must understand that:

① the administration should not exceed 25 mg/min.
② the therapeutic serum concentration level is 25–30 mg/ml.
③ the medication should be reconstituted with 5% dextrose.
④ the solution will be unclear after reconstitution.

10.17 Which comment made by a client would indicate the client's ability for safe care during the last trimester of pregnancy? The client states, "I will:

    ① report any shortness of breath to my physician."
    ② report any headaches or blurred vision to my physician."
    ③ limit my fluid intake after 3 p.m."
    ④ limit my salt intake during this time."

10.18 What would the nurse look for in assessing pain in an 8-month-old infant?

    ① Decreased pulse rate
    ② Fluid intake increased
    ③ Respiratory rate decreased
    ④ Rubbing a body part and crying

10.19 How would the nurse position the ear of a 2-year-old while initiating ear drops?

    ① Pull the ear up and back.
    ② Pull the ear down and back.
    ③ Open the canal with an otoscope.
    ④ Position the client's head off the bed.

10.20 A child requires resuscitation secondary to a respiratory arrest. Which route would be most appropriate for the nurse to administer the epinephrine?

    ① IV
    ② Endotracheal
    ③ Indradermal
    ④ Subcutaneous

10.21 A client is admitted to the emergency room in severe emotional distress. Respirations are 42/min. and the blood gasses reveal a pH of 7.5 and a pCO_2 of 34. The nurse should first:

    ① instruct the client to breathe into a paper bag.
    ② start an IV of D_5W STAT.
    ③ administer 0_2 immediately.
    ④ place the client's head between his knees.

10.22 Which statement, made by the client during the admission interview, would be most indicative that this client is in an abusive relationship?

    ① "My husband does not need to know that I am pregnant."
    ② "I will give my prescription to my husband to be filled."
    ③ "I got this bruise when I fell off the step ladder."
    ④ "My husband and father don't get along so I am not allowed to visit my family."

10.23 During a non-stress test (NST), the nurse observes a decrease in fetal heart rate with any fetal movement. Which nursing action is the most appropriate?

    ① Reposition the mother on her right side.
    ② Notify the physician for further evaluation.
    ③ Document results in the nursing notes.
    ④ Stop the oxytocin (Pitocin) immediately.

10.24 An elderly client constantly screams out. The nursing staff is planning a behavior modification technique to deal with the screaming. Which initial nursing assessment is necessary in establishing a successful program?

    ① Monitor ability to complete activities of daily living (ADL).
    ② Assess levels of pain and correlate with response to analgesia.
    ③ Observe behavior at regular intervals to obtain baseline information related to the screaming.
    ④ Ask why the client is screaming and document it on the nursing assessment record.

10.25 A 4-year-old client is unable to go to sleep at night in the hospital. Which nursing interventions may best help promote sleep for the child? A 4-year-old client is unable to go to sleep at night in the hospital. Which nursing interventions may best help promote sleep for the child?

    ① Turn out the room light and close the door.
    ② Tire the child during the evening with play exercises.
    ③ Identify the child's home bedtime rituals and follow them.
    ④ Encourage visitation by friends during the evening.

10.26 During a nursing history with a 16-year-old client, she states that she drinks "lots" of fluids and still feels thirsty. What additional information is particularly important for the nurse to obtain at this time?

① An overall pattern of weight loss or gain for past three months
② Use of narcotic medication and over-the-counter drugs
③ Medication and food allergies
④ Menstrual history and current menstrual status

10.27 At 7:00 a.m., which assessment finding would indicate rapid diuresis in a client who received 80 mg Lasix at 6:00 a.m.?

① Hypotension
② Bradycardia
③ Eupnea
④ Hypertension

10.28 A postoperative client is to receive caphalexin monohydrate (Keflex) 500 mg PO QID. When should the nurse schedule medication administration?

① Every 6 hours
② Prior to meals
③ Routine 9-1-5-9
④ After an antacid

10.29 The nurse observes a 10-year-old leukemic client with a large arm burn that appears oily. The client states it was burned on a iron and her mother put cooking fat on it so it would not blister. The nurse should:

① document the findings in the chart and suggest she use an ointment next time.
② call the physician immediately to advise him of injury.
③ teach the client that oil holds germs and infection is more likely.
④ wash the burn with soap and water to remove the oil.

10.30 Which statement made by the parent of a 4-year-old with sickle cell anemia indicates a need for further teaching?

① "When she complains of pain, I give her baby aspirin."
② "I try to keep her away from people with infections."
③ "I sometimes have to give her Meperidine (Demerol) for pain."
④ "I encourage her to drink a lot of water."

10.31 The nurse administers 75 mg Meperidine (Demerol) IM to a postoperative client. Thirty minutes later the nurse would:

① change the client's position in bed.
② elevate the client's head and put a pillow under shoulders.
③ observe the client for nonverbal behaviors indicating comfort.
④ ambulate the client.

10.32 There is an order for starting regular insulin sliding scale.

Blood glucose levels:	Insulin order:
< 170 mg/dl	No insulin
170-240 mg/dl	10 units regular insulin S.C.
241–300 mg/dl	20 units regular insulin S.C.
>300 mg/dl	Notify provider of care for order.

The AM blood glucose level is 178 mg/dl.

Point and click on the syringe, the appropriate amount that should be administered.

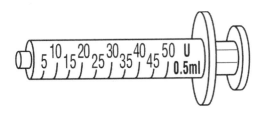

10.33 Your client is intubated and is receiving oxygen by T-piece at 50% FiO_2. You notice that the client has increasing secretions, anxiety and tachypnea. Your first action will be to:

① call the physician.
② increase the FiO_2.
③ administer a sedative as ordered.
④ assess lung sounds, suction PRN.

10.34 A physician has written an order for an HIV positive infant to receive her oral polio immunization. Which nursing actions are most appropriate?

① Wear gloves and a gown when administering the immunization.
② Administer the immunization as the infant is being discharged.
③ Call the physician and discuss the rationale for the immunization.
④ Administer the medication in the same manner as you would any other infant.

10.35 An adult client with a nasogastric tube has orders to receive acetaminophen (Tylenol) 650 mg PRN for a temperature greater than 101°F. Which measure should be included in the administration of this drug?

① The tablets should be swallowed carefully with sips of water.
② The medication should be withheld until the nasogastric tube is removed.
③ Placement of the nasogastric tube should be checked prior to giving medication.
④ Powdered medication should be used and mixed with water to form a solution.

10.36 An elderly client tells the nurse that he is worried about his wife's impending colostomy surgery. The nurse would:

① review the wife's surgical procedure with the husband.
② offer the client the option to take a class explaining the discharge care.
③ encourage the client to discuss how he feels and his fears about the surgery.
④ explain the importance of his attendance to the teaching sessions offered by the interstomal therapist.

10.37 In planning care for an infant with congenital heart disease who becomes easily fatigued and whose vital signs increase during feedings, the nurse would:

① give small, frequent feedings.
② change diapers before feeding.
③ increase the caloric content of the feedings.
④ mix rice cereal in the formula.

10.38 A 4-month-old infant, who had a temperature of 100.3°F following the last DTP (Diphtheria, Tetanus, and Pertussis) vaccine, is seen in the clinic for another immunization administration. Prior to administering the DTP, which nursing action would be a priority?

① Withhold the immunization.
② Give half the dose this injection.
③ Consult with the physician on giving Pediatric DP (Diphtheria and Tetanus).
④ Instruct the parents to give acetaminophen (Tylenol) following administration of the full dose of DTP.

10.39 During an examination with a mother in her last trimester, the nurse would identify which sign to indicate placenta previa?

① Painful vaginal bleeding
② Fetal bradycardia
③ Painless vaginal bleeding
④ Irritability of the uterus

10.40 Following the administration of an incorrect dose of medication, which statement would best describe the incident on a variance report

① Due to illegible physician order, 9 mg of gentamycin (Garamycin) was given IV at 0200 instead of 7 mg IV.
② At 0200, gentamycin (Garamycin) 9 mg was given IV instead of 7 mg IV as ordered.
③ At 0200, client received 2 mg more of gentamycin (Garamycin) than was ordered.
④ Gentamycin (Garamycin) 9 mg IV was given at 0200. Physician's order to decrease dose was not transcribed to the Kardex by previous shift RN.

10.41 The nursing evaluation of the neurological status of a newly-admitted client who has suffered a cerebral vascular accident would include:

① equality of pulses in all four extremities.
② orientation to person, place, and time.
③ regularity of neuromuscular claudication.
④ presence of Chadwick's sign.

10.42 Which laboratory test result would suggest that the anorexic client is at risk for developing renal calculi?

    ① High serum calcium levels
    ② Low serum potassium
    ③ High serum osmolality
    ④ AST (SGOT) elevation

10.43 Following the initiation of an IV oxytocin (Pitocin) drip, which would be the most appropriate nursing action?

    ① Assess vital signs every 15 minutes.
    ② Check the frequency and duration of contractions.
    ③ Determine blood pressure every 4 hours.
    ④ Monitor urine output for polyuria.

10.44 To maintain asepsis, the client on home peritoneal dialysis should be taught to:

    ① drink only distilled water.
    ② cap the Tenchkoff catheter when not in use.
    ③ boil the dialysate one hour prior to a pass.
    ④ clean the arteriovenous fistula site with hydrogen peroxide daily.

10.45 A client receiving a monoamine oxidase inhibitor (MAO) medication for treatment of depression should be instructed to avoid:

    ① tropical vacations.
    ② aged cheeses and Chianti wine.
    ③ ice cream sundaes.
    ④ driving a car.

10.46 Which action describes the best method for obtaining an infant's vital signs?

    ① Take an axillary temperature first because this is the most important measurement.
    ② Count respirations for 15 seconds and multiply the number by 4.
    ③ Count respirations for a minute prior to arousing the infant.
    ④ Use a stethoscope with a one and a half inch diaphragm for counting the apical pulse.

10.47 Which plan should be priority for a hypertensive client on Captopril (Capoten)?

    ① Encourage client to take medicine with meals.
    ② Discuss the need for a potassium supplement.
    ③ If client misses a dose, take 2 doses at next scheduled time.
    ④ Instruct client to take this drug one hour before meals.

10.48 A client taking trifluoperazine (Stelazine) should be instructed to notify the nurse if he experiences:

    ① nasal stuffiness.
    ② heat intolerance.
    ③ hand and arm tremors.
    ④ weight loss and diarrhea

10.49 Which statement made by the parents of a 9-year-old client with an ostomy would indicate they are proving quality home care?

    ① "We change the bag at least once a week, and we carefully inspect the stoma at that time."
    ② "We change the bag every day so we can inspect the stoma and the skin."
    ③ "We encourage our daughter to watch TV while we change her ostomy bag."
    ④ "We only have to change the ostomy bag every ten days."

10.50 Which statement by the client best indicates an emotional readiness for surgery?

    ① "I know the physician isn't telling me everything, but at this point, I can't do anything about it."
    ② "I've never heard of this specialist before. Does he do much work here?"
    ③ "I'm glad the trapeze is on my bed so I can start working on my exercises as soon as I wake up."
    ④ "Can you please check my record to be sure it says I'm diabetic?"

10.51 To prepare an adolescent client for a lumbar puncture, which instruction should the nurse include in her teaching?

    ① general anesthetic will be used.
    ② Fluids will be restricted for 8 hours before the test.
    ③ The client will need to remain flat in bed for 8 hours after the test.
    ④ A compression bandage will be in place for 10 hours after the test.

10.52 A nurse can be instrumental in diffusing a client's escalating aggressive/violent behavior by:

   ① utilizing an organized team to place the client in seclusion.
   ② leaving the client alone in his/her room to identify feelings of anger.
   ③ redirecting the client to a quiet activity to divert his/her attention and not disturb the other clients.
   ④ assisting the client in identifying and expressing his/her feelings of increasing anxiety, frustration and anger.

10.53 Which medication can be given intravenously to reverse the effects of a narcotic overdose?

   ① Hydromorphine (Dilaudid)
   ② Disulfiram (Antabuse)
   ③ Benztropine (Cogentin)
   ④ Naloxone (Narcan)

10.54 Two days after the placement of a pleural chest tube, the chest tube is accidentally pulled out of the intrapleural space. The nurse should first:

   ① replace the tube, using sterile gloves.
   ② apply a dressing immediately over the site, taping on 3 sides.
   ③ instruct the client to cough to expand the lung.
   ④ auscultate lung to determine if it is collapsed.

10.55 Metoprolol (Lopressor) 12.5 mg is prescribed and available are 50 mg tables. Point to the correct dosage.

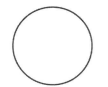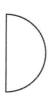

10.56 A 75-year-old hospitalized man uses a walker for ambulation support. He is receiving a diuretic and must use the bathroom several times during the night. Which of these actions would be a priority in promoting safety for this client?

   ① Maintain the side rails in the upward position.
   ② Leave the bedroom light on at all times.
   ③ Hold the diuretic medication.
   ④ Provide the client with a bedside commode.

10.57 In preparing the teaching plan for a prenatal client who is eight week's gestation with a positive VDRL, which instruction would be most appropriate for the nurse to include?

   ① Refrain from taking any medications to prevent damage to the fetus.
   ② Take the penicillin for the prescribed time.
   ③ Refrain from sexual activity.
   ④ Maintain the confidentiality of sexual partners.

10.58 Which nursing action offers the most support to a child and family in the terminal stage of the child's illness?

   ① Encourage the family to avoid any reference to death to not upset the child.
   ② Limit the amount of visiting time so the child does not become over-exhausted.
   ③ Assure the ongoing participation of all disciplines in the child's care, even after discharge if needed.
   ④ Limit the amount of information and explanations given to parents who are already overloaded at this time.

10.59 In assessing a one-month-old with respiratory distress, the nurse would anticipate which finding?

   ① Respiratory rate greater than 60
   ② Heart rate less than 100
   ③ Temperature less than 98°F
   ④ Systolic blood pressure greater than 110

10.60 Which plan would be a priority for a newly admitted client with meningitis due to Hemophilus influenza?

   ① Place in reverse isolation for at least 24 hours.
   ② Monitor vital signs and neurological checks every 4 to 6 hours.
   ③ Dim lights in the room and minimize environmental stimuli.
   ④ Encourage PO fluids to decrease the fever.

10.61 Prior to discharging a client after a mastectomy, the documentation in the chart should indicate that the client has been educated regarding which plan?

① Use a heating pad under the shoulder every other night.
② Wear a sling on the affected forearm for 4 weeks after surgery.
③ Attend the support group—RESOLVE.
④ Avoid use of the affected arm for blood pressure evaluation or for any needle sticks.

10.62 The charge nurse notices that whenever a client is admitted with a history of sexual abuse, the 3–11 nurse, subtly and sometimes overtly, verbally attacks the client. Further investigation reveals that the 3–11 nurse was sexually abused as a child. In making assignments, the charge nurse must:

① assign the nurse to this client to promote therapeutic feedback to the client about his behavior from someone who has been "on the other side."
② assign the nurse to the client and insist that the nurse begin therapy to work on unresolved feelings.
③ assign someone else to the client because the nurse is not ready to cope with this and may be detrimental to the client.
④ assign someone else to the client but do not inform the nurse of your rationale for doing so.

10.63 Several clients are admitted to the medical unit at the same time. Each client has an order for an IV to be started. Which case would the manager assign as priority for an IV start? A client with:

① abdominal pain.
② vaso-occlusive cell crisis.
③ mild dehydration.
④ surgery scheduled in the morning.

10.64 Prior to removing a nasogastric tube, the nurse aspirates 350cc of fluid. The nurse should now:

① return the 350cc through the tube to the client's stomach.
② remove the tube and have the client drink 350cc of a clear liquid.
③ chart the findings after removing the tube.
④ notify the physician after removing the tube.

10.65 Which factor would be most important for the rehabilitation nurse to assess during the admission of a new client? The client's:

① expectations of family members.
② understanding of available supportive services.
③ personal goals for rehabilitation.
④ past experiences in the hospital.

10.66 Two days after admission, a client's sputum culture is reported as positive for tuberculosis. While awaiting orders from the physician, the nurse should:

① initiate measures to transfer the client to a tuberculosis unit.
② institute measures to initiate respiratory isolation in the hospital.
③ arrange for all of the client's personal effects to be decontaminated.
④ notify the client's family that they have been exposed to a highly contagious disease.

10.67 Which plan would the nurse anticipate being most useful for the nursing home client with organic brain syndrome?

① Encourage verbalization of feelings regarding the relationship with family who initiated his nursing home placement.
② Help client express favorite pastimes and enjoyable activities.
③ Orient client to present time and assist in being alert when family visits.
④ Direct conversations to assist client to reminisce and talk about important past events in his life.

10.68 A client with peptic ulcer disease (PUD) is seen in your clinic for pain associated with gout. Which medication order should be questioned by the nurse?

① Colchicine
② Allopurinol
③ Probenecid
④ Indomethacin

10.69 A client has an order for antacids for his peptic ulcer disease (PUD). Which statement by the client indicates an understanding of how to take antacids? "I take them:

① with food."
② 30 minutes before and after meals."
③ 1 hour after meals."
④ with my other medications."

10.70 Which interventions will be most appropriate when obtaining urine from an indwelling catheter for culture and sensitivity?

① Unclamp the drainage spout from the urine bag, wipe it with alcohol, and collect the specimen in a sterile container.
② Clamp the catheter tubing, swab the injection port with alcohol, and aspirate urine into a syringe.
③ Remove the indwelling urinary catheter, insert a new one and obtain urine from the new sterile bag.
④ Don sterile gloves, disconnect the catheter from the drainage tubing, and drain the urine directly into a sterile container.

10.71 Which assistive care device should the nurse plan on having available for an elderly client who has a below-the-knee amputation?

① crutches
② 4-point walker
③ A cane
④ wheelchair

10.72 Prior to administering aspirin, the nurse will notify the physician if a client has which medical diagnosis?

① Peptic ulcer disease (PUD)
② CVA
③ Osteoarthritis
④ Rheumatoid arthritis

10.73 The nurse would identify which situation as an indication for the nursing assistant to participate in a clinical skills lab?

① Anchoring a Foley catheter bag on the side of the bed rail
② Elevating the head of the bed for a client receiving a tube feeding
③ Using gloves to empty urine from a graduated cylinder
④ Turning a client who is bed-ridden every two hours to prevent skin breakdown

10.74 A CVA client begins to choke and cough on a piece of meat. Which action would be a priority for the nurse to implement with the client?

① Provide blows to the back.
② Assist with expelling the meat immediately.
③ Avoid interfering with his attempt to expel the meat.
④ Administer 5 abdominal thrusts followed by a blind finger sweep.

10.75 The physician begins methotrexate on a client with rheumatoid arthritis. Which lab test should be done monthly?

① Liver function tests
② Erythrocyte sedimentation rate (ESR)
③ Urinalysis
④ Serum pH.

SENDING LOVE
Since we're unable to meet,
I thought it would be neat,
to send something to keep,
to show my love is deep.

—Margaret S. Wright
(Sylvia's Mom 1914–2003)

Answers & Rationales

10.1 ① This is a priority to prevent accidental countershock. Option #2 is incorrect because the equipment should be checked every 8 hours. Option #3 is incorrect because the equipment should remain plugged in at all times. Option #4 is correct information but is not a priority.

10.2 ④ Protecting the client's safety is a priority for the nursing care plan. Options #1, #2, and #3 are not necessary for this client and do not address safety.

10.3 ② A high pitched cry in infants is a sign of increased intracranial pressure. Option #1 does not indicate any immediate problem. As pressure increases, pupils may be dilated. Options #3 and #4 do not reflect complications with increased intracranial pressure.

10.4 ④ Protecting the client's safety is a priority for the nursing care plan. Options #1, #2, and #3 are not necessary for this client and do not address safety.

10.5 ① It is important to communicate with everyone on the unit about budget management because this will affect the unit as a whole. Options #2, #3, and #4 will not be useful.

10.6 ② The transmission of Chlamydia may or may not have been made clear to both partners so the nurse would have to assess this first. Chlamydia is a reported sexually-transmitted disease. Option #1 may be part of the follow-up. Option #3 is a possibility, but most cultures used today have few false positives. Option #4 would be done later in the nursing assessment.

10.7 ① It is a sign of hemorrhage. Options #2 and #3 are correct, but not priority to Option #1. Option #4 is incorrect because it is a sign of normal healing.

10.8 ① Option #1 is correct. The client is stable and the lowest acuity. Options #2, #3, and #4 would be inappropriate for the CNA.

10.9 ② Complications of thrombolytic therapy include bleeding which can occur with intramuscular injections. The nurse should confer with the physician about the appropriateness of the order. Options #1 and #4 are not necessary. Option #3 will be monitored but is not a priority action in this instance.

10.10 ① Option #1 is correct. Fatigue is a useful guide in gauging activity tolerance in patients with decreased cardiac output. Option #2 is incorrect. The patient is not asking for specific dos and don'ts, but rather a general guide to use for activity in general. This may indicate that the nurse is abdicating client-teaching responsibilities. Option #3 may indicate developing pulmonary edema, and the client should discontinue activity at this point. Option #4 is inaccurate and may cause the client to lose independence.

10.11 ③ This is the most concrete evidence of aggressive behavior. Options #1, #2, and #4 are less directly related to aggression.

10.12 ④ The information indicates the woman is in transition phase. Analgesics cause depressed respirations in the baby. Options #1 and #2 contain correct information but not for this situation. Option #3 does not address the immediate problem.

10.13 ③ Adequate hydration is a priority for any client in sickle cell crisis. Option #1 may be correct for the situation but is not a priority to Option #3. Options #2 and #4 are not priority actions for this client.

10.14 ① More health promotion is necessary since these medications should be taken with meals because they can cause GI distress. Option #2 is imperative since NSAIDs reduce platelet adhesiveness predisposing clients to bleeding, especially after surgery. Routinely, clients will stop the NSAIDs two weeks prior to surgery. There is no need for more teaching. Option #3 must be reported. It is an adverse reaction from these medications. There is no indication for more teaching. Option #4 indicates the client understands this is a problem. Dark and tarry stools indicate blood or bleeding from the GI tract.

10.15 ④ Option #4 is correct. S. Viridans can enter the blood steam if forceful brushing, oral care, or dental work causes bleeding gums. Options #1 and #2 are incorrect as S. Viridans is normal flora in the mouth. Option #3 is unnecessary.

10.16 ① The rate of administration is very important. At this rate, toxicity should be decreased. Several complications, most commonly experienced by the elderly, include cardiotoxicity, atrial ventricular conduction depression and ventricular fibrillation. Option #2 is incorrect because the therapeutic range is 10-20 mg/ml. Option #3 can cause precipitation. Normal saline is the fluid of choice. Option #4 is unsafe because the solution must be clear.

10.17 ② Signs of advanced pregnancy induced hypertension are headaches, blurred vision, and epigastric pain which are imperative to report to the physician. Option #1 is expected due to the enlarged uterus causing pressure on the lungs. Options #3 and #4 are not appropriate.

10.18 ④ Since infants cannot talk, the nurse needs to be aware of nonverbal signs of pain such as rubbing his ear because of an earache. Option #1 would increase. Option #2 is non-specific regarding pain. Option #3 does not reflect pain.

10.19 ② The correct positioning of the child's ear while instilling ear drops is to pull the ear down and back. This will assist in accessing the auditory canal. Option #1 is correct for an adult client. Options #3 and #4 contain inaccurate information.

10.20 ② The quickest and most effective route would be via endotracheal tube. Remember ELAIN to assist in recalling the drugs that can be given via the endotracheal tube (Epinephrine, Lidocaine, Atropine, Isuprel and Narcan). Option #1 would be slower than #2, and the other distracters are incorrect.

10.21 ① Because of hyperventilation, the client is in alkalosis so having him re-breathe his own CO_2 will reverse his blood gases. Option #2 does not address the problem. Option #3 is incorrect because the client is not hypoxic. Option #4 is for a client who feels faint.

10.22 ④ Option #4 is correct. This is indicative that the client is secluded from family which is a sign of abuse. Option #1 is the client's right to privacy. Option #2 is not indicative of abuse. Option #3 is not an indicative sign of abuse.

10.23 ② A decrease in the fetal heart rate (FHR) during the NST should be immediately evaluated by the physician. Options #1 and #3 do not resolve the immediate problem. Option #4 is incorrect because Oxytocin (Pitocin) is not used for the non-stress test.

10.24 ③ In designing an effective behavior modification program, an accurate baseline data about the target behavior in relation to frequency, amount, time, and precipitating factors must first be collected. Options #1 and #2 are incorrect because each option assesses only one area of behavior that may related to the target behavior of screaming and does not provide comprehensive data for developing a behavior management program. Option #4 will most likely give inaccurate information.

10.25 ③ Preschool-aged children require bedtime rituals which should be followed in the hospital if possible. Option #1 would increase child's fear. Options #2 and #4 would not promote sleep.

10.26 ① Excessive thirst and weight loss are two notable symptoms of diabetes mellitus. Options #2, #3, and #4 do not provide useful information related to the assessment information.

10.27 ① A decreasing pre-load caused by rapid diuresis can cause a significant change in cardiac output that can decrease systemic blood pressure. Options #2, #3, and #4 do not reflect diuresis.

10.28 ① A blood level must be achieved and maintained for antibiotics to be effective. Therefore, the medication is scheduled around the clock. Options #2 and #3 are inappropriate. Option #4 is unnecessary.

10.29 ④ Because leukemic clients are immuno-suppressed, they are more susceptible to infections. Cooking fat applied to an open wound increases the possibility of infection. Burns should be immediately rinsed with tap water to reduce the heat in the burn. Options #1 and #3 do not address the immediate problem of cleansing the wound. Option #2 is not necessary at this time based on the information presented.

10.30 ① Aspirin can cause hemorrhage during a sickle cell crisis and definitely indicates a need for further teaching. Options #2 and #4 are important aspects in the case of a sickle cell client to prevent sickling crisis. Option #3 is an appropriate medication used to decrease the client's pain.

10.31 ③ In evaluating the effectiveness of pain medication, the nurse must first identify actual outcomes of the client's sense of well-being and comfort. Options #1 and #2 would be helpful in promoting comfort for the client. However, the priority is to determine pain medication effectiveness. Option #4 would be done after the client has some pain relief.

10.32 Point and click on the syringe the appropriate amount that should be administered.

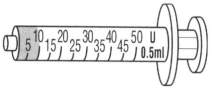

Answer: Syringe—gray up to 10.

10.33 ④ Additional assessment data helps define the problem. Suctioning can relieve distress and restore airway patency. Option #1 will delay nursing intervention to treat the problem. Option #2 will not be useful if the airway is not patent. Option #3 is inappropriate and could lead to CO_2 retention.

10.34 ③ Polio is a live virus and should not be given to children who are immunocompromised. Options #1, #2, and #4 do not address the identified problem of the compromised immune system.

10.35 ③ Liquid acetaminophen may be administered via the nasogastric tube after tube placement has been checked. Option #1 is incorrect because the client is NPO so nothing can be taken orally. Option #2 is incorrect since medication should not be withheld. Option #4 is incorrect because Tylenol does not come in powdered form at this time.

10.36 ③ This is a common cause related to anxiety. Encouraging the client to talk about his fears will assist in alleviating this anxiety. Other options are secondary.

10.37 ① Feeding small amounts more frequently will not cause as much fatigue and cardiovascular stress. Option #2 is important, but it does not relate to fatigue with feedings. Options #3 and #4 will not reduce fatigability.

10.38 ④ Low-grade fever may occur after a DTP. An antipyretic is useful prior to and after immunizations. Option #1 is not indicated. Option #2 is incorrect because the child would still receive the Pertussis which would probably cause another febrile reaction. Option #3 would be correct if there was a concern with seizures.

10.39 ③ This is a sign of placenta previa. Option #1 could be a sign of abruptio placenta. Option #2 indicates fetal distress. Option #4 is not specific of any disorder.

10.40 ② This is a factual account of exactly what happened. A variance report should be factual and objective. Option #1 is incorrect because this statement blames the physician's handwriting. Option #3, while true, does not present all of the information. It simply states a conclusion which cannot be verified without further investigation. Option #4 does not present all the facts and places blame.

10.41 ② This is an integral part of the neurological evaluation. In addition, assessments of motor activity, eyes, and pupil equality are part of the neurological work-up. Option #1 is irrelevant for a neurological assessment. Option #3 is not a correct statement. Option #4 is a probable sign of pregnancy.

10.42 ① This indicates that osteoporosis is occurring and may lead to renal calculi. Option #2 does not respond to renal calculi. Options #3 and #4 are more likely to be seen in a client who is being treated for a chemical dependency.

10.43 ② Oxytocin is given to stimulate contraction of uterine muscle fibers. It is important to assess the contractions due to potential hypertonia and possible rupture of the uterus. Options #1 and #3 do not assess for the desired response to the medication. Option #4 is not the desired response as Pitocin has a mild antidiuretic effect.

10.44 ② Capping the peritoneal catheter when not in use keeps the catheter sterile. Option #1 is unnecessary. Option #3 is unnecessary and probably harmful to the solution. Option #4 is incorrect because there is no arteriovenous fistula in peritoneal dialysis. This is hemodialysis access and does not require daily cleaning with hydrogen peroxide.

10.45 ② MAO inhibitors, when combined with certain foods containing tyramine (especially aged and processed foods), cause a significant increase in blood pressure. Option #1 would be more appropriate when advising a client taking antipsychotic medications about the problem with photosensitivity. Option #3 is not relevant. Option #4 is more appropriate when advising a client taking antianxiety medications.

10.46 ③ Respirations should be counted for one full minute prior to arousing the infant with a temperature probe or stethoscope. After the infant is stimulated, the crying interferes with accurate evaluation. Option #4 is incorrect because observations should be done first.

10.47 ④ Food reduces absorption by 30-40%. Option #1 is incorrect due to the absorption reduction by food. Option #2 is incorrect because it may cause potassium toxicity. Option #3 may cause an overdose.

10.48 ③ These are major side effects of Stelazine. Extrapyramidal reactions should be reported immediately. Options #1, #2, and #4 represent possible side effects of antipsychotic medications and may not require immediate intervention.

10.49 ① Ostomy bags should be changed at least once a week. This is a good time for the stoma to be closely inspected. Option #2 is incorrect because the bag should be changed only when the seal around the stoma is loose or leaking. Option #3 does not encourage client participation or foster independence. Option #4 is incorrect because the bag should be changed more often.

10.50 ③ This statement indicates acceptance and a readiness to participate in postoperative care. Option #1 indicates feelings of fear and helplessness. Option #2 indicates fear and lack of trust. Option #4 indicates fear that something will be missed.

10.51 ③ To prevent a post-lumbar puncture headache, the client should remain flat in bed for 8 hours after the test. Options #1 and #2 are not protocol for this test. Option #4 is inappropriate for procedure.

10.52 ④ As the client begins to escalate his anger, the nurse can be very helpful in using psychological/communication strategies. Option #1 is incorrect because it would be more useful to try Option #4 first. Option #2 can become potentially dangerous to the client and property. Option #3 might further escalate his frustration and anger because his ability to focus and concentrate is diminished due to an elevated anxiety level.

10.53 ④ Narcan blocks the neuroreceptors affected by opiates to reverse the effects. Option #1 is a narcotic analgesic. Option #2 is used with alcoholic clients. Option #3 is an anti-Parkinson medication.

10.54 ② Option #2 is correct as this decreases the change of atmospheric air entering the pleura but still allows for the escape of pleural air. Option #1 chest tube insertion is a medical procedure. The old tube is contaminated. Option #3 will not be useful. Deep breathing associated with coughing can increase the amount of atmospheric air entering the pleural space. Option #4 should be reevaluated after emergency measures are instituted.

10.55

Rationale: 12.5 milligrams is 1/4 of a 50 mg table.

10.56 ④ Option #4 is a priority for promoting safety for this client who must get up to void during the night. Option #1 would create a safety issue for this client. Option #2 does not address the nursing concept. Option #3 is not an alternative for the client.

10.57 ② It is vitally important to complete all the penicillin. Option #1 is a true statement concerning the pregnant client not taking over-the-counter medications unless directed by a physician but is not a priority for this client. Option #3 may be unrealistic. She needs to inform others and ideally, for the present time, refrain from sexual activity. Option #4 is incorrect because communicable diseases are reportable, and partners of contacts need to be notified so they may be treated.

10.58 ③ The care of a child who has been this ill involves many disciplines, and the family will continue to need support long after discharge. Option #1 is incorrect because they should be helped to openly deal with whatever issue the child raises. Option #2 is critical at this stage. Don't limit the time; help them use it fully. Option #4 is incorrect because one of the nurse's major functions is to keep the family well informed.

10.59 ① Tachypnea is a classic sign of respiratory distress. The normal range of respirations for an infant is 30-60 per minute. Option #2 represents bradycardia which is not an expected finding in this situation. Options #3 and #4 are not relevant to evaluating respiratory distress.

10.60 ③ This will prevent complications with seizures which can occur. Option #1 is incorrect because clients with meningitis are placed in respiratory isolation for at least 24 hours. Option #2 is incorrect because these assessments should be done more frequently. Option #4 is incorrect because many clients will be on fluid restriction due to potential increased intracranial pressure.

10.61 ④ No blood pressure or needle sticks are done on the affected arm because of potential circulatory impairment or infection. Option #1 is unnecessary. Option #2 is avoided. Gentle exercise started early in the postoperative course helps decrease muscle tension as well as repair muscle function more quickly. Option #3 is incorrect because the appropriate support group for a post-mastectomy client is Reach to Recovery.

10.62 ③ In the selection of client assignments, it is important for the charge nurse to consider the abilities of each staff member. When a nurse is having difficulty coping with certain types of clients, she needs to be reassigned until she is able to deal with them in a therapeutic way. Options #1 and #2 are not appropriate for the situation. Option #4 is incorrect because it would be important for the charge nurse to address her concerns to the 3-11 nurse.

10.63 ② The client with vaso-occlusive crisis is a priority for hydration due to the physiological clumping of the RBCs. With hydration, the circulation improves, decreases discomfort, and promotes adequate oxygenation. Option #1 is incorrect because an IV may not be indicated. Option #3 may not require an IV. Option #4 will have the IV for surgery started appropriately prior to surgery.

10.64 ① Option #1 is correct. The stomach contents should be returned to the stomach so that valuable electrolytes will not be lost. Option #2—NG tubes are ordinarily utilized for stomach decompression or nausea. The nurse would not force 350cc of fluid on a client that has just had the tube removed. Option #3—This distracter does not address the question. Option #4—This is an unnecessary action at this point.

10.65 ③ It is important for the nurse to understand what the client expects from the rehabilitation program for future success. Options #1, #2 and #4 are important to assess, but they are not as crucial for future success as the client's goals.

10.66 ② All clients with tuberculosis are placed in respiratory isolation in the hospital and the nurse should begin preparations for this immediately. Option #1 is unnecessary at this time. When indicated, the physician will write appropriate transfer orders. Option #3 is incorrect because the personal effects do not have to be decontaminated. Option #4 is secondary.

10.67 ④ The geriatric client should be encouraged to talk about his life and important things in the past because he has recent memory loss. Option #1 is incorrect because he may not remember why or where he is. Option #2 is not as important as Option #4. Option #3 is incorrect because even with orientation, the client soon forgets.

10.68 ④ Indomethacin is an NSAID and is contraindicated in clients with peptic ulcer disease. It would also be contraindicated in clients with renal insufficiency. Options #1, #2, and #3 are potential orders for gout. Colchicine has an anti-inflammatory action limited to crystal-induced inflammation. Allopurinol inhibits the enzyme xanthine oxidase and blocks the formation of uric acid. Probenecid is an uriosuric drug which acts to inhibit renal tubular reabsorption of uric acid.

10.69 ③ When antacids are given 1 hour after eating, gastric acidity is minimized for another 1-2 hours, countering the food-induced stimulation of acid secretion. Options #1 and #2 are incorrect because if given with a meal, the antacid is wasted since food is an adequate buffer. Option #4 is incorrect because they interact with the medications and decrease the effectiveness.

10.70 ② Option #2 is the correct method that ensures a fresh, uncontaminated sample. Option #1 is incorrect. Urine obtained from the bag has been standing and will not give a reliable culture result. Option #3 is inappropriate and results in additional trauma to tissues. Option #4—urine collected from the bag—is not a reliable source for a culture.

10.71 ④ The client will be safest in a wheelchair. Option #1 is unsafe for an elderly client with a below-the-knee amputation. Options #2 and #3 are unmanageable without the assistance of a prosthesis.

10.72 ① Aspirin works by inhibiting prostaglandin production. As a result, a major side effect is gastric mucosal injury resulting in ulceration. Bleeding occasionally occurs from gastritis or ulceration. If PUD is already a problem, this client is predisposed to complications. Options #2, #3, and #4 would necessitate the use of aspirin.

10.73 ① This action would indicate a need for further clinical training. Anchoring a Foley catheter bag to the side of the bedrail can result in a reflux of urine back in the bladder. Options #2, #3, and #4 are appropriate actions.

10.74 ③ If the adult client is coughing forcefully, do not interfere with the client's attempt to expel the foreign body. Options #1, #2, and #4 are inappropriate.

10.75 ① Short-term, low-dose therapy is well tolerated but hepatocellular injury can occur. Careful monitoring of the LFTs is required. Option #2 is increased in the presence of abnormal plasma proteins associated with inflammatory conditions. Option #3 is incorrect because this drug does not usually affect the kidneys. Option #4 is not a concern with this drug.

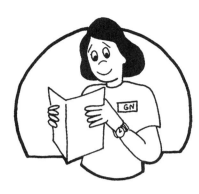

Congratulations!
You're almost through!

Category Analysis – Post-test #1

1. Fluid-Gas	26. Nutrition	51. Sensory-Perception-Mobility
2. Elimination	27. Pharmacology	52. Psycho-Social
3. Sensory-Perception-Mobility	28. Pharmacology	53. Pharmacology
4. Psycho-Social	29. Safe Effective Care	54. Fluid-Gas
5. Safe Effective Care	30. Health Promotion	55. Pharmacology
6. Health Promotion	31. Pharmacology	56. Sensory-Perception-Mobility
7. Fluid-Gas	32. Pharmacology	57. Safe Effective Care
8. Safe Effective Care	33. Fluid-Gas	58. Psycho-Social
9. Safe Effective Care	34. Health Promotion	59. Health Promotion
10. Health Promotion	35. Pharmacology	60. Sensory-Perception-Mobility
11. Psycho-Social	36. Psycho-Social	61. Safe Effective Care
12. Health Promotion	37. Nutrition	62. Safe Effective Care
13. Health Promotion	38. Pharmacology	63. Safe Effective Care
14. Pharmacology	39. Health Promotion	64. Nutrition
15. Safe Effective Care	40. Safe Effective Care	65. Psycho-Social
16. Pharmacology	41. Sensory-Perception-Mobility	66. Safe Effective Care
17. Health Promotion	42. Elimination	67. Psycho-Social
18. Sensory-Perception-Mobility	43. Pharmacology	68. Elimination
19. Pharmacology	44. Safe Effective Care	69. Elimination
20. Pharmacology	45. Pharmacology	70. Elimination
21. Fluid-Gas	46. Nutrition	71. Sensory-Perception-Mobility
22. Psycho-Social	47. Pharmacology	72. Pharmacology
23. Fluid-Gas	48. Pharmacology	73. Safe Effective Care
24. Psycho-Social	49. Elimination	74. Fluid-Gas
25. Health Promotion	50. Psycho-Social	75. Pharmacology

Directions

1. Determine questions missed by checking answers.
2. Write the number of the questions missed across the top line marked "item missed."
3. Check category analysis page to determine category of question.
4. Put a check mark under item missed and beside content.
5. Count check marks in each row and write the number in totals column.
6. Use this information to:
   - identify areas for further study.
   - determine which content test to take next.

We recommend studying content where most items are missed—then taking that content test.

Number of the Questions Incorrectly Answered

Post-test #1	Items Missed																													Totals
C Safe Effective Care																														
O Health Promotion and Maintenance																														
N Psycho-Social Integrity																														
T Physiological Adaptation: Fluid Gas																														
E Reduction of Risk Potential: Sensory-Perception-Mobility																														
N Basic Care and Comfort: Elimination																														
T Physiological Adaptation: Nutrition																														
Pharmacological and Parenteral Therapies																														

Post-test #2

It's the action, not the fruit of the action that's important.
You have to do the right thing...You may never know
What results come from your action,
But if you do nothing, there will be no result.
—*Ghandi*

✔ **Clarification of this test...**

Just keep on working on your testing practice and study. Here are some more questions to help you identify your study needs.

11.1 Select all that apply when doing a dressing change on a client with an abdominal wound.

① Wash your hands.
② Squeeze antibiotic ointment directly on the wound.
③ Pour antiseptic cleaning agent from an unsterile bottle after putting on sterile gloves.
④ Saturate cotton balls with the cleaning agent.
⑤ Work from the top of the incision, wiping once to the bottom, and then discard the pad.
⑥ If client has a surgical drain, clean drain surface first.

11.2 Which of these interventions would be most appropriate when performing glucose testing with One-Touch or Accu-Chek? Select all that apply.

① Dilate the capillaries by applying a coo, moist compress to the area for about 3 minutes.
② Wipe the puncture site with an alcohol sponge, and dry it thoroughly with a gauze pad.
③ Make the puncture on the end of the fingertip.
④ After puncturing finger, squeeze site to facilitate blood flow.
⑤ Touch a drop of blood to the reagent patch on the strip making sure to cover the entire patch.
⑥ Leave the blood on the strip for exactly 30 seconds.

11.3 Which of these would be the most appropriate to assign to the LPN? Select all that apply. A client who:

① has the diagnosis of myasthenia gravis.
② is receiving chemotherapy.
③ is a new admission with chest pain.
④ is being discharged and needs new diabetic teaching.
⑤ is in Buck's traction.

11.4 To promote client safety, which pieces of equipment should be readily available at the bedside when client has a seizure disorder? Select all that apply.

① oral airway
② nasogastric tube
③ suction
④ ventilator
⑤ tracheostomy set

11.5 Which client will the nurse identify as most at risk for neglect?

① A 3-day-old infant of a single mother with no source of income.
② A 99-year-old woman cared for in a nursing home.
③ A 35-year-old disabled adult male living with his elderly mother.
④ A 40-year-old drug addict living in a group housing center.

11.6 Which of these home environmental assessments would present the highest risk for injury to a client with Parkinson's Disease?

① Throw rugs on carpet in a formal living room.
② Nightlight between bedroom and bathroom.
③ Eats meals and snacks in the kitchen at the bar and uses high bar stools.
④ Uses a cane for ambulation.

11.7 To promote safety, the nurse would implement which action in obtaining a blood specimen from a client with hepatitis B?

① Clean area with antiseptic solution.
② Wear a pair of clean gloves.
③ Apply pressure to site for 5 seconds.
④ Recap needle to avoid carrying exposed needle.

11.8 Which observation would be most important during the first 48 hours after the admission of a client with severe anxiety?

① What is important to the client?
② How does the client view self?
③ In what situations does the client get anxious?
④ Who in the client's family has had mental problems?

11.9 A 72-year-old client has an order for digoxin (Lanoxin) 0.25 mg PO in the morning. At 7:00 a.m., the nurse reviews the following information:
- apical pulse, 68
- respirations, 16
- plasma digoxin level, 2.2 ng/ml

Based on this assessment, which nursing action is appropriate?

① Give the medication on time.
② Withhold the medication, notify the physician.
③ Administer epinephrine 1:1000 stat.
④ Check the client's blood pressure.

11.10 A client is ordered cefoxitin (Mefoxin) 2 gm. IV piggyback in 100 cc 5% Dextrose in water. The primary IV is 5% Dextrose in lactated ringers infusing by gravity. Which safety measure should be included in the administration of this medication?

① The medication should be administered slowly at 20–25 cc/hr.
② The primary IV solution should be changed.
③ The piggyback infusion bag should be hung higher than the primary infusion.
④ An infusion pump must be obtained prior to administration.

11.11 When exploring ways to effectively manage the budget, the nurse will most likely find that she will have to set goals for the unit. What would be an appropriate goal for the unit?

① Decrease overhead by limiting supplies utilized to operate the unit.
② Stabilize the total work force by utilizing only part-time employees with limited working hours.
③ Develop an incentive program that will demonstrate cost-effective measures to maintain the overall budget.
④ Participate in open-forums to discuss the issues of budget management on a consistent basis.

11.12 A client is to be taking the tricyclic antidepressant medication imipramine (Tofranil) at home following discharge. The nurse should instruct the client to report which symptoms immediately?

① Sore throat, fever, increased fatigue, vomiting, diarrhea
② Dry mouth, nasal stuffiness, weight gain
③ Rapid heartbeat, frequent headaches, yellowing of eyes or skin
④ Weakness, staggering gait, tremor, feeling of being drunk

11.13 The physician has just informed a client that an amputation of the leg is needed. The client is crying as you enter the room. Which technique that the nurse can utilize is the most therapeutic?

① Sit with client quietly until crying stops; then inquire about feelings.
② Ask what is causing client to feel so badly.
③ Comfort by hugging and tell client not to worry.
④ Try to distract by talking about her family.

11.14 The client is admitted with cerebrovascular accident (CVA) and has facial paralysis. Nursing care should be planned to prevent which complication?

① Inability to talk
② Inability to swallow
③ Inability to open the affected eye
④ Corneal abrasion

11.15 Which statement by a client indicates an understanding of the cause of herpes zoster?

① "I will avoid exposure to children with German measles."
② "I had the chickenpox in grammar school."
③ "Using a condom during intercourse will be necessary."
④ "I will bathe more often than in the past."

11.16 The nurse has been caring for a schizophrenic client receiving haloperidol (Haldol) IM. She notices the following new symptoms in the client:
- high fever
- tachycardia
- muscle rigidity
- incontinence

These findings suggest that the client is experiencing:

① tardive dyskinesia.
② Parkinson's syndrome.
③ acute dystonic reaction.
④ neuroleptic malignant syndrome.

11.17 Which technique is best for obtaining a urine specimen for a culture and sensitivity from a client with an existing indwelling catheter?

① Clean the drain of the collection bag with an antiseptic before filling the specimen container.
② Obtain the specimen from the drainage bag in the morning.
③ Using a sterile syringe with a small gauge needle, aspirate urine from the catheter port.
④ If the catheter has been in place for 48 hours, replace it before obtaining the specimen.

11.18 A client is ordered to take metronidazole (Flagyl) PO TID at home. Which client statement indicates a knowledge deficit and need for teaching?

① "I'll be sure to take this medication with meals."
② "I'll call my physician if my skin becomes itchy."
③ "I'll limit my alcohol intake to two drinks per day."
④ "I understand that my urine may become brown-colored and is normal."

11.19 The nurse's assessment of a client who abuses cocaine includes:

① bradycardia, miosis, hypertension.
② mydriasis, abdominal cramps, excessive salivation.
③ hypotension, bradycardia, abdominal cramps.
④ hypertension, tachycardia, tremor.

11.20 Which technique should be used in the administration of heparin sodium (Heparin)?

① Gently massage the injection site.
② Do not aspirate after inserting the needle.
③ Use a 1-inch, 18–20 gauge needle.
④ Administer the medication at the deltoid muscle.

11.21 A nursing unit is implementing a project involving changes in the way the unit is managed. The nursing manager on the unit continues to have problems with a team member that has been very disruptive regarding the implementation of the project. What is the best approach for the nurse manager in handling this situation?

① Call the unit supervisor and advise her of the problems with the team member and ask her how to handle the situation.
② Privately meet with the team member, review her behavior, and determine if she is aware of the impact her behavior has on the unit.
③ Involve the other members of the team in attempting to discourage the disruptive team member's behavior.
④ Counsel with the disruptive team member and ask her why she is not happy working on this unit.

11.22 A client is experiencing a severe panic attack and has threatened to hurt another client on the unit. The nurse would expect to administer which PRN medication as ordered?

① Chlorpromazine (Thorazine)
② Lithium carbonate (Lithane)
③ Haloperidol (Haldol)
④ Phenytoin (Dilantin)

11.23 The nurse should teach the mother of a newborn which concept regarding umbilical cord care?

① Apply a sterile gauze dressing with petroleum jelly to cord.
② Position diaper over the umbilicus to maintain dryness.
③ Clean cord with alcohol several times a day and expose to air frequently.
④ Apply erythromycin ointment to cord several times a day to prevent infection.

11.24 An extremely agitated client is receiving rapid neuroleptization with haloperidol (Haldol) IM every 30 minutes while in the psychiatric emergency room. The most important nursing intervention is to:

① monitor vital signs, especially blood pressure every 30 minutes.
② remain at client's side for reassurance.
③ tell client name of medication and its effect.
④ monitor anticholinergic effects of medication.

11.25 You are caring for a client who is two days post op abdominal surgery. Which assessment data, on the following intake and output sheet (I&O), would require further action by the nurse?

Source	7a-7p	7p-a
P.O.	0 ml	0 ml
IV	1500 ml	1500 ml
Urine	900 ml	1000 ml
Nasogastric tube	500 ml	50 ml

① P.O. intake
② Intravenous fluid balance
③ Urine output
④ Nasogastric suction drainage

11.26 What is the nurse's next action when a client states, "I am going to end it all, myself."

① Ask the client, "Do you have a plan to kill yourself?"
② Tell the client, "Suicide is not the answer. Let's talk about what has brought you to this decision."
③ Call the physician and tell him what the client has said.
④ Ask the client, "Have you ever felt this way before?"

11.27 Which action by the nurse is most appropriate when a client requests that a nurse on a previous shift not care for him again.

① Document the issue on an incident report.
② Inform the nurse manager of the incident.
③ Explain to the client the nurse was having a bad day.
④ Address the client's concerns with the charge nurse.

11.28 Which assessment would be important to include in the history of a 7-year-old with glomerulonephritis?

① Strep throat 12 days ago
② Weight loss with diarrhea
③ Increase in fluid intake and voiding frequently
④ Decrease in energy with an increased need for sleep

11.29 Which vital sign recorded on a 2-month-old infant should be discussed with the pediatrician?

① Heart rate of 120 beats per minute (bpm).
② Rectal temperature of 101.5°F.
③ Respiratory rate of 40.
④ Blood pressure of 90/60.

11.30 A client is receiving furosemide (Lasix) 40 mg IV bid. Prior to administering the medication, the nurse should check for:

① muscle weakness.
② metabolic acidosis.
③ hyperkalemia.
④ hypertension.

11.31 The nurse's best response to a preschool child who asks if he is going to die is:

① "Everyone dies sometime."
② "Don't be silly. You get stronger every day."
③ "You sound concerned. Tell me what made you ask that question."
④ "You are eating so much better and getting out of bed sometimes."

11.32 The infant had a myelomeningocele repair. The parents' acceptance is observed by the home care nurse when they:

① state the infant will outgrow this problem in time.
② have the neighbor do bladder expression.
③ measure the head circumference daily.
④ discuss the expectation of child walking in one year.

11.33 Before administering the MMR (Measles, Mumps and Rubella) vaccine to a 15-month-old toddler, the nurse should check with the mother about:

① sibling reaction to immunizations.
② allergies to eggs or neomycin.
③ allergies in family members to medications.
④ diarrhea in this client a week ago without temperature.

11.34 When assessing orientation to person, place and time for an elderly hospitalized client, which principle should be understood by the nurse?

① Short-term memory is more efficient than long-term memory.
② The stress of an unfamiliar environment may cause confusion.
③ A decline in mental status is a normal part of aging.
④ Learning ability is reduced during.

11.35 Which nursing action is a priority for a child admitted with a positive stool culture for Salmonella?

① Change diet to clear liquids.
② Initiate intravenous fluids.
③ Place child in enteric isolation.
④ Apply cloth diapers.

11.36 After a client is admitted with pregnancy-induced hypertension (PIH), which is the most important nursing action?

① Start an IV.
② Measure vital signs.
③ Administer magnesium sulfate.
④ Notify lab to draw the blood.

11.37 The nurse is aware that which of the following assessment findings would support a diagnosis of Cushing's syndrome?

① Hypotension
② Thin facial features
③ Well-developed arm and leg muscles
④ Central or truncal-type obesity.

11.38 A nurse would anticipate assessing which initial side effects from a client undergoing chemotherapy?

① Alopecia and purpura
② Anorexia and weight loss
③ Nausea and vomiting
④ Coughing and shortness of breath.

11.39 For the immobile client, which nursing assessment indicates a need for intervention?

① Drainage from the Foley catheter is clear, with a pH of 6.5.
② The client's skin blanches over the scapular areas.
③ Bilateral chest excursion is present.
④ The client drinks three glasses of orange juice every day.

11.40 To evaluate for adverse reactions of a narcotic injection, the nurse would observe:

① elevated temperature.
② hypertension.
③ decreased pulse rate.
④ increased respirations.

11.41 What would be the most appropriate action for the nurse to take after noting the sudden appearance of a fixed and dilated pupil in a neuro client?

① Reassess in five minutes.
② Check client's visual acuity.
③ Lower the head of the client's bed.
④ Call the physician.

11.42 In developing discharge plans with the family of the client in stage four Parkinson's disease, it is most important for the nurse to include which activities?

① Ambulate twice daily.
② ROM to all extremities four times a day.
③ Hobbies and games such as knitting and putting puzzles together.
④ Encourage and provide writing materials.

11.43 Which statement made by the client in sickle cell crisis indicates a need for further teaching?

① "My pain is from poor circulation due to sickling of the cells."
② "I will need to see a genetic counselor when I get married."
③ "I have a trip planned to snow ski in 3 weeks."
④ "I need to stay away from strenuous activities."

11.44 Which statement made by a client who is prescribed Allopurinol (Zyloprin) has an appropriate understanding of how to safely take the medication? "I will:

① take the medication 60 minutes prior to meals."
② drink 2.5–3 liters of fluid per day."
③ increase my intake of vitamin C."
④ continue eating oatmeal and a slice of whole wheat toast for breakfast."

11.45 Which statement made by the client indicates a correct understanding of client-controlled epidural analgesia (PCA)?

① "If I start feeling drowsy, I should notify the nurse."
② "This button will give me enough to kill the pain whenever I want it."
③ "If I start itching, I need to call the nurse."
④ "This medicine will make me feel no pain."

11.46 What is the initial nursing priority for an infant admitted to the pediatric unit with possible Hemophilus influenzae meningitis?

① Encourage fluids to prevent dehydration.
② Restrain child appropriately to maintain integrity of IV site.
③ Place child in respiratory isolation.
④ Encourage parents to hold and rock infant to promote comfort.

11.47 Which statement by a client indicates that the client is using the defense mechanism of conversion?

① "I love my family with all my heart, even though they don't love me."
② "I could not take my final exams because I was unable to write."
③ "I don't believe I have diabetes. I feel perfectly fine."
④ "If my wife was a better housekeeper, I wouldn't have such a problem."

11.48 Which statement indicates parental understanding about the cause of their newborn's diagnosis of cystic fibrosis?

① "The gene came from my husband's side of the family."
② "The gene came from my wife's side of the family."
③ "There is a 50 percent chance that our next child will have the disease."
④ "Both my husband and I carry a recessive trait for cystic fibrosis."

11.49 Prior to mixing different types of insulin, the nurse should:

① rotate the vial at least 1 minute between both hands.
② gently shake each vial for at least 1 minute.
③ throw away all cloudy color insulin.
④ take the vials out of the refrigerator for 30 minutes.

11.50 Which diversional activity is most appropriate for a 12-year-old client recovering from a sickle-cell crisis?

① Walking in the hall 20 minutes 2 times a day
② Watching the cartoon channel all day
③ Talking to best friend on the telephone
④ Putting together large-pieced wooden puzzles

11.51 Which nursing observation indicates an early complication of hypoxemia in a child with epiglottitis?

① Tachycardia
② Cyanosis
③ Circumoral pallor
④ Difficulty swallowing

11.52 Which action observed by the nurse would indicate a client's ability to care for his own colostomy?

① Irrigating the colostomy with 2000 ml of warm tap water
② Changing the appliance twice a day
③ Inserting the irrigating tube 6" into the stoma
④ Fitting the appliance securely around the edge of the stoma

11.53 Which nursing action is most appropriate when an infant is admitted for fever, poor feeding, irritability, and a bulging fontanel?

① Perform neuro checks every four hours.
② Place the client in respiratory isolation.
③ Monitor client's urine output closely.
④ Encourage fluid intake.

11.54 Which nursing action is a priority for a newborn with a myelomeningocele?

① Elevate the head of the bed to decrease intracranial pressure.
② Immediately intubate the infant to decrease the potential for respiratory distress.
③ Position the infant supine to prevent damage to the sac.
④ Cover the sac with sterile, warm, moist compresses to maintain asepsis.

11.55 Which statement made by a client indicates a correct understanding of the side effects of phenazopyridine hydrochloride (Pyridium)? "My medicine:

① will make me urinate more frequently."
② should be taken only at bedtime."
③ will cause my urine to become orange."
④ should be taken before meals."

11.56 Which recommendation by the nurse would offer the greatest support to a newly diagnosed AIDS client and his family?

① Avoid all contact with anyone except immediate family.
② Speak to a representative from the local AIDS support group.
③ Stop all sexual activity immediately.
④ Begin chemotherapy as soon as possible.

11.57 Which question would best aid the nurse in assessing the orientation of a client on the psychiatric unit?

① "Who is the president of the United States?"
② "Do you remember my name?"
③ "What is your name?"
④ "What time is it?"

11.58 In performing a nursing audit, the nurse is evaluating the nursing documentation. Which should be present in the charting for a clinet receiving total parenteral nutrition (TPN)?

  ① Weight, blood glucose, I&O
  ② Amount of blood withdrawn for lab studies
  ③ Position during dressing change
  ④ CVP reading obtained during infusion to TPN

11.59 Which client statement indicates a need for more information regarding oral contraceptives?

  ① "I will need check-ups every six months."
  ② "I should take the pill the same time each day."
  ③ "If I forget a pill one day, I should take it when I remember. Then take the next pill as scheduled the next day."
  ④ "If I miss 2 pills, I will take them when I remember and continue the normal schedule."

11.60 Which assessment would be most important regarding safety for a client receiving vincristine sulfate (Oncovin)?

  ① Fatigue and nausea.
  ② Polyphagia and polydipsia.
  ③ Hypotension and alopecia.
  ④ Paresthesia and difficulties in gait.

11.61 During morning assignments, a nurse is assigned to several clients. Which would be first to receive morning care?

  ① A client with a recent appendectomy
  ② A client with infectious meningitis
  ③ An immunosuppressed client
  ④ A client with COPD

11.62 Care of a 70-year-old woman with symptoms including temperature of 103.4°F, moderate dehydration, bilateral rales in lower lobes of lungs, and disorientation to time and place, would be based on understanding that:

  ① the client is experiencing temporary delirium secondary to the infectious process.
  ② the client is probably displaying early symptoms of Alzheimer's Disease.
  ③ old people get confused often as a normal part of the aging process.
  ④ a referral to a nursing home for continuing care will be necessary for this client.

11.63 A client in the ER is displaying the following symptoms:
  • elevated vital signs
  • hallucinations
  • aggressive behavior.
The client's friend says she thinks he has been using hallucinogenic drugs. The appropriate nursing action would be to:

  ① put the client in full restraints.
  ② decrease environmental stimulation.
  ③ call the security guards.
  ④ administer a PRN dose of chlorpromazine (Thorazine).

11.64 The nurse is caring for a client who is taking Disulfiram (Antabuse). The nurse should caution the client to avoid the intake of which of the following?

  ① Aged cheeses
  ② Liquid cough medicines
  ③ Chicken or beef liver
  ④ Yogurt or sour cream

11.65 The nurse does not know the answer to a question asked by the client. What is the most appropriate response to assist in developing a trusting relationship?

  ① "Why don't you ask your physician this question?"
  ② "Here is some written information that will answer your question."
  ③ "I don't know the answer, but will find out and let you know in 30 minutes."
  ④ "Don't worry about this issue; it should never happen to you."

11.66 The nurse is caring for a client who is extremely flirtatious, charming, and willing to manipulate others. Which measure should the nurse take?

  ① Limit the client's behavior and share that information with nursing staff on all three shifts.
  ② Ask another nurse to care for this particular client.
  ③ Document the client's behavior so that the physician will order medication to control his behavior.
  ④ Listen empathetically and help meet the client's needs.

11.67 One of the goals the nurse and client with Post Traumatic Stress Disorder (PTSD) mutually agreed upon is an increase in participation in "out of the apartment" activities. Which recommendation will be the most therapeutic while achieving that goal?

  ① Take a day trip with a friend.
  ② Take an 11-minute bus ride alone.
  ③ Join a support group and participate in a victim assistance organization.
  ④ Take a 10-minute walk with spouse around the block.

11.68 Which client would be the first to receive morning care? A client with a diagnosis of:

  ① appendectomy.
  ② infectious meningitis.
  ③ AIDS.
  ④ COPD.

11.69 A charge nurse is developing the assignment for the evening shift. In a semi-private room, Client A has neutropenia. Client B has a tracheostomy with purulent drainage and a pending C&S. Which assignment is the most appropriate?

  ① Assign an experienced nurse to care for both clients in the same room.
  ② Assign two nurses—one nurse for Client A, and another nurse for Client B—in the same room.
  ③ Place Client A in a private room. Assign the same nurse to care for Client A and Client B.
  ④ Place Client A in a private room. Assign different nurses to care for Client A and Client B.

11.70 A 6-month-old infant is on Isomil and weighs fifteen pounds. Which nursing observation on a home visit would indicate a need for further teaching?

  ① The infant is sucking a pacifier.
  ② The infant is crawling on the floor.
  ③ The father speaks sternly to the infant for pulling books from the bookcase.
  ④ The father gives the baby a bottle with whole milk.

11.71 An 11-month-old baby is having trouble gaining weight after discharge from the hospital. To best assess the problem, the nurse would:

  ① observe the child at mealtime.
  ② inquire regarding the child's eating pattern.
  ③ weigh the baby each month.
  ④ try to feed the baby for the mother.

11.72 A client has been receiving morphine sulfate 15 mg IV push for several days as pain management for severe burns. Nursing assessment reveals a decrease in bowel sounds and slight abdominal distention. Which nursing action is the most appropriate?

  ① Recommend morphine dose be decreased.
  ② Withhold pain medication.
  ③ Administer medication by another route.
  ④ Explore alternative pain management techniques.

11.73 Which assessment would be a priority for evaluating the status of a pleurevac connected to a right middle lobe chest tube?

  ① Incentive spirometry
  ② Breath sounds
  ③ Chest tube drainage
  ④ Chest X-ray

11.74 Following hip replacement surgery, an elderly client is ordered to begin ambulation with a walker. In planning nursing care, which statement by the nurse will best help this client?

  ① "Sit in a low chair for ease in getting up to the walker."
  ② "Make sure rubber caps are present on all four legs of the walker."
  ③ "Begin weight-bearing on the affected hip as soon as possible."
  ④ "Practice tying your own shoes before using the walker."

11.75 An elderly client with mild osteoarthritis needs instruction on exercising. In planning nursing care, which instruction would best help this client?

  ① Swimming is the only helpful exercise for osteoarthritis.
  ② Warm-up exercises should be done prior to exercising.
  ③ Exercises should be done routinely even if joint pain occurs.
  ④ Isometric exercises are most helpful to prevent contractures.

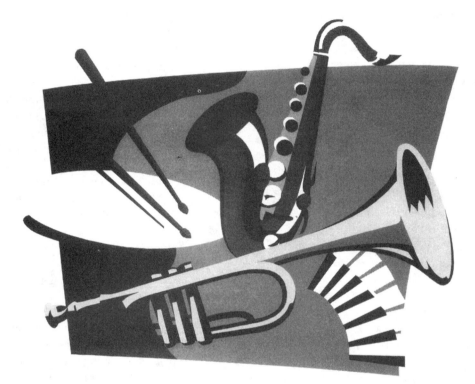

Celebrate *Your* Great *Work!*
Congratulations!

Answers & Rationales

11.1 ① Options #1 and #5 are correct. Option #2
        ⑤ should be squeezed directly onto the sterile
            field. Option #3 has contaminated gloves
            as currently reads. Sterile gloves should be
            placed on after unsterile bottle has been ma-
            nipulated. Option #4 should be sterile gauze
            pad. Avoid using cotton balls because they
            may shed fibers in the wound, causing irrita-
            tion, infection, or adhesion. Option #6 should
            be cleansed last since most drainage promotes
            bacterial growth. This drain is considered
            most contaminated area.

11.2 ② Options #2 and #5 are correct. Option
        ⑤ #1—dilation should be done with warm,
            moist compresses. Option #3 is incorrect.
            The puncture should be on the sides of the
            fingertip and position the lancet perpendicular
            to the lines of the client's fingerprints.

11.3 ① Options #1 and #5 are correct because they
        ⑤ require general nursing care that is congru-
            ent with the Nurse Practice Act. Option #2
            would require IV management and special-
            ized assessment skills. Option #3 would
            require initial assessment. LPNs can do
            ongoing assessments, but it is not in the scope
            of practice to complete the initial assessment.
            Option #4 is incorrect because it requires
            initial teaching. The LPN can reinforce
            teaching but it is currently not in the scope of
            practice to do the initial teaching.

11.4 ① Airway is a priority after a seizure. Do not
        ③ attempt to force anything into client's mouth
            if jaws are clenched shut. If jaws are not
            clenched, place an airway in client's mouth.
            This protects the tongue and also provides a
            method of suctioning the airway should client
            vomit. Evaluate respiratory status. If vomit-
            ing occurs, be prepared to suction the client
            to clear the airway and prevent aspiration.

11.5 ① This client is most at risk for neglect. Op-
            tions #2, #3, and #4 are lower risk than Op-
            tion #1.

11.6 ③ The bar stools present the highest risk factor
            for falls to this client. Option #1 is a concern
            but not a priority over Option #3. Options #2
            and #4 may assist client versus being a risk
            factor.

11.7 ② Clean gloves should be worn at all times
            when handling any client's body fluids.
            Option #1 is correct but not a higher prior-
            ity over Option #2. Option #3 is incorrect
            because venipuncture sites of clients with
            hepatitis B should be held for a longer period
            of time due to possibility of increased bleed-
            ing associated with an impaired liver. Option
            #4 is unsafe.

11.8 ③ This will provide necessary information in
            the baseline assessment of the client's anxi-
            ety. Options #1, #2, and #4 are helpful data
            which can be collected during treatment, but
            do not take priority during the first 48 hours.

11.9 ② Withhold the medication and notify the physi-
            cian because the therapeutic plasma level of
            digoxin is 0.5-2.0 ng/ml. Option #3 is not
            necessary at this time. Option #4 is not a
            priority.

11.10 ③ When using a gravity drip, the piggyback
            fluid level should be higher than the primary
            infusion. Option #1 is incorrect because the
            antibiotic should be administered within one
            hour. Options #2 and #4 are not necessary for
            safe infusion.

11.11 ③ Developing an incentive program to maintain
            revenue will involve the whole unit. This
            will also give accountability and responsibil-
            ity back to the staff on the unit. Option #1
            may be counter-productive. Option #2 may
            decrease quality of care. Option #4 may be
            useful and secondary to Option #3.

11.12 ① These are possible side effects of Tofranil which can be resolved by changing the dosage or changing the medication. Option #2 describes side effects of antidepressants which the client can learn to manage at home without changing the medication. Options #3 and #4 describe side effects of a different category of medications.

11.13 ① "Being with" the client as acknowledgement and dealing with impending loss demonstrates the nurse's acceptance of the client's need to grieve. Allowing the client time to cry and then asking to describe feelings demonstrates the nurse is willing to listen and validate the client's feelings. Option #2 is not acknowledging the situation requiring an amputation. Option #3 might be somewhat premature and uncomfortable unless both participants in the relationship find touching acceptable. It is inappropriate to tell her not to worry. Option #4 is avoidance of the situation.

11.14 ④ The client will be unable to close his eye voluntarily. When the facial nerve (cranial nerve VII) is affected, the lacrimal gland will no longer supply secretions that protect the eye. Options #1, #2, and #3 may occur, but nursing care cannot prevent them.

11.15 ② Herpes zoster (shingles) is a reactivation of latent varicella (chickenpox) which has an increased frequency rate among adults with weakened immune systems. Option #1 is not correlated with measles. Option #3 is incorrect because this is not a sexually-transmitted disease. Option #4 is incorrect because the problem is not related to hygiene.

11.16 ④ This severe reaction to antipsychotic medication occurs in clients who are severely ill as a result of dopamine blockage in the hypothalamus. Option #1 would be characterized by abnormal facial and tongue movements. Option #2 would be characterized by tremors, rigidity, and shuffling gait. Option #3 would be characterized by severe muscle contractions of the head and neck.

11.17 ③ Indwelling catheters have a port for the withdrawal of sterile urine specimens. Options #1 and #2 will not provide a sterile specimen from the collection bag. Option #4 is not necessary.

11.18 ③ Metronidazole (Flagyl) will produce a disulfiram-like (Antabuse) reaction if any form of alcohol is used. Options #1, #2, and #4 indicate an understanding of the concepts related to taking this medication.

11.19 ④ Cocaine elevates the blood pressure and pulse along with causing a fine tremor. Cardiac arrhythmias can occur, especially with the use of crack cocaine. Excessive salivation and bradycardia are not found with cocaine abuse.

11.20 ② Aspirating the syringe with a subcutaneous heparin solution can cause bruising. Option #1 is incorrect because the heparin injection site should not be rubbed. Option #3 is incorrect because the needle is too long. Option #4 is incorrect because the medication should be given subcutaneously.

11.21 ② It is important to determine what the problem is with the disruptive team member. The best way to do that is in private. Review with her the disruptive behavior and attempt to determine the source of the problem. If this does not solve the situation, then the supervisor should be notified. Option #2 better describes the solution than does Option #4. Other team members should not be brought into the situation.

11.22 ③ Haldol is particularly effective in reducing assaultive behavior associated with severe anxiety. Option #1 is more likely to be used as a PRN when a client is experiencing agitation associated with schizophrenia. Option #2 is an antimanic drug. Option #4 is an anticonvulsant medication.

11.23 ③ This will encourage drying and assist in preventing infection. Option #1 is appropriate for circumcision care. Option #2 will keep the area moist. Diaper should be placed below the umbilicus. Option #4 is incorrect because the antibiotic ointment is not necessary.

11.24 ① While all of these nursing interventions are necessary during rapid neuroleptization, monitoring vital signs is of utmost importance to assure client safety and physiological integrity. Rapid neuroleptization is a pharmacological intervention used to rapidly diminish severe symptoms which accompany acute psychosis. The alpha-adrenergic blockade of peripheral vascular system lowers blood pressure and causes postural hypotension. Options #2 and #4 are secondary. Option #3 may be done later.

11.25 ④ Option #4 is correct. Sudden cessation or drastic decrease of nasogastric drainage indicates blockage or disruption of the drainage system. Normal gastric production is 1-1.5 L daily. 500 mL per twelve-hour shift is expected. Option #1 is incorrect because the client has a draining nasogastric tube. P.O. intake is not expected. Option #2 demonstrates that the I.V. fluid balance is appropriate. Option #3 is incorrect because the urine output is slightly more than intake and is not a cause of concern.

11.26 ① Option #1 is priority to identify if the client has a plan for suicide before proceeding to intervention. Options #2, #3, and #4 do not assess if the client has a plan which is priority if a client mentions suicide intent.

11.27 ④ As a client advocate, the nurse needs to intervene to assure the client's request is met. The issue needs to be discussed with the charge nurse so that accurate communication occurs between the shifts and personnel involved. Option #1 is inappropriate. Option #2 should occur, but after the charge nurse is advised of the situation. Option #3 is making excuses and not addressing the issue.

11.28 ① There is a 10-14 day latent period between group A beta hemolytic streptococcal infection and the onset of signs of glomerulonephritis. Option #2 includes signs of hypovolemia. Option #3 includes signs of diabetes mellitus. Option #4 is not specific to a particular diagnosis.

11.29 ② Option #2 is correct because a temperature above 101.3°F rectally in a child less than 3 months old is abnormal and can signify a serious infection. Options #1, #3 and #4 are normal in a 2-month-old infant.

11.30 ① The major symptoms of hypokalemia are muscle weakness and atony. Option #2 is incorrect because hypokalemia accompanies metabolic alkalosis. Option #3 is incorrect because hypokalemia would be the problem. Option #4 is not a side effect.

11.31 ③ Exploring what happened to cause the client to ask the question would assist the nurse in answering questions. Options #1, #2 and #4 do not explore the client's feelings.

11.32 ③ Parents' participation in care may be the first sign of acceptance. Measuring the head circumference is important due to the risk of hydrocephalus following surgery, but even simple care like bathing the child, could bring acceptance. Option #1 is incorrect because the child has a chronic problem. Option #2 indicates parents' lack of interest and inability to care for child. Option #4 shows a lack of understanding about myelomeningocele.

11.33 ② Allergies to MMR come from egg, foul, and neomycin due to the growth of the live virus on egg embryo. Option #1 is incorrect because there is no absolute relationship between the siblings' allergic responses. Option #3 is not relevant to this vaccination. Option #4 is more significant for oral polio administration.

11.34 ② The stress of an unfamiliar situation or environment may lead to confusion among the elderly. Option #1 is incorrect because long-term memory is more efficient than short-term. Options #3 and #4 are not affected by aging. The elderly client may be slower at doing things.

11.35 ③ Enteric isolation prevents the transmission of Salmonella to other individuals. Options #1, #2, and #4 may be appropriate but are not a priority over Option #3 which will prevent transmission.

11.36 ② It is imperative to do a baseline assessment in order to successfully evaluate the treatment. Options #1 and #4 are not priority actions. Option #3 is correct but not a priority to Option #2.

11.37 ④ The client with Cushing's will have abnormal fat distribution which causes a central or truncal type obesity. Option #1 is incorrect because the client tends to have increased blood pressure. Option #2 is incorrect because the client will have a "moon" face. Option #3 is incorrect because the extremities will be thin.

11.38 ③ The most common side effects of chemotherapy are nausea and vomiting. Options #1 and #4 are typically later findings. Option #2 can be a result of Option #3.

11.39 ② Blanching or hyperemia that does not disappear in a short time is a warning sign of pressure ulcers. Option #1 is normal urine. Option #3 is a normal respiratory assessment finding. Option #4 is irrelevant.

11.40 ③ Narcotics can cause a decrease in heart rate. Option #1 is irrelevant. Option #2 is incorrect because hypotension will result. Option #4 is incorrect because respiratory depression will result.

11.41 ④ A fixed and dilated pupil represents a neurological emergency. Option #1 does not take action necessary for the immediate situation. Option #2 cannot accurately be evaluated with increased ICP. Option #3 would increase the intracranial pressure.

11.42 ② In stage four Parkinson's disease, the client is immobile. Option #1 is incorrect because the client would be unable to ambulate. Options #3 and #4 are incorrect because the client cannot perform activities which require small muscle dexterity.

11.43 ③ The mountains are low in oxygen concentration which, along with increased activity, would contribute to sickling of the cells. Options #1, #2, and #4 indicate a correct understanding.

11.44 ② Fluids are imperative to decrease the side effects of a gout attack or renal stones. Option #1 is incorrect because the drug should be taken following meals due to nausea and vomiting. Option #3 will increase the likelihood of renal calculi formation. Option #4 is high in purine which is a precursor to uric acid. This counteracts the purpose of administering the medication.

11.45 ③ A common side effect of narcotics used in epidural pain management is itching. Options #2 and #4 are incorrect. Option #1 is secondary.

11.46 ③ To prevent the spread of the infection, the client is placed in respiratory isolation for at least 24 hours after implementation of antibiotic therapy. Option #1 is incorrect because the fluids are determined by client status. Fluids are usually limited to prevent cerebral edema. Option #2 is appropriate but is not a priority to Option #3. Option #4 would cause discomfort to the client's head.

11.47 ② The client has converted his anxiety over school performance into a physical symptom that interferes with his ability to perform. Option #1 may be reaction formation. Option #3 is denial. Option #4 is projection.

11.48 ④ Cystic fibrosis is inherited by an autosomal recessive trait. Both parents are carriers of the abnormal gene. There is a 25 percent chance of passing the gene on to any of their offspring. Options #1, #2, and #3 are inaccurate.

11.49 ① Rotating resuspends the modified insulin preparations and helps to warm the medication. Option #2 causes bubbles and foam which can alter the dose. Option #3 is incorrect because longer acting insulins are supposed to be cloudy. Option #4 is incorrect because insulin does not have to be refrigerated as long as it is at normal room temperature.

11.50 ③ This will conserve energy and still meet psychosocial needs of peer involvement. Option #1 will not conserve much needed energy. Option #2 is an isolating activity and is not age appropriate. Option #4 is appropriate for preschool children.

11.51 ① Option #1 is correct. The heart rate correlates with hypoxemia and is an early finding along with restlessness. Options #2 and #3 would be late signs. Option #4 is a sign of epiglottitis.

11.52 ④ The appliance should fit easily around the stoma and protect the skin. Option #1 is incorrect because no more than 1000 ml of irrigation fluid should ever be used. Option #2 is incorrect because the appliance should only be changed when it begins to leak or becomes dislodged. Option #3 is incorrect because the catheter should not be inserted over 4" into the stoma.

11.53 ② These are classic signs of meningitis, and the client should be isolated from other clients. Options #1 and #3 are appropriate but are not a priority over Option #2 when the client is first admitted. Option #4 is inappropriate for this situation.

11.54 ④ Prevention of infection is critical for this infant. The head of the infant's bed should remain flat unless otherwise ordered. Option #2 is irrelevant to this situation. Option #3 is of utmost importance, but to do this, the infant must be prone or on his side.

11.55 ③ The drug may change the urine to an orange color. Option #1 is not accurate because this drug is not a diuretic. It has a local anesthetic action on the urinary tract mucosa. Options #2 and #4 are incorrect because the drug should be taken after meals.

11.56 ② The establishment of a support system from the beginning is very important to any terminally ill client, especially with a disease like AIDS that is associated with a social stigma. Option #1 is incorrect because general isolation is not necessary. The client does need education regarding exposure to infectious agents. Option #3 is not necessary as long as precautions are taken to prevent spreading the disease. Option #4 is inappropriate to the situation.

11.57 ③ This is a specific question related to the orientation of the person. Option #1 is incorrect because some well-oriented people do not know the answer to this question depending upon their age, educational level, etc. Option #2 is irrelevant. Option #4 is incorrect because without consulting a watch or clock, most well-oriented people cannot answer this question.

11.58 ① Daily weights, blood glucose, and I&O evaluate the effectiveness of TPN. Option #2 is unnecessary. Option #3 may be charted but is secondary to #1. Option #4 is incorrect. The CVP should not be determined with TPN infusing.

11.59 ④ If 2 pills are missed, they should be taken. However, another form of contraception for the remainder of the month should be used. Options #1, #2, and #3 are correct and do not require more information.

11.60 ④ These assessments indicate a problem with peripheral neuropathy. These can result in difficulties with safety and will mandate a change in the plan of care. Option #1 does occur but is not a priority over Option #4. Option #2 includes signs of diabetes. Option #3 is not a priority over Option #4.

11.61 ③ WBCs are usually decreased in the immunosuppressed client which predisposes to infection. AM care should be completed on this client first, especially before the client with meningitis. Option #1: the nurse may find it useful to provide time for a PRN for pain to work before she begins AM care on this client. Option #4: this client would need care done slowly so as not to fatigue him.

11.62 ① Delirium, accompanied by some disorientation, is often caused by a systemic infection such as pneumonia, especially in an older person who may be more vulnerable to illness. Options #2, #3, and #4 are premature assumptions and are not based on the data presented.

11.63 ② The symptoms may subside with time and decreased stimulation. Options #1 and #3 are not necessary at this time. Option #4 is inappropriate.

11.64 ② Many liquid cough medicines have an alcohol base which will interact with the Antabuse to produce nausea and vomiting. Options #1, #3, and #4 are foods which interact with MAO inhibitor medications.

11.65 ③ Option #3 is most appropriate in developing a trusting relationship. Option #1 is practicing nurse avoidance. Option #2 is only providing information. Option #4 provides false reassurance.

11.66 ① A manipulative client needs firm limits, and those limits must be known and followed by all the nursing staff. If not, client will be able to split the staff into opposing forces. Options #2, #3, and #4 are inappropriate nursing actions with this client.

11.67 ③ Support groups of people who have suffered similar acts of violence can be helpful and supportive in teaching clients how to deal with the traumatizing situation and the emotional aftermath. Options #1, #2, and #4 are all reasonable recommendations to begin utilizing in a systematic desensitization program after the crisis period is alleviated.

11.68 ③ In an immunosuppressed client, the WBCs are usually decreased which predisposes the client to infections. It would be important to do this client's AM care first, especially before the client with meningitis. Option #2 care is given after Option #3. Option #1 is incorrect, but the nurse might find it helpful to medicate the client prior to giving AM care. Option #4 would need care done in a way not to cause fatigue increase the hypoxia.

11.69 ④ Infection in a neutropenic individual may cause morbidity and fatality if untreated. Place neutropenic client in a private room. Limit and screen visitors and hospital staff with potentially communicable illnesses. Options #1, #2, and #3 may be harmful to client A.

11.70 ④ A 6-month-old on a soy-based formula is probably allergic to cow milk products. Many children who are sensitive to cow's milk cannot tolerate it until the age of 2. Options #1, #2, and #3 are acceptable activities in caring for this age child.

11.71 ① Direct observation of a typical mealtime will give the most information. Option #2 may or may not secure an accurate picture. The weight should be obtained more often or on each visit as opposed to Option #3. Option #4 circumvents the routine patterns of behavior surrounding feeding times.

11.72 ④ Morphine is the drug of choice for burn pain management. When a side effect becomes apparent, exploration of alternative techniques such as visualization become important. Option #1 might be used, but with a possible impending ileus suspected, this option is not ideal. Options #2 and #3 are inappropriate.

11.73 ④ The chest x-ray will be able to visualize fluid and air in the pleural space. Options #1, #2, and #3 would be beneficial to evaluate but are not as inclusive as Option #4.

11.74 ② Intact rubber caps should be present on walker legs to prevent accidents. Options #1, #3, and #4 should be avoided for 4-6 weeks.

11.75 ② Warm-up or stretching exercises should always be done prior to and after exercising. Option #1 is only one helpful exercise. Option #3 is incorrect because painful joints should not be exercised. Option #4 does not involve joint movements.

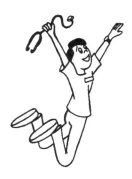

Good job! Only the
Simulated Exam to go!

Those who have one foot in the canoe and one foot in the boat are going to fall in the water.

—Tuscarora Indian Proverb

Category Analysis – Post-test #2

1. Safe Effective Care	26. Psycho-Social	51. Health Promotion
2. Nutrition	27. Safe Effective Care	52. Elimination
3. Safe Effective Care	28. Health Promotion	53. Health Promotion
4. Safe Effective Care	29. Health Promotion	54. Health Promotion
5. Psycho-Social	30. Pharmacology	55. Pharmacology
6. Sensory-Perception-Mobility	31. Psycho-Social	56. Psycho-Social
7. Safe Effective Care	32. Health Promotion	57. Psycho-Social
8. Psycho-Social	33. Health Promotion	58. Safe Effective Care
9. Pharmacology	34. Health Promotion	59. Health Promotion
10. Pharmacology	35. Safe Effective Care	60. Pharmacology
11. Safe Effective Care	36. Health Promotion	61. Safe Effective Care
12. Pharmacology	37. Nutrition	62. Fluid-Gas
13. Psycho-Social	38. Nutrition	63. Psycho-Social
14. Sensory-Perception-Mobility	39. Sensory-Perception-Mobility	64. Pharmacology
15. Health Promotion	40. Pharmacology	65. Psycho-Social
16. Psycho-Social	41. Sensory-Perception-Mobility	66. Psycho-Social
17. Safe Effective Care	42. Sensory-Perception-Mobility	67. Psycho-Social
18. Pharmacology	43. Fluid-Gas	68. Safe Effective Care
19. Safe Effective Care	44. Pharmacology	69. Safe Effective Care
20. Pharmacology	45. Pharmacology	70. Health Promotion
21. Safe Effective Care	46. Sensory-Perception-Mobility	71. Health Promotion
22. Psycho-Social	47. Psycho-Social	72. Elimination
23. Health Promotion	48. Health Promotion	73. Fluid-Gas
24. Pharmacology	49. Nutrition	74. Health Promotion
25. Fluid-Gas	50. Health Promotion	75. Health Promotion

Directions

1. Determine questions missed by checking answers.
2. Write the number of the questions missed across the top line marked "item missed."
3. Check category analysis page to determine category of question.
4. Put a check mark under item missed and beside content.

5. Count check marks in each row and write the number in totals column.
6. Use this information to:
   - identify areas for further study.
   - determine which content test to take next.

We recommend studying content where most items are missed—then taking that content test.

Number of the Questions Incorrectly Answered

Post-test #2	Items Missed																						Totals
C Safe Effective Care																							
O Health Promotion and Maintenance																							
Psycho-Social Integrity																							
N Physiological Adaptation: Fluid Gas																							
T Reduction of Risk Potential: Sensory-Perception-Mobility																							
E Basic Care and Comfort: Elimination																							
N Physiological Adaptation: Nutrition																							
T Pharmacological and Parenteral Therapies																							

Practice Exam

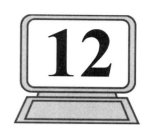

Remember Edison's remark: "If we did all the things we are capable of doing we would literally astonish ourselves." Astonish yourself!

✔ **Clarification of this test...**

The Practice Exam has been designed to be comparable to NCLEX® with

☞ Approximately 43–67% of the items representing Physiological Integrity

☞ Approximately 21–33% of the items representing Safe Effective Care Environment

☞ Approximately 6–12% of the items representing Psycho-Social Integrity

☞ Approximately 6–12% of the items representing Health Promotion

☞ Each phase of the Nursing Process is represented.

The majority of the items are decision-making questions. We believe if you master the top NCLEX® behaviors and concepts listed at the beginning of the chapters, you will HAVE IT MADE!!

12.1 A 5-year-old client admitted 3 days ago with a fractured femur develops varicella. Select all the possible plans that would be appropriate for this client.

  ① Place client in a private room that has monitored negative pressure in relation to surrounding area.
  ② Wear gowns and masks when entering room.
  ③ Wear gloves when entering room.
  ④ Wear respiratory protection (mask or face shield) when entering the room.
  ⑤ Use standard precautions and place with another 5-year-old with a fractured radius.

12.2 Which parts of the body would the nurse use to measure the pulse oximeter reading?

  ① finger and toe
  ② finger and earlobe
  ③ finger and chest
  ④ earlobe and toe

12.3 The nurse is caring for a client who has neisseria meningitis. Which of the following infection control precautions should the nurse implement? Select all that apply.

  ① Wear gloves when entering client's room.
  ② Request client's visitors to wear a gown when in the room.
  ③ Wear a mask when working within 3 feet of the client.
  ④ Keep visitors 3 feet from infected client.
  ⑤ Limit movement of the client from the room.
  ⑥ If the client must leave the room, have him wear a surgical mask, if possible.

12.4 A client with a history of heart failure and hypertension is taking a variety of medications at home. In teaching the client about the blood pressure lowering effects of the medications, which of the client's medications will she include in the discussion? Select all correct answers.

① Hydrochlorothiazide (HCTZ)
② Simvastatin (Zocor)
③ Lisinopril (Zestril)
④ Nizatidine (Axid)
⑤ Atenolol (Tenormin)

12.5 A client is receiving a magnesium antacid 15 cc via nasogastric tube every 4 hours. The nurse should assess which side effect?

① constipation
② diarrhea
③ nausea
④ oral thrush

12.6 During hospital rounds, a nursing supervisor smells smoke coming from a client's bathroom. She opens the bathroom door and finds the client unresponsive on the floor and the waste can on fire. Which is her most appropriate response?

① Drag the client from the bathroom and close the door.
② Activate the fire alarm located outside the client's room.
③ Move the waste can to the shower and turn the shower on.
④ Call for help from other staff members.

12.7 During a cardiac assessment, where should the nurse place the stethoscope to accurately evaluate the aortic heart sound?

① the second intercostal space right of the sternum
② the second intercostal space left of the
③ the fifth intercostal space at the left mid-clavicular line
④ the third intercostal space right of the sternum

12.8 A nurse observes another nurse contaminate a Foley catheter. An appropriate nursing action would be to:

① report the incident to the supervisor.
② clean the catheter with Betadine and continue with procedure.
③ ignore the incident.
④ offer to assist and get another sterile catheter.

12.9 The client is returning from surgery with a chest tube after a lobectomy. Select all the equipment that should be at the bedside for this client.

① Clamp
② Sterile gauze
③ Sterile gloves
④ IV cut-down tray
⑤ Suction equipment

12.10 While performing an electrocardiogram (ECG), which of the interventions would be most appropriate to implement?

① Use alcohol or acetone pads on the client's fleshy areas and secure electrodes.
② Have the client lie in the Semi-Fowler's position for the procedure.
③ Encourage client to breathe deeply during procedure.
④ If client has excess hair on his chest, shave the area, rub area with alcohol, and dry it before placing the electrodes.

12.11 During suctioning of a client with an endotracheal tube, the heart rate decreases from 100 to 50 beats per minute. What would be the priority nursing action?

① Continue suctioning client.
② Administer epinephrine to increase the HR.
③ Stop procedure and evaluate the breath sounds.
④ Discontinue the procedure and reconnect client to the ventilator.

12.12 In evaluating the effectiveness of teaching a client with a permanent-demand pacemaker, the client should state that feelings of fainting, dizziness and a slow irregular pulse most likely indicate:

① failure of the pacemaker battery.
② competition between the heart and the pacemaker.
③ occurrence of pericardial tamponade.
④ a rejection of the foreign body.

12.13 In preparing for a traumatic wound debridement, what intervention would be most appropriate?

① Pack the wound with Betadine soaks prior to debridement.
② Prior to procedure, clean wound with alcohol.
③ Irrigate wound in preparation for debridement with 10 psi.
④ Pack the wound with gauze pads soaked in normal saline solution until debridement.

12.14 The nurse indicates she has an appropriate understanding of prioritizing her workload when she implements which client's plan of care first?

① A 7-year-old in a sickle cell crisis
② An 8-year-old admitted for shunt revision
③ A 17-year-old with a fractured femur
④ A 20-year-old with pelvic inflammatory disease

12.15 What would be the best flow rate of O_2 for a client with COPD?

① 2 liters per minute.
② 5 liters per minute.
③ 6 liters per minute.
④ 9 liters per minute.

12.16 Which parameter most affects the accuracy of a measurement made on a pulse oximeter?

① Hypothermia
② Irritability
③ Oxygen intake
④ Digit used

12.17 A thirty-five-year-old client is being monitored for increased intracranial pressure after sustaining a closed head injury. An arterial blood gas is performed on the client, and the results include a $PaCO^2$ of 33 mm Hg. It is most important for the nurse to:

① Advise the provider of care that the client needs supplemental oxygen.
② Auscultate the client's lungs and suction if indicated.
③ Document the results from the procedure and continue to monitor for signs of increasing intracranial pressure.
④ Encourage the client to decrease his breathing rate.

12.18 Which of these assessments would be a priority for the nurse to report to the physician 6 hours after a cast has been applied to the left leg?

① The pedal pulse is stronger on the left foot.
② The left foot is cool to touch.
③ There is an alteration in the sensation to the left foot.
④ The capillary refill to the toes is less than 2 seconds.

12.19 On the fourth postoperative day after GI surgery, the nurse assesses a client shaking, diaphoretic, with a temperature of 103.6°F. The physician is called for antibiotic orders. The most important assessment the nurse would want now is:

① client's weight.
② vital signs.
③ blood and urine cultures.
④ neurological evaluation.

12.20 After evaluating the circulation in an arm in a cast, which assessment requires physician notification?

① Apical pulse of 88
② Tingling, cold fingers
③ Lack of cooperativeness by the client
④ Warm fingers with an alteration in capillary refill

12.21 While evaluating a quality indicator of client room placement, which of the following client transfers from the medical/surgical units to the maternity unit would indicate the nurses know how to safely manage room placement for clients?

   ① A client with rubella
   ② A client with chronic hepatitis B
   ③ A client with RSV
   ④ A client with systemic lupus erythematosus

12.22 A client is to undergo an emergency appendectomy. Which assessment would be a priority before the anesthesia is administered?

   ① Location, intensity, and duration of the pain
   ② Last time client ate any solid food
   ③ Evaluation of vital signs
   ④ History of previous surgeries

12.23 A 30-hour-old newborn begins to exhibit a high-pitched cry, irritability, diarrhea, sneezing, and frequent tremors. The priority assessment by the nurse is to evaluate for:

   ① history of maternal drug abuse.
   ② newborn sepsis.
   ③ cardiac arrhythmias.
   ④ maternal sepsis.

12.24 Which nursing plan would be the highest priority for a client after a grand mal seizure?

   ① Elevate the head of the bed.
   ② Place an oxygen mask on the client.
   ③ Report the characteristics and the length of the seizure.
   ④ Administer valium IV push.

12.25 Which nursing action has the highest priority in preparing a sterile field?

   ① Place the field below the waist.
   ② Face the sterile field.
   ③ Position drape prior to applying gloves.
   ④ Reapply gloves after opening equipment.

12.26 A nurse through restraints uses physical force to prevent departure of the client. This is an example of:

   ① false imprisonment
   ② malpractice
   ③ negligence
   ④ coercion

12.27 A radium implant is found in the bed of a client who is being treated for cervical cancer. The appropriate plan for the nurse to include in her care is:

   ① reposition the implant immediately in the cervix with the physician's assistance.
   ② remove it from the bed and discard in the unit's biohazardous materials container.
   ③ remove it from the bed using tongs, discard in the biohazardous materials container in the room, and notify Radiology.
   ④ remove it from the room after notifying the physician.

12.28 The nurse has administered sublingual nitroglycerin (Nitrostat) to a client complaining of chest pain. Which observation is most important for the nurse to report to the next shift?

   ① The client indicates a need to urinate frequently.
   ② Blood pressure has decreased from 140/80 to 98/62.
   ③ Respiratory rate has increased from 16 to 24.
   ④ The client indicates the chest pain has subsided.

12.29 A client was admitted for regulation of her insulin. She takes 15 units of Humulin N insulin at 8:00 a.m. every day. At 4:00 p.m., which nursing observation would indicate a complication due to the insulin?

   ① Acetone odor to breath, polyuria, and flushed skin
   ② Irritability, tachycardia., and diaphoresis
   ③ Headache, nervousness, and polydipsia
   ④ Tenseness, tachycardia, and anorexia.

12.30 After abdominal surgery, a client is admitted from the recovery room with intravenous fluid infusing wide open. He receives 850 cc in less than 60 minutes. Which observation would indicate a problem?

   ① CVP reading of 12 and bradycardia
   ② Tachycardia and hypotension
   ③ Dyspnea and oliguria
   ④ Rales and tachycardia

12.31 During the initial assessment of a client with myxedema, the nurse would carefully observe for which symptoms?

   ① Tachycardia, fatigue, and intolerance to heat
   ② Polyphagia, nervousness, and dry hair
   ③ Lethargy, weight gain, and intolerance to cold
   ④ Tachycardia, hypertension, and tachypnea

12.32 An 80-year-old client is admitted with a possible fractured right hip. During the initial nursing assessment, which of the following observations of the right leg would validate or support this diagnosis?

   ① The leg appears shortened, is abducted, and externally rotated.
   ② Plantar flexion is observed with sciatic pain occurring down the leg.
   ③ From the hip, the leg appears longer and is externally rotated.
   ④ There is evidence of paresis with decreased sensation and limited mobility.

12.33 Which of the following instructions given to the client taking warfarin sodium (Coumadin) indicate the nurse is negligent? Client is instructed to:

   ① notify provider of care if stool becomes tarry.
   ② eat a diet high in green leafy vegetables.
   ③ return to the clinic for periodic blood tests.
   ④ discontinue taking ginseng while taking Coumadin.

12.34 A client develops acute renal failure and is on continuous peritoneal dialysis. Which assessment finding would indicate the most common complication associated with this procedure?

   ① Hypotension
   ② Hypertension
   ③ Pruitis
   ④ Bradycardia

12.35 A client is admitted for a series of tests to verify the diagnosis of Cushing's syndrome. Which assessment findings would support this diagnosis?

   ① Buffalo hump, hyperglycemia, and hypernatremia
   ② Nervousness, tachycardia, and intolerance to heat
   ③ Lethargy, weight gain, and intolerance to cold
   ④ Renal calculi, lethargy, and constipation

12.36 Which reflex would be abnormal to observe in a 6-month-old child?

   ① Presence of a positive Babinski reflex
   ② Extrusion reflex occurs when feeding.
   ③ Able to voluntarily grasp objects
   ④ Rolls from abdomen to back at will.

12.37 A client is admitted to the emergency room with a gunshot wound in the chest and in severe respiratory distress. Which nursing action has the highest priority when managing the emergency?

   ① Establish and maintain an open airway.
   ② Start cardiopulmonary resuscitation.
   ③ Initiate oxygen therapy.
   ④ Obtain an arterial blood gas.

12.38 A toddler admitted with an elevated blood lead level is to be treated with intramuscular injections of calcium disodium edentate (EDTA) and dimercaprol (BAL). Which nursing action would have the highest priority?

   ① Keep a tongue blade at the bedside.
   ② Encourage the child to participate in play therapy.
   ③ Apply cool soaks to the injection site.
   ④ Rotate the injection site.

12.39 Which assessment finding would indicate gentamycin (Garamycin) toxicity?

   ① Decreased hearing
   ② Blurred vision
   ③ Nausea and vomiting
   ④ Macular rash

12.40 Which assessment would document an allergic blood transfusion reaction?

   ① Hypotension
   ② Chills
   ③ Respiratory wheezing
   ④ Lower back discomfort.

12.41 Prior to administering Atenolol (Tenormin) and digoxin (Lanoxin), which assessment would be most important to report and document?

   ① Bradycardia
   ② Tachycardia
   ③ Hypertension
   ④ Serum potassium – 3.8 meg/l

12.42 A client is admitted to the outpatient oncology unit for his routine chemotherapy transfusion. His current lab report is WBC 2500/mm³, RBC 5.1 x 10⁶/mm³, and calcium 5 mEq/L. Which nursing diagnosis would be the priority? A potential for:

    ① fatigue related to decrease in red cells.
    ② infection related to low white cell count.
    ③ anxiety secondary to hypoparathyroid disease.
    ④ fluid volume deficit due to decreased fluid intake materials.

12.43 A urinalysis has been done on a client who has been complaining of dysuria, urinary frequency, and discomfort in the suprapubic area. After evaluation the results, the nurse would order a repeat urinalysis based on:

    ① negative glucose.
    ② RBCs present.
    ③ no WBCs or RBCs reported.
    ④ specific gravity 1.018.

12.44 In planning care for a client in Buck's traction, the nurse would:

    ① turn the client every two hours to the unaffected side.
    ② maintain client in a supine position.
    ③ encourage client to use a bedside commode.
    ④ prevent foot drop by placing a foot board to the bed.

12.45 Which assignment would be most appropriate for the nursing assistant?

    ① Doing a sterile dressing change on a 60-year-old male admitted for skin grafts.
    ② Obtaining a temperature on a 70-year-old client receiving the final 40 minutes of a blood transfusion.
    ③ Assisting a client newly diagnosed with a CVA to eat his dinner.
    ④ Completing the initial vital signs on an 80-year-old who has just returned to her room after having abdominal surgery.

12.46 The primary goal of nursing interventions for a client who has Multiple Sclerosis with a progressive disability should be to:

    ① maintain a cheerful, positive outlook.
    ② remain physically active and independent.
    ③ maintain good personal hygiene.
    ④ remain in a quiet environment to decrease stimuli.

12.47 A client is admitted to the emergency room after an acute asthmatic attack. Vital signs on admission include:
    • Pulse 98
    • Respiratory rate 40 with substernal retracting.
Immediate care by the nurse should include placing the client in which position?

    ① High Fowler's
    ② Supine position
    ③ Trendelenburg
    ④ Sim's position

12.48 A 19-year-old client is seen in the emergency room for an overdose of acetylsalicylic acid (Aspirin). Which plan represents correct care in the Emergency Room?

    ① If aspirin was ingested within the last two hours, administer activated charcoal powder.
    ② Initiate an intravenous infusion and administer Protamine sulfate.
    ③ Since aspirin overdose will cause bleeding, Vitamin K (AquaMephyton) should be given.
    ④ Obtain an arterial blood gas and request respiratory therapy to begin respiratory support.

12.49 Which client condition may precipitate a toxic reaction to Phenytoin (Dilantin)?

    ① Impaired liver function
    ② Decreased hemoglobin and hematocrit
    ③ White blood count of 10,000/mm³ and serum sodium of 140 mEq/L
    ④ Depressed neurological functioning.

12.50 An infant is admitted for vomiting and diarrhea. The anterior fontanelle is depressed and a fever of 103.2°F is noted. Which plan would be most appropriate initially to assist with rehydration?

① Determine daily weights and evaluate weight loss.
② Evaluate child's ability to take in fluids.
③ Place a full bottle of Pedialyte at bedside.
④ Start an intravenous infusion.

12.51 The best action while assisting the physician with the spinal tap on a 4-month-old would be to:

① restrain the child appropriately.
② instruct parents about procedure.
③ provide support to the child.
④ elevate the head of the bed.

12.52 After abdominal surgery, a client has a nasogastric tube to low suctioning. The client becomes nauseated, and the nurse observed a decrease in the flow of gastric secretions. Which nursing intervention would be most appropriate?

① Irrigate the nasogastric tube with distilled water.
② Aspirate the gastric contents with a syringe.
③ Administer an antiemetic medication.
④ Insert a new nasogastric tube.

12.53 Which teaching would be appropriate regarding wearing anti-embolism stockings following surgery?

① Wear them when legs are cramping.
② Wear them the entire time client is in the hospital.
③ Put stockings on in the evening prior to going to bed.
④ Put stockings on after client has been out of bed and walked around.

12.54 A child is in Bryant's traction. During the neurovascular assessment, the nurse notes that the foot of the uninjured leg feels warmer to touch than that of the broken leg. What action should the nurse implement now?

① Recognize that as long as the foot of the injured leg is warm to touch, circulation is doing well.
② Encourage child to move his foot by playing a toe-moving game with him.
③ Cover the colder foot with a sock and check its temperature in one hour.
④ Recognize that the strapping may be too snug and notify the physician.

12.55 The nurse would administer AquaMephyton (Vitamin K) to a neonate by:

① an injection into the vastus lateralis.
② mixing it in the formula.
③ drops into the inner canthus.
④ subcutaneously into the anterior thigh

12.56 Which plan would be a priority in an emergency wound evisceration?

① Maintain moisture to the wound.
② Start an IV and begin antibiotics.
③ Keep a sterile dressing over the wound.
④ Irrigate the wound with normal saline.

12.57 During chemotherapy of an outpatient who is lethargic, weak, and pale, which intervention would be most important for the nurse to implement?

① Establish emotional support.
② Position for physical comfort.
③ Maintain respiratory isolation.
④ Hand washing prior to care

12.58 Which response to mannitol (Osmitrol) is desired for decreasing the intracranial pressure of a client with a closed head injury?

① The blood pressure increases to 150/90.
② Urinary output increases to 175 cc/hour.
③ Decrease in the level of activity
④ Absence of fine tremors of the fingers

12.59 A 28-year-old client, gravida 2, para 1, in her third trimester of pregnancy has had diabetes since age 12. Which statement made by the client indicates an understanding regarding the insulin requirements during the third trimester?

   ① "I cannot continue to exercise as this will increase my insulin needs."
   ② "I understand my insulin requirements will increase as my pregnancy progresses."
   ③ "Since the baby has a normal pancreas, my insulin needs will not change."
   ④ "The more weight I gain, the more insulin I will need to take."

12.60 Which observation indicates the client has an understanding of appropriate crutch walking?

   ① Weight bearing is under the arm on the axillary area.
   ② The crutches are placed about 18–20 inches in front of him with each step.
   ③ The weight of the body is being transferred to the hands and the arms.
   ④ Leather sole shoes are worn to increase the smooth motion across the floor.

12.61 Which statement would indicate a need for further teaching for a client discharged on warfarin sodium (Coumadin)?

   ① "I need to observe my bowel movements for blood."
   ② "I am going to return for periodic blood tests."
   ③ "I will need to use an electric razor for shaving."
   ④ "I understand I need to decrease my sodium intake."

12.62 A client is currently hospitalized with renal failure and has 3+ pitting edema of the lower extremities. Which nursing observation would indicate a therapeutic response to therapy for the edema?

   ① Potassium level of 4.0 mEq/L.
   ② Serum glucose of 140 mg/dL.
   ③ Increased specific gravity of the urine
   ④ Weight loss of 5 lbs. over last 2 days.

12.63 Several days after a myocardial infarction, a client was placed on a 2 Gm sodium diet. Which selection would indicate compliance with the diet?

   ① Scrambled egg, orange slices and milk
   ② Instant oatmeal, toast, and orange juice
   ③ Poached egg, bacon, and milk
   ④ Biscuit, fruit cup, and sausage.

12.64 Which heart sound is indicative of ventricular overload and poor contractility?

   ① S1
   ② S2
   ③ S3
   ④ S4

12.65 Which would be most responsible for prolonging wound healing in the older client?

   ① Depression
   ② Increased social contacts
   ③ An increase in the adipose tissue
   ④ An intake of 20 to 35 g. of fiber per day

12.66 In the immediate postoperative period, which nursing assessment would be a priority in a client with a pneumonectomy?

   ① Presence of breath sounds bilaterally
   ② Position of trachea in sternal notch
   ③ Amount and consistency of sputum
   ④ An increase in the pulse pressure

12.67 The most important assessment the nurse must do on a primipara in early labor with ruptured membranes is:

   ① determine the pH of the amniotic fluid.
   ② evaluate the mother's blood pressure.
   ③ with the next contraction, check the monitor for an early deceleration.
   ④ observe the perineal area for evidence of a prolapsed cord.

12.68 Which diet selections should be included in the teaching plan of the client with osteoporosis?

   ① Steak and baked potato
   ② A glass of skim milk and a toasted cheese sandwich
   ③ Chicken and salad
   ④ Fish and French fries

12.69 A client is in labor and is receiving magnesium sulfate IV. Which assessment is most important to report to the nurse on the next shift?

①   Respiratory rate change from 13/min. to 15/min.
②   Increase in anxiety and hyperactivity
③   Presence of nausea and refusal to take clear liquids
④   Urine output change from 60 cc/hr to 40 cc/hr

12.70 A child is requiring resuscitation secondary to a respiratory arrest. Which route would be most appropriate for the nurse to administer the epinephrine?

①   IV
②   Endotracheal
③   Intradermal
④   Subcutaneous

12.71 Which action would be of highest priority when starting an intravenous line on a client admitted to the ER?

①   Put gloves on prior to beginning the procedure.
②   Wear a gown during the procedure.
③   Wash hands vigorously after the procedure.
④   Put on gloves, gown, and mask prior to approaching client.

12.72 A baby is born with a meningomyelocele. Prior to surgery, which nursing action has the highest priority?

①   Protect the sac from injury.
②   Encourage parental bonding.
③   Prevent contracture.
④   Provide tactile stimuli.

12.73 In the crowded hospital cafeteria, a nurse overhears a nursing assistant openly discussing a client with her peers. Which nursing action would have the highest priority?

①   Report the nursing assistant's behavior to the Director of Nursing.
②   Complete an incident report regarding the behavior.
③   Discuss with the nursing assistant the importance and implications of client confidentiality.
④   Report the incident to the evening charge nurse.

12.74 The charge nurse is making the morning assignment for a group of clients including several who are HIV positive, or who have AIDS. There are 3 unlicensed nursing assistants to assist with morning care. One of the nursing assistants states: "I am not going to take care of anyone who has AIDS." What is the best nursing action for the charge nurse to take regarding the assignment of the morning?

①   Tell the nursing assistant that when she was hired she was advised about HIV positive clients, and she does not have a choice in the type of assignments she receives.
②   Respect the nursing assistant's request and assign all of the HIV positive clients to the other two nursing assistants.
③   Determine what type of education the nursing assistant received regarding standard precautions, and evaluate her ability to follow the precautions.
④   Discuss with the nursing assistant in private that it is necessary for her to provide care to these clients and attempt to determine the source of fear.

12.75 What information is important for the nurse to explain to the mother whose child has been discharged on Tylenol?

①   Acetaminophen is the generic name for Tylenol; any acetaminophen product in the children's strength is okay for her to use.
②   The mother may purchase Tylenol in the children's or infant's strength for her child.
③   Determine if the mother has any acetaminophen at home either in the adult strength or in the children's strength for her child.
④   Tylenol is the generic name for the brand names of Advil or Motrin. Either of these in the children's strength may be used.

12.76 What would be most important to have at the bedside of a 36-month-old client with a fever of 103.4°F, respirations at 49/min. with suprasternal retractions present, drooling, and an enlarged epiglottis?

①   Defibrillator
②   Tracheostomy set-up
③   Tongue blade
④   IVAC pump

12.77 A client is given his Aminophylline (Somophyllin) capsule 4 hours too early. This incident is discovered 30 minutes after administration. Which plan would be the most appropriate?

① Document the event on an incident report, and notify the physician.
② Change time for next medication administration.
③ Assess for bradycardia and lethargy, and notify physician.
④ Skip the next dose of medication.

12.78 A client at 38 weeks gestation is admitted in active labor. The nursing assessment reveals a decreased blood pressure to 90/50 and the FHR is 130 and regular. Which nursing action would be most important?

① Call the physician and advise him of the decrease in blood pressure.
② Elevate the head of the bed to facilitate respirations.
③ Check the client's blood pressure and FHT every 30 minutes for the next 2 hours.
④ Place the client on her left side and reevaluate the blood pressure.

12.79 The client has an order for IV fluid of D5.2 normal saline, 1000 cc to run from 9 a.m. to 9 p.m. The drip factor on the delivery tubing is 15 gtts/cc. The nurse would adjust the IV to infuse at what rate?

① 21 gtt/min.
② 12 gtt/min.
③ 25 gtt/min.
④ 31 gtt/min.

12.80 After a right radical mastectomy, which position would be the most appropriate for a client?

① Left side with right arm protected in a sling
② Right side with right arm elevated
③ Semi-Fowler's position with right arm elevated
④ Prone position with right arm elevated

12.81 Which nursing assessment would be a priority for an elderly client who is very confused and disoriented when admitted from a long-term care facility?

① Determine level of mobility regarding safe walking.
② Evaluate teeth and determine appropriate diet.
③ Determine if a family member can remain at bedside.
④ Assess the respiratory status and evaluate for hypoxia.

12.82 A client is admitted to the Emergency Room with second and third-degree burns to the anterior chest, both arms, and right leg. Priority information to determine at the time of admission would include:

① percentage of burned surface area.
② amount of IV fluid necessary for fluid resuscitation.
③ any evidence of heat inhalation or airway problems.
④ circumstances surrounding the burn and contamination of the area.

12.83 Which nursing action is correct regarding the initial infusion of oxytocin (Pitocin)?

① Mix Pitocin in D_5W, begin at 5 mg/cc as primary IV to gravity flow.
② Decrease the rate/flow of Pitocin if fetal heart rate is below 150.
③ Piggyback the Pitocin into mainline IV and maintain flow by gravity.
④ Start an IV line and piggyback the Pitocin with an infusion pump.

12.84 The nurse is caring for a client who vigorously follows several rituals daily, including frequent hand-washing. The client's hands are now reddened and sensitive to touch. Which nursing action would be least helpful initially?

① Provide special skin care.
② Give positive reinforcement for nonritualistic behavior.
③ Limit the amount of time the client may use to wash hands.
④ Protect the client from ridicule by other clients on the unit.

12.85 A client is admitted for a total abdominal hysterectomy. When you give her the operative consent, she refuses to sign it. Which documentation in the chart would be appropriate?

① The surgeon was notified and stated he would return to speak with the client.
② The client was informed about the importance of signing the consent, and she should call the physician.
③ The husband was notified and gave a telephone consent.
④ The operating room was notified and surgery was canceled.

12.86 During a well-baby check-up on a 6-month-old, what would the nurse expect on assessment?

① Pincer grasp
② Sit with support
③ Birth weight tripled
④ Presence of the posterior fontanelle

12.87 Which nursing assessment would be indicative of a positive tuberculin skin test reaction?

① Induration of 10 mm at the site
② A pruitic rash of 5 mm at the site
③ High fever and congested cough
④ Erythema and inflammation at the site

12.88 To assess the right middle lobe (RML) of the lung, the nurse would auscultate at which location?

① Posterior and anterior base of right side
② Right anterior chest between the fourth and sixth intercostal
③ Left of the sternum, midclavicular at fifth intercostal space
④ Posterior chest wall, midaxillary right side

12.89 1000 cc. 5% dextrose in .45 saline is to be administered IV over 8 hours using an infusion pump for an adult client. What is the correct rate setting on the IV infusion pump?

① 125 cc/hr.
② 32 gtt/min.
③ 100 cc/hr.
④ 250 gtt/hr.

12.90 The parents of a newborn with a meningocele have been grieving the loss of their perfect child. After 3 days of grieving, progress in their emotional status would be indicated by which comment made by the parents?

① "When will it be safe for us to hold our baby?"
② "We would rather you feed our baby."
③ "What did we do to cause this problem?"
④ "When do you anticipate our baby going home?"

12.91 The nurse is assigned to work with the parents of a retarded child. With regard to the parents, which nursing action would be included in the care plan?

① Need to interpret the grieving process for the parents.
② Discuss the reality of institutional placement.
③ Assist the parents in making decisions and long-term plans for the child.
④ Perform a family assessment to assist

12.92 Which statement made by the client indicates a correct understanding of patient-controlled epidural analgesia (PCA)?

① "If I start feeling drowsy, I should notify the nurse."
② "This button will give me enough to kill the pain whenever I want it."
③ "If I start itching, I need to call the nurse."
④ "This medicine will make me feel no pain."

12.93 A woman being evaluated for infertility is given clomiphene citrate (Clomid) 50 mg daily to take for 5 days. She asks the nurse the purpose of the medicine. The nurse should instruct her that the action of clomiphene citrate (Clomid) is to:

① induce ovulation by changing the hormone effects on the ovary.
② change the uterine lining to be more conducive to implantation.
③ alter the vaginal pH to increase sperm motility.
④ produce multiple pregnancies for those who desire twins.

12.94 During the initial prenatal visit, the physician orders an iron supplement to be taken throughout the client's pregnancy. What information would be important for the nurse to tell the client regarding the iron?

  ① The medication should be taken with orange juice.
  ② Take the medication with antacids to decrease gastric distress.
  ③ Drinking 8 ounces of water will enhance absorption of the medication.
  ④ Notify the physician if stools become dark or loose.

12.95 A client with Addison's disease has been placed on Prednisone (Deltasone). Which comment by the client would indicate an understanding of how to take the medication?

  ① "I should take the medication one hour before meals."
  ② "It is important to take the medication with my meals."
  ③ "I will take the medication on an empty stomach."
  ④ "I will not drink milk right after I take my medicine."

12.96 A client has an order for a low sodium, low cholesterol diet. Which selection would reflect the client's compliance?

  ① Vegetable soup, applesauce, and hot chocolate
  ② Cheeseburger, French fries, and milk
  ③ Tomato and lettuce salad, and roasted chicken
  ④ Tuna fish sandwich, cottage cheese, and a coke

12.97 Which statement made by a client indicates a correct understanding of the care for an ileostomy?

  ① "I will not irrigate my ileostomy."
  ② "I will change the skin appliance very day."
  ③ "I will need to decrease my fluid intake."
  ④ "I will apply a cream around my stoma."

12.98 Which evaluation would indicate a therapeutic response to volume replacement in hypovolemic shock?

  ① Urine output increased to 50 cc per hour.
  ② Blood glucose of 180, serum potassium of 4.0 mEq/L.
  ③ CVP of 5 cm water, pupils equal and reactive
  ④ Pulse rate of 110 with no arrhythmias

12.99 A postoperative client has returned to his room from the surgical recovery area. The client is sleeping and is disoriented when aroused. Nursing actions to promote this client's safety would include:

  ① placing the call bell within the client's reach.
  ② staying with the client until totally oriented.
  ③ restraining all four extremities until client is oriented.
  ④ placing the side rails up until the client is fully awake.

12.100 The nurse is assessing an infant who is postoperative for repair of a cleft lip and palate. The respiratory assessment reveals the infant to have upper airway congestion and slightly labored respirations. Which nursing action would be most appropriate?

  ① Elevate the head of the bed.
  ② Suction the infant's nose.
  ③ Position the infant on his side.
  ④ Administer oxygen until breathing is easier.

12.101 Which assessment would indicate a client is disoriented? The client:

  ① cannot provide the name of her physician.
  ② is unable to list her current medications.
  ③ does not know where she is or what day it is.
  ④ asks repeatedly to be allowed to go home.

12.102 An unaccompanied client, who is six months pregnant, is admitted to the nursing unit with vaginal bleeding. Which comment made by the client would indicate a need for the nurse to assess the adequacy of the client's emotional support?

  ① "My husband will be so angry with me if I lose this baby."
  ② "I'm afraid I am going to lose my baby."
  ③ "I can't stay here. I don't have any insurance."
  ④ "I feel so guilty. I didn't want to get pregnant."

12.103 On a home health visit, an elderly client states, "This neighborhood has really gone down. I feel like a prisoner in my own home with all the trouble out there." Which nursing response would be best?

① "Have you and your neighbors formed a Neighborhood Watch?"
② "It must be very difficult for you to live in this neighborhood."
③ "I see a lot of police cars. You should be pretty safe."
④ "Tell me what has happened to make you feel that you are not safe."

12.104 A client is experiencing septic shock and the provider wants dosing of medications to be regulated so that a mean arterial pressure (MAP) between 65 and 75 mm Hg is maintained. Which of the client's blood pressure readings meet this goal?

① 135/90
② 125/80
③ 115/70
④ 105/60

12.105 The evening nurse on the psychiatric unit observed a client crying in her room following a visit from her physician. Which nursing documentation would be the most appropriate regarding this observation?

① Depressed following visit with the physician
② Appeared depressed after the visit from Dr. Brown
③ Crying in her room following Dr. Brown's visit
④ Upset with the physician after his visit

12.106 Prior to pushing any IV drugs during a "code blue," which assessment would be mandatory for safe care?

① Review the orders with the chart.
② Inspect the IV site for infiltration.
③ Evaluate the peripheral pulses.
④ Flush with dextrose between drugs.

12.107 A newly widowed, elderly client has been hospitalized following a suicide attempt. Which behavior most clearly indicates the client remains a suicide risk?

① He admits having vague suicidal ideas in the past.
② His history indicated difficulty forming relationships with caregivers.
③ He becomes emotional and cries when talking about his late wife.
④ He begins to give away some of his most prized possessions.

12.108 The nurse is caring for a client who is one day postoperative for a thoracotomy. Nursing actions on the care plan include:

① promoting ventilation and prevent respiratory acidosis.
② increasing oxygenation and removal of secretions.
③ increasing pH and facilitate balance of bicarbonate.
④ preventing respiratory alkalosis by increasing oxygenation.

12.109 Which nursing observation indicates a therapeutic response to the treatment for pneumonia?

① oral temperature of 101°F, increased chest pain with non-productive cough.
② cough productive of thick green sputum and complaints of feeling tired.
③ respirations at 20, no complaints of dyspnea, moderate amount of thin white sputum.
④ white cell count of 10,000/mm³, urine output at 40 cc/hour, decreasing amount of sputum.

12.110 The nurse is planning care for clients on a medical unit. Care needs to be provided for a pneumonia client and an AIDS client. Which plan represents the most appropriate assignments?

 ① The AIDS client and the pneumonia client should be assigned to one room with one nurse.
 ② The pneumonia and the AIDS client should be assigned to the same room, but assign the care to two different nurses.
 ③ The pneumonia and the AIDS client should be assigned to private rooms, and the care for both clients should be assigned to one nurse.
 ④ Both the pneumonia client and the AIDS client should have private rooms and care assigned to two different nurses.

12.111 In planning the diet teaching for a child in the early stages of nephritic syndrome, the nurse would discuss with the parents the following dietary changes:

 ① adequate protein intake, low sodium.
 ② low protein, low potassium.
 ③ low potassium, low calorie.
 ④ limited protein, high carbohydrate.

12.112 After a client is started on haloperidol (Haldol) 5 mg TID, which would be a priority for the nurse to discuss with the client?

 ① Stay away from foods high in tyramine.
 ② Move slowly to a standing position.
 ③ May experience a dry mouth
 ④ Limit salt intake.

12.113 Upon auscultation of a client's bowel sounds, the nurse notes soft gurgling sounds occurring every 5–20 seconds. This indicates:

 ① excessive intestinal motility.
 ② reduced intestinal peristalsis.
 ③ normal sounds.
 ④ rapid gastric emptying.

12.114 A client with chronic bronchitis is receiving supplemental oxygen via nasal cannula and orders state that the SpO_2 should be maintained at 90 percent or higher. During her nursing assessment, the nurse notices that the oxygen delivery is set at 7 liters per minute with an SpO_2 of 88 percent. The nurse should:

 ① Reduce the oxygen delivery to her no more than 2 liters per minute and stay with the client.
 ② Change the method of oxygen delivery to a simple mask or face tent.
 ③ Validate the SpO_2 value and further assess the client for possible causes of hypoxemia.
 ④ Investigate if the client, a significant other or a staff member set the oxygen at 7 liters.

12.115 After a client has returned to the floor from thyroidectomy surgery, which nursing intervention would have the highest priority?

 ① Monitor vital signs every four hours.
 ② Monitor for hemorrhaging by observing frequent swallowing.
 ③ Monitor signs of respiratory distress frequently.
 ④ Position client in supine position.

12.116 When assisting with a bone marrow aspiration, the nurse would plan to handle supplies by:

 ① handling additional supplies by dropping them onto a sterile tray.
 ② having all sterile packs unwrapped for the procedure in case needed.
 ③ reaching over the tray to remove contaminated supplies.
 ④ placing the bottle of sterile liquid on the sterile receptacle to avoid splashing.

12.117 Which is the best way for a nurse to determine the degree of edema in a limb?

 ① Estimate diameter of both limbs and compare.
 ② Depress skin and rank degree of pitting.
 ③ Describe swelling in affected area.
 ④ Pinch skin and note how quickly it returns to normal.

12.118 Before administering scheduled oral medications to a client following a bronchoscopy, which nursing assessment would be most important?

   ①   Auditory crackles and wheezes
   ②   Ability to cough and deep breathe
   ③   Bilateral thoracic expansion
   ④   Presence of a gag reflex

12.119 A client is admitted with the following symptoms: dependent pitting edema, abdominal distension, and a recent 10-lb. weight gain. The client has received 80 mg of furosemide (Lasix). Which nursing observation is most important to report to the next shift?

   ①   Complaining of nausea and vomiting
   ②   Urine output of 200 cc in 2 hours
   ③   Quiet and withdrawn behavior after lunch
   ④   Blood pressure was 160/90 and now is 140/90.

120.120 The nurse is caring for a client in labor. The nurse palpates a firm round form in the uterine fundus. On the client's right side, small parts are palpated, and on the left side, a long, smooth curved section is palpated. Which location should the nurse anticipate ausculating the fetal heart?

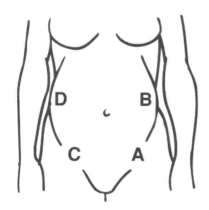

Category Analysis – Simulated Exam

1.	Safe Effective Care	28.	Pharmacology	55.	Pharmacology
2.	Fluid Gas	29.	Pharmacology	56.	Basic Care & Comfort
3.	Safe Effective Care	30.	Fluid-Gas	57.	Safe Effective Care
4.	Pharmacology	31.	Sensory-Perception-Mobility	58.	Pharmacology
5.	Pharmacology	32.	Sensory-Perception-Mobility	59.	Health Promotion
6.	Safe Effective Care	33.	Pharmacology	60.	Basic Care & Comfort
7.	Fluid-Gas	34.	Elimination	61.	Pharmacology
8.	Safe Effective Care	35.	Sensory-Perception-Mobility	62.	Fluid-Gas
9.	Safe Effective Care	36.	Health Promotion	63.	Nutrition
10.	Fluid Gas	37.	Fluid-Gas	64.	Fluid-Gas
11.	Fluid-Gas	38.	Pharmacology	65.	Psycho-Social
12.	Fluid-Gas	39.	Pharmacology	66.	Fluid-Gas
13.	Elimination	40.	Pharmacology	67.	Health Promotion
14.	Safe Effective Care	41.	Pharmacology	68.	Nutrition
15.	Fluid-Gas	42.	Safe Effective Care	69.	Pharmacology
16.	Fluid-Gas	43.	Elimination	70.	Pharmacology
17.	Sensory-Perception-Mobility	44.	Sensory-Perception-Mobility	71.	Fluid-Gas
18.	Sensory-Perception-Mobility	45.	Safe Effective Care	72.	Sensory-Perception-Mobility
19.	Safe Effective Care	46.	Sensory-Perception-Mobility	73.	Safe Effective Care
20.	Sensory-Perception-Mobility	47.	Fluid-Gas	74.	Safe Effective Care
21.	Safe Effective Care	48.	Pharmacology	75.	Pharmacology
22.	Elimination	49.	Pharmacology	76.	Fluid-Gas
23.	Sensory-Perception-Mobility	50.	Basic Care & Comfort	77.	Pharmacology
24.	Sensory-Perception-Mobility	51.	Sensory-Perception-Mobility	78.	Health Promotion
25.	Safe Effective Care	52.	Elimination	79.	Pharmacology
26.	Safe Effective Care	53.	Basic Care & Comfort	80.	Sensory-Perception-Mobility
27.	Safe Effective Care	54.	Sensory-Perception-Mobility	81.	Psycho-Social

82.	Fluid-Gas	95.	Pharmacology	108.	Fluid-Gas
83.	Pharmacology	96.	Nutrition	109.	Fluid-Gas
84.	Psycho-Social	97.	Elimination	110.	Safe Effective Care
85.	Safe Effective Care	98.	Fluid-Gas	111.	Nutrition
86.	Health Promotion	99.	Safe Effective Care	112.	Pharmacology
87.	Safe Effective Care	100.	Fluid-Gas	113.	Elimination
88.	Fluid-Gas	101.	Psycho-Social	114.	Fluid-Gas
89.	Fluid-Gas	102.	Psycho-Social	115.	Fluid-Gas
90.	Psycho-Social	103.	Health Promotion	116.	Safe Effective Care
91.	Psycho-Social	104.	Fluid-Gas	117.	Fluid-Gas
92.	Pharmacology	105.	Psycho-Social	118.	Fluid-Gas
93.	Pharmacology	106.	Pharmacology	119.	Fluid-Gas
94.	Nutrition	107.	Psycho-Social	120.	Safe Effective Care

Directions

1. Determine questions missed by checking answers.
2. Write the number of the questions missed across the top line marked "item missed."
3. Check category analysis page to determine category of question.
4. Put a check mark under item missed and beside content.
5. Count check marks in each row and write the number in totals column.
6. Use this information to:
   - identify areas for further study.
   - determine which content test to take next.

We recommend studying content where most items are missed—then taking that content test.

Number of the Questions Incorrectly Answered

Practice Exam	Items Missed																								Totals
C Safe Effective Care																									
O Health Promotion and Maintenance																									
N Psycho-Social Integrity																									
T Physiological Adaptation: Fluid Gas																									
E Reduction of Risk Potential: Sensory-Perception-Mobility																									
N Basic Care and Comfort: Elimination																									
T Physiological Adaptation: Nutrition																									
Pharmacological and Parenteral Therapies																									

Answers & Rationales

12.1 ①④ The client should be in airborne transmission-based precautions. Options #1 and #4 are correct for these precautions. Options #2 and #3 are not necessary. Option #5 is unsafe with varicella.

12.2 ② Option #2 is correct. These parts of the body would provide the most accurate reading for this value. Options #1, #3 and #4 are incorrect. For the answer to be correct, both body parts must be accurate.

12.3 ③④⑤⑥ Options #3, #4, #5, and #6 are appropriate for a client in droplet transmission-based precautions. Option #1 is appropriate for contact transmission-based precautions. Option #2 is incorrect. It would be correct for contact transmission-based precautions if clothing was going to have extensive contact with the client.

12.4 ①③⑤ Options #1, #3, and #5 are correct. Hydrochlorothiazide (HCTZ) is a thiazide diuretic that lowers the blood pressure by removing excess water from the blood. Lisinopril (Zestril) is an ACE inhibitor that lowers blood pressure by vasodilation. Atenolol, a beta antagonist, lowers the blood pressure by vasodilation and heart rate reduction. Simvastatin (Zocor), an antilipemic, and Nizatidine (Axid), a histamine antagonist, do not lower the blood pressure.

12.5 ② Option #2 is correct. Option #1 can occur with clients taking aluminum-based antacids. Option #3 can occur with many antibiotics and many other medications. Option #4 may occur with steroid inhalers.

12.6 ① Option #1 is correct. When confronted with a fire, the most important response from a nurse is to rescue the client. In order of priority, the proper responses are: 1) rescue; 2) alarm; 3) confine the fire; and 4) evacuate.

12.7 ① Option #1 is correct. Option #2 would be appropriate position to auscultate the pulmonic heart sound. Option #3 would be the appropriate location to auscultate the PMI. Option #4 is incorrect.

12.8 ④ This is being a client advocate. The observed nurse may need some assistance, and this would be an excellent opportunity to provide education regarding this procedure. Options #1 and #3 do not address the problem. Option #2 is unsafe practice and can lead to infection.

12.9 ①②③ Options #1, #2, and #3 are correct. Options #4 and #5 are not necessary for this procedure.

12.10 ④ Option #4 is correct. Alcohol or healer acetone pads in place of the electrode paste or gel may impair electrode contact with the skin and diminish the transmission quality of electrical impulses. Option #2—the client should be instructed to lie in a supine position. Option #3 is incorrect. Client should breathe normally.

12.11 ④ Option #4 is correct. The client is getting hypoxic and needs oxygen. Options #1 and #2 are incorrect. Option #1 is unsafe. Option #3 is partially correct. Stopping procedure is correct, but evaluating breath sounds is not a priority in this clinical situation over Option #4.

12.12 ① Battery failure will cause the pacemaker to be inoperable. The client may experience a heart block, or the signs presented in this situation. Pacing spikes will not occur if the pacemaker is not firing. Options #2, #3, and #4 are incorrect.

12.13 ④ Option #4 is correct. Option #1 is incorrect. Betadine is an inappropriate option. Option #2 is incorrect. Avoid using alcohol because it causes pain and tissue dehydration. Hydrogen peroxide may be used. The foaming action facilitates debris removal. However, peroxide should never be instilled into a deep wound because of the risk of embolism from evolving gases. Option #3 is incorrect when irrigating a traumatic wound. Avoid using more than 8 psi of pressure. High-pressure irrigation can seriously interfere with healing, kill healthy cells, and allow bacteria to infiltrate the tissue.

12.14 ① The sickle cell crisis would be a priority due to the need to start IV fluids for hydration purposes. The hypoxia must be corrected immediately with IV fluids and oxygen. Option #2 would only be a preparation prior to surgery. Options #3 and #4 are important but not priorities to Option #1.

12.15 ① Oxygen must be administered in low concentrations to maintain the stimulus to breathe. Increased oxygen levels decrease the stimulation to breathe which will result in CO_2 narcosis. Options #2, #3, and #4 are settings that are too high.

12.16 ① Hypothermia may result in vasoconstriction which will not provide an accurate reading. It is important to keep the digit and extremity warm. Though irritability will increase the oxygen demand, Option #2 is incorrect because the reading will remain accurate. Option #3 is incorrect because it is the parameter that is being evaluated. Option #4 is insignificant as long as the digit and extremity are kept warm.

12.17 ③ Option #3 is correct. A lower-than-normal $PaCO_2$ can actually benefit the client because it reduces intracranial pressure by preventing cerebral vasodilation. The results should be reported to the physician and monitoring for signs of increased intracranial pressure should continue. Option #1 is incorrect. There is no evidence that supplemental oxygen is needed. Option #2 is incorrect. There is no evidence that suction is indicated. Suctioning elevates intracranial pressure and therefore should be minimal. Option #4—instructing the client to slow his breathing rate is inappropriate because it could elevate the $PaCO_2$ which could increase intracranial pressure.

12.18 ③ Option #3 is the priority due to potential risk of compartmental syndrome. This is a sign of potential nerve involvement which can result in permanent damage. Option #1 presents no problem. Option #2 makes no comparison to the right foot. Option #4 is no problem.

12.19 ③ The problem is probably infection, and laboratory tests should be completed prior to antibiotic therapy. Options #1 and #4 are not specific to this case. Option #2 has already been evaluated.

12.20 ② This is indicative of an alteration in the circulation from the cast being too tight causing an unsafe evaluation that could result with the client losing part of his extremity. Option #1 is irrelevant. Option #3 is important, but is not the priority as Option #2. Option #4 is partially acceptable. The capillary refill can lead to Option #2. Therefore, Option #2 is the priority of concern with alteration in perfusion.

12.21 ④ Option #4 is correct. Options #1, #2, and #3 are dangerous for a maternity client since these diseases are communicable. Infection control is the priority concern here.

12.22 ② This is a priority due to the possibility of aspiration. While it is important to complete Options #1, #3, and #4, they are not a priority over Option #2.

12.23 ① This is the priority assessment since the signs of drug withdrawal are more frequently associated with central nervous system alterations, gastrointestinal disturbances, and tachypnea. Options #2, #3, and #4 are secondary.

12.24 ③ It is important to monitor the beginning, the behaviors during the seizure, and the duration of the seizure. This will assist the neurologist in determining a more specific location and cause of the seizures. Option #1 is incorrect because the client should be positioned on his side to facilitate the draining of oral secretions and minimize aspiration. Option #2 is incorrect since this is not an automatic protocol, and there is not enough data to substantiate this action. Option #4 is incorrect after the seizure is over.

12.25 ② Never turn the back to a sterile field. Maintain it above the level of the waist. Options #1, #3, and #4 are incorrect.

12.26 ① Option #1 is correct. False imprisonment is unlawful detention. Implied false imprisonment is the use of words, threats, or gestures to restrain client. An example of this is refusing to allow client to leave hospital until bill is paid or refusing to release newborn until bill is paid. Option #2—malpractice—is a professional practice which injures someone through failure to meet the proper standard of care. Option #3—negligence—is unintentional harm to another which occurs through failure to act in a reasonable and prudent manner. Option #4—coercion—is to accomplish something by force or threat.

12.27 ③ This is the safest plan for the radioactive material. Safety is a priority when dealing with implants—the client's, the nurse's, and the visitor's. Option #1 is inappropriate. Option #2 does not clarify how to remove it from the bed. Option #4 is incomplete and is unsafe for any radioactive material.

12.28 ② Hypotension is a significant side effect of nitroglycerin. While the effect may be transient, the client's blood pressure needs to be closely observed to assure that it does not continue to fall. Options #1 and #3 are not relevant to this medication. Option #4 is an expected outcome.

12.29 ② Humulin N insulin is an intermediate insulin that peaks from 8-12 hours after onset. This is when signs and symptoms of hypoglycemia occur. Options #1, #3, and #4 are signs of hyperglycemia.

12.30 ④ Rales and tachycardia would indicate a cardiovascular fluid overload. Option #1 is a normal CVP reading. Options #2 and #3 do not contain information relevant to fluid overload.

12.31 ③ These are signs and symptoms of hypo-function of the thyroid. Some other assessments would include dry hair, facial expression mask-like, thickened skin, enlarged tongue, and drooling. Options #1 and #4 contains signs of hyperfunction of the thyroid. Option #2 contains signs of hyperthyroidism.

12.32 ① These are accurate assessments of the position of a fractured hip prior to repair. Option #2 occurs with foot drop. Option #3 is incorrect because the leg will not appear longer. Option #4 occurs with injury to the lumbar disc area.

12.33 ② Option #2 is correct. Green, leafy vegetables are high in vitamin K, and this is the antidote for coumadin. Options #1, #3 and #4 are correct instructions. Option #1 would be indicative of bleeding. Option #3—client will need to have pT and/or INR evaluated. Option #4—Ginseng and coumadin will increase the risk for bleeding.

12.34 ① As with hemodialysis, hypotension is most likely to result from rapid removal of fluid from the intravascular space. Options #2, #3, and #4 are not complications associated with this procedure.

12.35 ① Cushing's Syndrome is characteristic of these assessments, as well as weight gain, moon-like face, purple striae, osteoporosis, mood swings, and high susceptibility to infections. Option #2 contains symptoms of hyperthyroidism. Option #3 contains symptoms of hypothyroidism. Option #4 includes symptoms of hyperparathyroidism.

12.36 ② The extrusion reflex disappears between 3-4 months of age. Option #1 disappears at approximately 1 year. Options #3 and #4 are normal occurrences at this age level.

12.37 ① The first action is to establish an airway. If there is no airway, any other resuscitation will not be helpful. Since the client hasn't had a cardiac arrest, Option #2 is inappropriate. Option #3 does not deal with the problem of the severe dyspnea. Option #4 is not a priority.

12.38 ④ The highest priority is to prevent tissue damage and promote tissue absorption of the medicine which is accomplished through rotation of the injection sites. Option #1 is ineffective. It is important to have seizure precautions and emergency respiratory equipment available. Option #2 is important to implement but is not a priority. Option #3 contains incorrect information.

12.39 ① Decreased hearing and vertigo occur as a result of involvement of the 8th cranial nerve which is caused from gentamycin (Garamycin) toxicity. Options #2, #3, and #4 are not toxic effects of this antibiotic.

12.40 ③ Allergic reaction is characterized by wheezing, urticaria (hives), facial flushing, and epiglottal edema. Options #1, #2, and #4 are indicative of a hemolytic transfusion reaction.

12.41 ① Option #1 is correct. When clients take beta blockers concurrently with cardiac glycoside and/or calcium channel blockers, there is an increased risk for bradycardia. Options #2, #3, and #4 are not correct for this situation. Option #4 is a therapeutic lab value.

12.42 ② Clients with a low WBC count are susceptible to infection. Option #1 contains incorrect information. The RBCs are not decreased. Option #3 is not correctly stated as a nursing diagnosis. Option #4 is a potential but not a priority.

12.43 ③ With the client complaints, WBCs and RBCs should not be present. WBCs are a response to the inflammation process and irritation of the urethra. RBCs are increased when the bladder mucosa is irritated and bleeding. Option #1 is not a primary component in determining urinary tract infections. Option #2 is not as complete a response as Option #3. Option #4 indicates the concentration of the urine for this specimen and is not specifically associated with a urinary tract infection.

12.44 ① Immobility is a leading cause of problems with Buck's traction. It is important to turn client to the unaffected side. Option #2 is incorrect because the head of the bed can be elevated 15 to 20 degrees since the supine position can increase problems with immobility. Option #3 is incorrect because the client is on strict bed rest. Option #4 would interfere with the traction.

12.45 ② Option #2 is correct since it is in final time of transfusion. Option #1 is not appropriate. Option #3 is newly diagnosed. Option #4 is initial and would be inappropriate.

12.46 ② The goal of care for this disease is to maintain independence as long as client is able. Options #1 and #3 are not primary goals, but are included in the care plan. Option #4 is inappropriate for this client.

12.47 ① This will facilitate maximum expansion of the lungs and will decrease the pulmonary workload. Options #2, #3, and #4 would not improve the quality of respirations and would increase client anxiety.

12.48 ① The charcoal, if given within two hours, will absorb the particles of salicylate. Option #2 is an antidote for Heparin. Option #3 is an antidote for warfarin (Coumadin). Option #4 may be necessary later after evaluating the response to charcoal.

12.49 ① Phenytoin (Dilantin) is metabolized and excreted by the liver. Elderly clients frequently have some degree of liver impairment and are a high risk for the toxic reaction. Options #2 and #3 are not affected by Dilantin. Option #4 is incorrect.

12.50 ② This will assist in determining if hydration can be done through oral fluids alone. Option #1 is done but is not to assist with rehydration. It evaluates rehydration. Option #3 does not solve the problem since it doesn't guarantee the child is taking fluids. Option #4 may be implemented later.

12.51 ① The safest objective is to prevent trauma to the child during the procedure so the child must be restrained. Option #2 would be done prior to obtaining consent and performing the procedure. Option #3 should be done before and/or after the procedure. Option #4 will not expose the spinal column of a 4-year-old.

12.52 ② The nurse should aspirate or inject a small amount of air while auscultating the rush of air over the epigastric area. Option #1 is incorrect because the tube would be irrigated with normal saline after the position of the tube was evaluated. Options #3 and #4 do not assess the status of the nasogastric tube.

12.53 ② The stockings should be worn the entire time the client is in the hospital. They should be removed with the bath and replaced after the skin is dry and prior to the client getting out of bed. Option #1 is incorrect because the stockings should be worn to prevent any discomfort and to increase the blood flow. Option #3 is incorrect because the stockings should be worn during the day and when the client is non-ambulatory. Option #4 is incorrect because the stockings should be applied prior to getting out of bed.

12.54 ④ The assessment indicates that the ace is too tight and it needs readjusting. Option #1 ignores the possibility of the ace being too tight. Options #2 and #3 do not relieve the circulation problem.

12.55 ① AquaMephyton (Vitamin K) is given in the vastus lateralis. Options #2, #3, and #4 are not correct routes of administration of this medication.

12.56 ① The priority is to maintain moisture to prevent the wound from drying out and becoming necrotic prior to returning to surgery. Option #2 is inappropriate. Option #3 needs to be moist in order to be correct. Option #4 needs to be continuous to be correct.

12.57 ④ Chemotherapy can lead to immunosuppression which predisposes the client to infection. Hand-washing is one of the most effective means of decreasing the infection transmission. Options #1 and #2 are appropriate but not a priority. Option #3 is not the correct isolation during chemotherapy.

12.58 ② Mannitol (Osmitrol) is an osmotic diuretic, thus increasing the urinary output. The diuresing effects facilitate the decrease in the intracranial pressure. Options #1, #3, and #4 are not indications of desired effects of the medication.

12.59 ② During both the second and third trimester, the need for insulin will increase due to insulin antagonism by the placental hormones. Option #1 is incorrect because the client is encouraged to continue to exercise. Option #3 is incorrect because the baby's pancreas is normal. However, the mother's insulin needs will increase. Option #4 is incorrect because weight gain in pregnancy and insulin needs do not correlate.

12.60 ③ The arms should be bent at 35 degree angle and weight should be placed on the hands and arms. Option #1 is incorrect because pressure placed on the axillae can damage the brachial plexus. Option #2 is incorrect because crutches should be placed 8-10 inches in front with each step. Option #4 is unsafe. Shoes should be non-slip soles.

12.61 ④ Sodium does not affect the action of Warfarin sodium (Coumadin) and indicates that the client has a misunderstanding. Options #1, #2, and #3 indicate an understanding of the potential side effect of hemorrhage. Coumadin is an anticoagulant. The client needs to return to be evaluated for any bleeding and have routine blood work done.

12.62 ④ Edema is a result of sodium and fluid retention. Weight loss should occur if therapy is effective. Options #1 and #2 do not relate to edema. Option #3 is inappropriate for this client.

12.63 ① All are low in sodium, and milk is allowed on a salt-restricted diet. Option #2 is incorrect because bacon is high in sodium. Option #4 is incorrect because all baked breads are high in sodium along with the sausage.

12.64 ③ S3 indicates congestive heart failure from ventricular overload and decreased muscle contractility. Options #1 and #2 are normal heart sounds and are not indicative of pathology. Option #4 would indicate hypertension.

12.65 ① Depression is a frequent cause of malnutrition in the older client. Psychological, sociological, and economic factors, chronic disease, and polypharmacy all contribute to the potential or actual problem of malnutrition which will prolong wound healing. Option #2 could be a contributing factor if said decrease in social contacts. Option #3 is a normal process with aging and is not responsible for prolonging wound healing unless it is an extreme increase. Option #4 is the recommendation from the American Cancer Association for dietary fiber. This may improve the intake of vitamins and minerals as well as being beneficial for glucose tolerance.

12.66 ② The position of the trachea should be evaluated. With a tracheal shift, an increase in pressure could occur in the operative side and cause pressure against the mediastinal area. Option #1 is incorrect because on the surgical side, breath sounds will be absent. Option #3 is important to observe, but not as high a priority as Option #2. Option #4 does not relate to the situation.

12.67 ④ The initial assessment is to check for a prolapsed cord. Option #1 is a useful assessment but inappropriate for this situation. It will determine if the fluid is urine (acidic) rather than amniotic fluid. Option #2 is incorrect because the mother's blood pressure is not affected by rupture of the membranes. Option #3 would read variable decelerations for a cord prolapse.

12.68 ② The calcium intake is important in minimizing the development of osteoporosis. Both of these contain calcium. The other options are not focused on calcium intake.

12.69 ④ Magnesium sulfate is a central nervous system depressant. A side effect is oliguria. Option #1 is not a concern because the respirations are increasing. Options #2 and #3 are not relevant for the medication.

12.70 ② The quickest and most effective route would be via endotracheal tube. Remember ELAIN to assist in recalling the drugs that can be given via the endotracheal tube (Epinephrine, Lidocaine, Atropine, Isuprel, and Narcan). Option #1 would be slower than Option #2 and the other distracters are incorrect.

12.71 ① The priority action is to put the gloves on prior to initiating any activity which would cause the nurse to come into contact with client's blood (universal precautions). Options #2 and #4 are unnecessary unless there is a high risk that blood is going to be splattered. Option #3 is always important in preventing infections but not as high a priority as Option #1.

12.72 ① Protecting the exposed sac to prevent infection and trauma is a priority. Options #2, #3, and #4 are correct, but not the highest priority.

12.73 ③ The nursing assistant needs to be re-educated about the importance of maintaining client confidentiality. Options #1, #2, and #4 are avoiding the current situation. If the behavior continues, then this must be communicated to a different level of authority.

12.74 ④ The charge nurse should discuss standard precautions (universal precautions) with the unit nursing assistant (UNA) and determine the nature of her problem. It may be easily solved with education, or the assistant may need to be transferred to another unit. Option #1 may cause the UNA to resign when she may be retrained. Option #2 does not show respect for other UNAs. Option #3 is not an issue.

12.75 ① The generic, children's-strength, acetaminophen is less expensive than the brand names (Tylenol) and may be used. Option #3, the mother should be instructed to use only the children's strength. The infant's strength of Tylenol is more concentrated. Option #4, acetaminophen, is not the generic name for Advil or Motrin. These are Ibuprofen.

12.76 ② An airway is a priority. Epiglottitis can cause a sudden total airway obstruction. Option #1 is not appropriate to this situation. Option #3 is incorrect because this client has airway problems, not a seizure problem, plus a padded tongue blade is no longer recommended. Option #4 is not specific for the potential emergency of airway obstruction.

12.77 ① Document the error on an incident report, assess for side effects, and notify the physician. Options #2 and #4 are unsafe, incorrect nursing interventions. Option #3 is incorrect information. Tachycardia and hyperactivity are signs of aminophylline overdose.

12.78 ④ The decrease in blood pressure is most likely due to pressure on the inferior vena cava which occurs in the supine position (vena-caval syndrome). By positioning the client on her side, the pressure is relieved and the blood pressure will increase. Option #1 may be necessary, but Option #4 should be done first. Option #2 does not address the problem of low blood pressure. Option #3 is incorrect because the problem needs to be addressed immediately.

12.79 ① The IV is to run in 12 hours, or 720 minutes. The formula is: volume to be infused is divided by 720 times 15. Another calculation may be used to determine the number of cc's per hour, then per minute and multiplied by the drip factor. Options #2, #3, and #4 are incorrect calculations.

12.80 ③ This position will facilitate the removal of fluid from the venous pathways and lymphatic system through gravity. The arm is elevated to enhance circulation and prevent edema. Option #1 is incorrect because a sling is not necessary; the arm needs to be elevated. Option #2 is incorrect because the right arm cannot be elevated from this position. Option #4 is incorrect because the prone position is inappropriate.

12.81 ④ The presence of hypoxia needs to be addressed immediately. The hypoxia also contributes to the confusion. Options #1, #2 and #3 are important to consider but are secondary to Option #4.

12.82 ③ The priority of care is to determine if any heat inhalation has occurred that would cause airway problems. Option #1 is secondary. Option #2 will be done as soon as Option #1 is completed. Option #4 will also be done, but Option #3 remains the priority.

12.83 ④ The Pitocin should always be a secondary infusion and the infusion controlled by an IV pump. Option #1 is incorrect because Pitocin should be a secondary infusion. Option #2 contains incorrect information. Normal range for fetal heart tones is 120 to 160 per minute. Option #3 is incorrect because the rate should be maintained by an infusion pump.

12.84 ③ Placing a limit on the ritual initially will only increase the client's anxiety and need for the rituals. Limits must be gradually instituted. Options #1, #2, and #4 are appropriate nursing actions.

12.85 ① The client and/or family must be informed about questions or concerns about the surgery prior to signing the consent. After notifying the physician, the physician's response should be documented. Options #2, #3, and #4 do not protect the client's rights.

12.86 ② A 6-month-old should sit with help. Option #1 is present at 9 months of age. Option 3 is present at 1 year. Option #4 is closed by 2-3 months.

12.87 ① A positive skin test is determined by the area of induration (raised) rather than the area of inflammation. This correctly describes a positive reaction to the skin test. Options #2 and #4 describe other types of inflammatory responses. Option #3 does not have anything to do with reading the skin test.

12.88 ② The RML is found right anterior between the fourth and sixth intercostal spaces. Options #1 and #4 are incorrect because the RML cannot be auscultated from the posterior. Option #3 is the point of maximum impulse or apical pulse.

12.89 ① Pump rates are always set in cc's per hour. 1000 cc divided by 8 hours equals 125 cc/hr. Option #2 is incorrect because there is not enough information to calculate gtts/min. Option #3 is in an incorrect calculation. Option #4 is too fast for any standard drop factor.

12.90 ① This comment indicates a desire to begin stroking and cuddling this baby. This must happen before parents can actually provide physical care. Option #2 indicates a fear or a sense of insecurity with the feedings. Option #3 indicates some feeling of guilt. Option #4 is a request for information and does not address the question.

12.91 ④ This will help the nurse know where the family is in regards to grieving, coping, etc. Options #1, #2, and #3 are inappropriate before the assessment. Actions can be taken only when the circumstances are known.

12.92 ③ A common side effect of narcotics used in epidural pain management is itching. Options #1 and #4 are incorrect. Option #2 may give false reassurance.

12.93 ① Clomiphene Citrate (Clomid) induces ovulation by altering the estrogen and stimulating follicular growth to produce a mature ovum. Options #2 and #3 are infertility problems, but Clomid does not affect them. Option #4 is not an appropriate use of the medication.

12.94 ① Vitamin C facilitates the absorption of iron. Option #2 is incorrect because antacids will decrease the absorption of the iron. Option #3 is incorrect because although the client needs increased fluids, fluids will not affect absorption. Option #4 is incorrect because dark stools are characteristic of iron therapy, and there is no need to notify the physician.

12.95 ② Prednisone (Deltasone) can cause ulcers. Administering it with meals or with milk will assist in protecting the GI mucosa. Options #1 and #3 do not protect the stomach. Option #4 is incorrect because the drug is recommended to be given with milk.

12.96 ③ Fresh fruits and vegetables are low sodium, and roasted chicken is low cholesterol. Option #1 is incorrect because canned foods contain increased salt, and milk contains cholesterol. Option #2 is incorrect because breads contain sodium, and frying increases the cholesterol. Option #4 is incorrect because bread and carbonated beverages contain sodium.

12.97 ① There is no need to irrigate an ileostomy. The stool remains loose and it cannot be controlled with irrigations. Option #2 is incorrect because appliances should only be changed when there is a leak. Option #3 is incorrect because the client needs to maintain a high fluid intake due to the loss through the ileostomy. Option #4 is incorrect because it will decrease the adherence of the appliance to the skin and increase the incidence of leaking.

12.98 ① The primary objective of fluid replacement is to perfuse the vital organs. The increase in urine output to a normal range indicates that the kidneys are adequately perfused. Therefore, other major organs are being perfused also. Option #2 does not give any indication of adequate fluid replacement. Option #3 is incorrect because although the CVP is an indicator of fluid balance, a CVP at 5 cm water is in the low range and does not indicate tissue perfusion. Option #4 is incorrect because the client is tachycardiac, and the absence of arrhythmias does not indicate tissue perfusion.

12.99 ④ Side rails should always be up for any disoriented client. Option #1 is appropriate but is not the safety priority. Option #2 is incorrect because it is not necessary to stay with the client, especially while he is sleeping. Option #3 is incorrect because restraints are not necessary at this time.

12.100 ② Suctioning the nose will help open the airway. Option #1 will not promote adequate drainage from the upper airway. Option #3 will facilitate drainage of mucous from the upper airway and will assist the adjustment to breathing through the nose, but is secondary to Option #2. Option #4 does not relieve the congestion.

12.101 ③ The ability to identify person, place, and time correctly are the cardinal signs of orientation status. Options #1 and #2 may be from memory loss and not disorientation. Option #4 is incorrect because the client may be very oriented and wants to go home.

12.102 ① The client's concern about her husband's feelings indicates that he may not be able to support her emotionally at this time. Option #2 reflects a reality-based concern. Option #3 indicates an economic concern. Option #4 indicates she needs to talk about her current feelings. It does not give any indication of level of emotional support.

12.103 ④ Assessing the basis for the client's fears and encouraging discussion about those fears are the first positive steps. Option #1 jumps to solutions without adequately defining the problem. Option #2 is an empathetic response but does not gain any more information, or encourage the client to continue. Option #3 provides false reassurance.

12.104 ④ Option #4 is correct. The formula for mean arterial pressure (MAP) is SBP + 2 DBP divided by 3. The blood pressure with mean arterial pressure between 65 and 75 is 105/60 (MAP = 75).

12.105 ③ An objective description of the client's mood and documentation of what actually occurred is the most appropriate nursing action. Options #1, #2, and #3 interpret the behavior, or make assumptions regarding the behavior, rather than describing the behavior.

12.106 ② It is imperative to push these potent resuscitation drugs into a vein versus the tissue because they will be ineffective in tissue and can cause tissue damage. Option #1 is incorrect during a "code" since orders will be verbal. Option #3 is incorrect since there are NO pulses which is the reason for resuscitation. Option #4 is inappropriate.

12.107 ④ Giving away prized possessions is an indication that he does not intend to be using them in the future and is considered a sign of suicidal intentions. Option #1 is of concern, but does not imply active suicidal ideation at the present time. Option #2 may be true but is not a sign of suicidal intent. Option #3 is a normal expression of grief.

12.108 ① The primary purpose of this nursing measure is to improve and/or maintain good gas exchange, especially the removal of CO_2 in order to prevent respiratory acidosis. Option #2 is correct, but Option #1 is better because it addresses ventilation rather than oxygenation. Option #3 is incorrect because increasing the pH is not desirable. Option #4 is incorrect because respiratory alkalosis is not prevented by this nursing measure.

12.109 ③ The sputum characteristics indicate a decrease in the pneumonia. This is supported by the respiratory status. Options #1 and #2 validate the infection is still present. Option #4 does not substantiate the status of the infection.

12.110 ④ To prevent the spread of infection, the clients should have private rooms with different nurses. Option #1 is incorrect because this assignment increases the potential for transmission of infection. Option #2 keeps the clients in the same room. Option #3 puts them in separate rooms; however, the same nurse is caring for them.

12.111 ① If the child can tolerate the protein intake, it is encouraged to increase healing. Sodium is usually restricted. Option #2 is indicated in later stages of renal failure. Option #3 does not address the protein at all. Option #4 may be appropriate if the child cannot tolerate the protein intake.

12.112 ② A side effect of Haldol is hypotension. Moving slowly to a standing position will decrease the problem with orthostatic hypotension. Option #1 would be appropriate for a monoamine oxidase inhibitor (MAO). Option #3 is incorrect because this medication does not cause anticholinergic effects. Option #4 is incorrect because salt does not have any effect on the medication.

12.113 ③ Option #3 is the correct description of bowel sounds. Options #1, #2, and #4 all reflect abnormal bowel sounds related to hypo or hyper motility of the GI tract.

12.114 ③ Option #3 is correct. Because of the risk of inaccuracy in SpO_2 assessment, an abnormal SpO_2 should always be validated with a second reading. Once this is accomplished, the client should be assessed for other causes of hypoxemia such as airway congestion or narrowing that can be seen in bronchitis. Option #1 is incorrect. It is true that an oxygen delivery of 7 liters per minute is too high for a client with chronic bronchitis because of the risk for respiratory depression, but simply reducing the delivery to 2 liters does not address the patient's hypoxemia. Option #2 is incorrect. This practice must be authorized by the provider and does not appropriately address the client's hypoxemia. Option #4 is incorrect. It is likely that the delivery of 7 liters per minute is an error, but this act is low priority in this clinical circumstance.

12.115 ③ After the surgery, swelling can occur which causes respiratory distress. Option #1 is not as specific to this surgery. Option #2 is for monitoring a postoperative tonsillectomy. Option #4 is unsafe. The head of bed should be elevated.

12.116 ① Sterile articles are to be dropped at a reasonable distance from the edge of the sterile area. Option #2 is incorrect because sterile packs should be opened only as needed. Option #3 is incorrect because an unsterile arm should never reach over a sterile field. Option #4 is incorrect because the outer lip of a bottle containing sterile liquid is not considered sterile.

12.117 ② The severity of edema is characterized by grading it 0 (2 mm pitting) to 4+ (8 mm pitting). Option #1 is inappropriate. Option #3 is not as objective. Option #4 is evaluating hydration.

12.118 ④ The oral pharynx is anesthetized with a local anesthetic that inhibits the gag reflex during the bronchoscopy. Return of the gag reflex is necessary in order to safely administer any oral fluids/medications. Options #1, #2, and #3 are important respiratory assessments, but are not the priority in this situation.

12.119 ② Furosemide is a diuretic which warrants close observation of the client's urine output. Option #1 may be a result of abdominal distention. Option #3 is subjective and doesn't address the question. Option #4 may occur as a result of volume loss but is not a priority to Option #2.

12.120 ✌ The fetal heart rate with the LOA position would be ausculated at point A. LOP-point B; ROA-point C; ROP-point D.

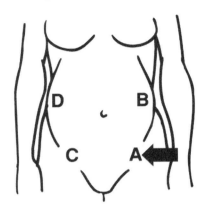

CGFNS™

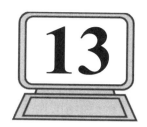

Human nature is the same all over the world.
—Earl of Chesterfield, 1747

The certification of Graduates of Foreign Nursing Schools has many steps. This chapter is provided for international nurses who are preparing for the CGFNS™ Qualifying Exam. This chapter has been written as a result of many requests from international nurses who have attended our review sessions.

Many of you have been practicing nursing for years in your home country. Now you are preparing for the CGFNS™ Qualifying Exam to assess your chances of passing the U.S. nurse licensing exam, the NCLEX-RN® examination. Due to our extensive experience in preparing international nurses for the NCLEX-RN®, we are very aware of your unique issues when preparing for both the CGFNS™ Qualifying Exam and the NCLEX-RN®.

The items in this book, and specifically in this chapter, have been written to prepare you to be successful and PASS the CGFNS™ Qualifying Exam by providing you the current information on the NCLEX-RN® exam.

Those preparing for NCLEX® can utilize these practice questions as a bonus.

NURSING PRACTICE IN THE USA

T TOTAL PATIENT CARE (Focus on how a patient will respond to an ill-

E EQUIPMENT (Responsible for caring for patients whose care involves high-tech equipment.)

A ACCOUNTABLE (Nurses are responsible for their actions.)
ASSERTIVE (Ask questions of health care professionals.)
ADVOCATES (Counsel patients, protect patient rights.)

C COMMUNICATION (Must communicate with patient, family members, and total health care team.)

H HEALTH PROMOTION (Help patients understand health care system, and assist in making health care decisions.)

P PREVENTION, PRACTICE ACT (Governs Legal Nursing Practice)

T TEACH (Responsible to teach patients and family members how to manage their health care needs)

MOST FREQUENTLY ASKED QUESTIONS

1. *Question:*
    What is the format used for the questions?

    a. Essay
    b. Multiple Choice
    c. Matching
    d. Fill in the blank

    Answer:
    b. Multiple Choice

2. *Question*:
    How will my score be determined?

    Answer:
    The total number of correct answers is calculated and converted to a scale. The CGFNS™ scale ranges from 1–800 with 400 required for passing. CGFNS™ will provide you with your scaled score as well as the passing score for the examination. You will also be provided with a graphic diagnostic profile of how well you performed in each area of client needs.

GOOD NEWS ALERT:
You only have to get around 50% correct to pass!

3. *Question*:
    When do I get my exam results?

    Answer:
    Eight to ten weeks after you take the CGFNS™ Qualifying Exam, you will be contacted by mail indicating if you passed or failed the CGFNS™ Qualifying Exam.

4. *Question*:
    Should I leave answers blank if I don't know, or should I guess at the answer?

    Answer:
    Credit is given for each correct answer. If you are uncertain which answer is correct, select the answer that seems the most correct. The score is based on the number of questions you answer correctly. It is best to guess rather than leave an answer blank.

5. *Question*:
    How many questions are on the CGFNS™ Qualifying Exam?

    Answer:
    Currently 271 questions.

6. *Question*:
How many parts are there to the exam?

Answer:
There are 2 parts. Part 1 includes 150 questions. This is given in the morning. You will have 2 hours and 30 minutes to complete this section. You will then take a lunch break. You will then take Part 2 which includes 121 questions. You will have 2 hours to answer these questions.

7. *Question:*
How much time should I take in answering a question?

Answer:
One minute—do not spend too much time on any one question. Complete as much of the CGFNS™ Qualifying Exam as you can in the designated time. No additional time will be allotted. After the proctor directs you to stop, you will not be given any additional time.

8. *Question*:
What are some of the nursing responsibilities in the USA that may be different from my current responsibilities as a nurse in my country?

Answer:
Refer to Nursing Practice in the USA.

9. *Question:*
Do you have any recommendations on how I can control my anxiety?

Answer:

A Anxiety is contagious; avoid contact with anxious people.

N No "crash study."

X X out negative thinking.

I Identify strengths and weaknesses.

E Eat a light and healthy meal—foods you usually eat.

T Take control by appropriate preparation and positive thinking.

Y YOU WILL PASS!!!!!

10. *Question*:
Do you have any hints on how to answer questions about therapeutic communication?

Answer:
Communication is a concept *evaluated* on the exam. Remember, "It is important to PULL information from the client." When answering these questions, select answers that do the following:

P Promote clarification regarding client's condition.

U Understand client's needs.

L Listen for client's feelings and respond in a nonjudgmental manner.

L Look for answers to be client focused (encourage client's family to reflect, think, talk.)

Just as **PULL** assists you with remembering effective communication, **BLOCKS** will assist you in remembering barriers, or **BLOCKS** to communication. Do not select these for answers!

B Behavior of client is disapproved.

L Looks at false reassurance ("Don't worry").

O Organize communication focusing on nurse versus patient.

C Closed-ended questions versus open-ended. "Do you have concerns about the exam?" versus "Tell me your concerns about the exam."

K Know what patient should do with no regard to feelings.

S Starts a question with Why.

THE BOTTOM LINE…This can be EASY!

E Each question is worth one minute of your time.

A Always use a test-taking strategy.

S Stop 10 minutes before time is up.

Y You fill in ALL blanks.

13.1 Two days after admission to the hospital, an elderly client reports that her hands are shaking, she cannot relax, and she feels "things moving around in her bed." The nurse assesses her pain level to be a 4 on a 10 scale. Which would be the best follow-up response from the nurse?

① "This hospitalization is causing you to be anxious."
② "What pain medication do you normally take at home?"
③ "Can you attribute your hands shaking to a particular event?"
④ "I'd like to review your drug and alcohol history with you."

13.2 The nurse finds the client on the floor next to her bed in a puddle of urine. She states, "I've been ringing to go to the bathroom and no one would come." The nurse should document:

① Client states "I needed to go to the bathroom and no one would answer call button."
② Client found lying on floor with no shoes on after falling out of bed.
③ Patient found lying on floor next to bed.
④ Client states that she couldn't reach the call button and had to use the restroom.

13.3 A client with severe chronic asthma has been taking 40 mg of prednisone daily for several months and has developed Cushing's syndrome. Because she is so uncomfortable with the effects of the prednisone, the client stops taking the medication and is admitted to the emergency department with respiratory failure and Addisonian crisis. Which medication should be administered to the client first?

① Epinephrine intravenously
② Albuterol (Proventil) by nebulizer
③ Methylprednisolone (Solu-Medrol) intravenously
④ Ipratropium (Atrovent) by nebulizer

13.4 A client with gastroesophageal reflux disease (GERD) has received extensive client teaching on the disease and related home care. Which statement by the client suggests that he is implementing the teaching?

① "I usually drink a small glass of water before bed."
② "I avoid food such as celery and bran cereal."
③ "I changed from butter to margarine."
④ "I quit drinking coffee and cola drinks."

13.5 During hospital rounds, a nursing supervisor smells smoke coming from a client's bathroom. She opens the bathroom door and finds the client unresponsive on the floor and the waste can on fire. Which is her most appropriate response?

① Drag the client from the bathroom and close the door.
② Activate the fire alarm located outside the client's room.
③ Move the waste can to the shower and turn the shower on.
④ Call for help from other staff members.

13.6 A nurse is providing a prostate cancer screening clinic for men over 50. During a visit to the clinic, clients are offered a prostate-specific antigen test. Which question is most appropriate for the nurse to ask clients before the blood sample is drawn?

① "Are you allergic to iodine or radiopaque dyes?"
② "Have you had rectal penetration in the last 48 hours?"
③ "Do you strain when you void or have a bowel movement?"
④ "Have you eaten red meat within 24 hours?"

13.7 A client with Parkinsonism is having problems with ambulation and is experiencing wavering and stumbling. Which client teaching would be most beneficial in preventing the client from falling?

① Keep the arms as still as possible when walking.
② Walk with the feet spaced at hip width.
③ Maintain a slightly forward-leaning position.
④ Focus eyes on the level of the horizon.

13.8 A client's thrombocyte count is 510,000. Which nursing intervention is most important?

① Observe for nosebleeds.
② Use a manual sphygmomanometer.
③ Encourage fluid intake.
④ Minimize physical activity.

13.9 A nurse is evaluating a client's ability to change the dressing on the left deltoid following an incision and drainage of an abscess. Which behavior by the client indicates further teaching is needed?

① Using clean gloves to remove the dressing
② Removing the tape by pulling away from the wound
③ Cleansing the wound with saline
④ Measuring the wound's length and width

13.10 Which assessment of the lungs by auscultation would the nurse expect to evaluate if a client has a left lower lobe consolidation?

① Absent breath sounds
② Bronchophony
③ Vesicular breath sounds
④ Wheezes

13.11 A client diagnosed with a lower GI bleed has an order for 1 unit of packed red blood cells. What information is most important to be documented during this procedure?

① Vital signs prior to procedure
② Confirmation that the nurse alone verified the blood label information
③ The total volume that is to be infused
④ Vital signs before, during, and after procedure, date and time started and completed

13.12 Which plan would be the most appropriate for a 34-week pregnant woman who is being treated with magnesium sulfate and bed rest for pregnancy induced hypertension?

① Assessing the equality of the pedal pulse
② Assessing the abdominal circumference
③ Assessing for an increase in the urine output
④ Obtaining the client's daily weight

13.13 A nurse is caring for a client who is in the first 24 hours following a renal transplantation and observes hematuria. What is the nurse's highest priority concern?

① Reporting evidence of transplant rejection to the provider
② Advising the provider that fluid intake should be increased
③ Continuing to monitor the urine's volume and appearance
④ Using a urine dipstick to check for proteinuria

13.14 A registered nurse (RN) is teamed with a practical nurse (PN) to provide care for a group of eight clients. The client that should most likely be assessed by the RN is the client:

① who started her menses within the last 24 hours.
② whose family insists she get the "best care available."
③ who is arriving as a transfer from a skilled nursing facility.
④ who is a newly diagnosed Type I diabetic with a blood sugar of 180 mg/dl.

13.15 A client with inflammatory bowel disease is placed on a daily dose of cyclosporine (Sandimmune) in an oral solution form. Which behavior by the client demonstrates knowledge of how to take the drug?

① He mixes it in a citrus juice and stirs it well.
② He waits at least 30 minutes to take the drug after mixing it in a solution.
③ After taking the medication, he adds water to the container and drinks that, too.
④ He uses a plastic or Styrofoam cup to mix the medication solution.

13.16 Six months after her vaginal hysterectomy, a client tells the nurse, "Sex with my husband is painful." Which is the most appropriate response from the nurse?

① "Are you using a water-soluble lubricant during intercourse?"
② "Tell me what aspect of sex is painful to you."
③ "It may be too early after surgery to be having sex."
④ "I will advise your surgeon to talk to you about this."

13.17 A client is one day post-operative after an abdominal hysterectomy and is being evaluated for discharge from the hospital. The nurse identifies edema in the client's left leg. The nurse should:

   ① instruct the client to increase the frequency of post-op leg exercises.
   ② consult the client's chart for a history of renal failure or heart failure.
   ③ evaluate the foot of the client's bed at least thirty degrees.
   ④ measure both legs at midthigh and midcalf.

13.18 The 72-year-old client is discharged to a rehab setting following hospitalization for carotid artery endarderectomy. He has an ongoing history of nocturnal disorientation. After receiving Ambien 10 mg po for sleep, he was found on the floor unconscious at 2:00 a.m. The best documentation should include which of the following?

   ① Patient found on floor face down unconscious with side rails down. Bleeding noted from a significant cut just over left brow. Called provider.
   ② Upon opening the door, patient was found face down non-responsive. Moderate bleeding was noted from his left forehead. Provider called.
   ③ The client sustained a cut of his left forehead. House supervisor paged and provider notified.
   ④ The client found on floor non-responsive. Assessment revealed 4-inch cut over left eyebrow bleeding moderately. Pressure dressing applied. Carotid and radial pulses present. V/S stable. House supervisor, provider, and family notified.

13.19 A 70-year-old client with herpes zoster is assigned to a practical nurse for total patient care. While the practical nurse is away from the unit, the patient requests pain medication and a registered nurse gives the client an intramuscular injection in the dorosogluteal site. When turning the client, the registered nurse notices a first degree pressure sore on the client's coccyx area. The practical nurse's charting from one hour previous states, "No skin breakdown." The registered nurse should:

   ① Talk to the practical nurse about the assessment when she returns to the unit.
   ② Correct the practical nurse's charting to address the pressure sore.
   ③ Document that there has been a change in the client's skin assessment.
   ④ Ask the client to state a time when the practical nurse did the skin assessment.

13.20 A client has right radius and ulna fractures following a motorcycle accident and has an external fixator. He develops loss of two-point discrimination in the fingers on his right hand. Before notifying the provider, the nurse should:

   ① elevate the right arm on pillows.
   ② place the right arm at heart level.
   ③ put the right arm in a dependent position.
   ④ vary the right arm position every 15 minutes.

13.21 A 35-year-old client who sustained a closed head injury is being monitored for increased intracranial pressure. An arterial blood gas is performed on the client, and the results include a $PaCO_2$ of 33 mm Hg. It is most important for the nurse to:

   ① encourage the client to slow his breathing rate.
   ② auscultate the client's lungs and suction if indicated.
   ③ advise the physician that the patient needs supplemental oxygen.
   ④ report the results and continue to monitor for signs of increasing intracranial pressure.

13.22 A 25-year old client with a recent history of sinusitis demonstrates a positive Brudzinski sign. The therapeutic approach by the nurse that has the highest priority is:

① controlling intracranial pressure.
② administering prescribed antibiotics.
③ adding pads to the side rails of the bed.
④ hydrating the patient with 0.45% saline.

13.23 When correcting a documentation made in the wrong chart, which of the following best describes the appropriate action by the nurse?

① Mark through the error with one line, and write above it "error" along with the nurse's initials.
② Mark through the statements with one line and write "wrong chart."
③ Write: "Late note. This was entered in error on the wrong chart."
④ If an instance occurs where a late entry is needed, it is better to start that day over on a fresh sheet by copying what had taken place prior to it, and therefore record it in the correct order.

13.24 The nurse observes that a fire has started in the client's room. Which action should the nurse take first?

① Confine the fire to the client's room.
② Extinguish the fire.
③ Pull the fire alarm.
④ Rescue the client.

13.25 A city council person is admitted to the hospital after experiencing chest pain at a ribbon-cutting ceremony. A journalist from the newspaper contacts the hospital's nursing supervisor and asks her for a report on the client's status. Prior to giving information to the journalist, it is most important for the supervisor to:

① Advise the journalist of HIPAA guidelines.
② Contact the hospital's chief executive officer.
③ Ensure the journalist is authorized to receive such information.
④ Obtain signed authorization from the client.

13.26 Which assignment would be appropriate for the Labor and Delivery (L&D) nurse who will be working for one shift on the Medical Surgical unit?

① A 3-year-old with croup
② A 30-year-old with malignant hypertension
③ A 40-year-old with unstable angina
④ A 50-year-old with congestive heart failure

13.27 After establishing IV access, what would be the best for the nurse to document immediately after procedure?

① The type of catheter used and number of venipuncture attempts.
② The type of IV fluid hung and equipment used.
③ The date, time, venipuncture site, type and gauge of catheter, and IV fluid hung.
④ Type, amount, and flow rate of IV fluid, condition of IV site.

13.28 What question would be most important to ask a male client who is in for a digital rectal examination?

① "Have you noticed a change in the force of the urinary stream?"
② "Have you noticed a change in tolerance of certain foods in your diet?"
③ "Do you notice polyuria in the AM?"
④ "Do you notice any burning with urination or any odor to the urine?"

13.29 Which statement made by the new mother indicates an understanding of screening for PKU for her newborn son who she is breastfeeding?

① "I will have him tested 24 hours after birth."
② "I will return to the clinic in 48 hours for the screening."
③ "I will return in 1 week to obtain blood samples."
④ "I will return in 1 month for the screening."

13.30 Which of these schedules would be the most appropriate to recommend to a pre-menopausal woman regarding her self breast exam?

① One week prior to the monthly period
② One week after the menstrual period
③ During every shower
④ The same day monthly

13.31 During the history, which information from a 20-year-old client would indicate a risk for development of testicular cancer?

① Genital Herpes
② Hydrocele
③ Measles
④ Undescended testicle

13.32 Which plan is most appropriate for meeting the needs for a Hindu family after the loved one has died?

① Allow the family to wash the body.
② Allow the priest to touch the body.
③ Allow chanting to be done during the "last rites."
④ Do not consult with family about organ donations since it is considered a sin.

13.33 A common side effect of positive end expiratory pressure (PEEP) is:

① increased blood pressure
② decreased cardiac output
③ decreased lung compliance
④ increased venous return to heart

13.34 Organize the following steps to suctioning in chronological order (with 1 being the first step in this procedure).

① Put on sterile glove.
② Lubricate catheter with normal saline.
③ Apply suction for 5-10 seconds.
④ Explain procedure to client.
⑤ Wash hands thoroughly.

13.35 Which findings would indicate that a client with Adult Respiratory Distress Syndrome (ARDS) is deteriorating?

① PaO_2-88%, R-24
① PaO_2-87%, HR-80
① PaO_2-58, HR-108
① PCO_2-47, R-32

13.36 The nurse is assessing a child with a tentative diagnosis of appendicitis. This diagnosis is most often manifested by:

① sharp pain with extreme gastric distention.
② rebound tenderness in the right lower abdominal quadrant, with decreased bowel sounds.
③ growing pain, radiating to the lower back.
④ pain on light palpation in epigastric area with diarrhea.

13.37 While the nurse is providing care for a client who is on a volume cycled positive pressure ventilator, the low volume alarm sounds. What assessment would you anticipate the nurse to make?

① Client is biting on the tubing.
② Excessive fluid is in the ventilator tubing.
③ A leak in the client's endotracheal tube cuff
④ Client is lying on the tubing.

13.38 Which of these documentations indicate the nurse understands how to accurately evaluate the client's stool for occult blood?

① Collect stool placed in a clean container to examine for pathological organisms.
② Remained on regular diet prior to test being done.
③ Stool sample obtained from one area of the stool.
④ Guaiac testing—positive for occult blood. Paper turned blue.

13.39 What is the priority of care after the urinary catheter is removed?

① Encourage client to eliminate fluid intake.
② Document size of catheter and client's tolerance of procedure.
③ Evaluate client for normal voiding.
④ Documentation of client teaching.

13.40 Which client is a likely candidate for developing acute renal failure?

① Young female with recent ileostomy due to ulcerative colitis.
② Middle-age male with elevated temperature and chronic pancreatitis.
③ Teenager in hypovolemic shock following a crushing injury to the chest.
④ Child with compound fracture of right femur and massive laceration to left arm.

13.41 Which of these statements made by a female client who has been abused by her spouse indicates the counseling has been effective?

① "I know my husband will never hurt me again."
② "I know it is my fault that he hits me."
③ "I promise I will get him to promise that he will not do it again."
④ "I have made arrangements to go to the battered women's shelter the next time he hits me."

13.42 Which clinical findings indicate a complication from diabetes insipidus?

① Urine specific gravity – 1.001
② Serum sodium - 135
③ Urine output greater than 200 cc/hr.
④ Weight loss of 2 lbs.

13.43 Which nursing action is most appropriate for a client receiving a tube feeding around the clock?

① Rinse the bag and change the formula every 4 hours.
② Rinse the bag and change the formula every shift.
③ Change the bag and formula every shift.
④ Rinse the bag and change the formula every 2 hours.

13.44 A 17-year-old is beginning chemotherapy for her malignancy. Which statement indicates she has a realistic perception of her health status?

① "I will be cured after my therapy is completed."
② "I may need to get a wig during my chemotherapy."
③ "I will be able to continue my current school schedule."
④ "I must have done something to cause this illness."

13.45 What nursing action is most appropriate when inserting a vaginal suppository?

① Remove the suppository from the wrapper and lubricate it with Vaseline.
② Instruct client to place in tampon after inserting the vaginal medication.
③ With an applicator on the forefinger of your free hand, insert the suppository about 2" (5 cm) into the vagina.
④ Direct the applicator up initially and then down and forward.

13.46 Which statement made by the client with a cast on his right leg indicates he understands how to safely walk up stairs with his crutches?

① "I will put my right leg up first."
② "I will put my left leg up first."
③ "I will put both of my crutches up first."
④ "I will put both of my legs up first."

13.47 The purpose of a continuous bladder irrigation (CBI) in a client first-day postoperative TURP is to:

① prevent urinary stasis and infection.
② maintain urinary dilution to prevent irritation.
③ keep urine flowing by preventing clot formation.
④ deliver medication directly to operative area.

13.48 What would the nurse ask the client to do when evaluating the cranial nerve XI?

① Ask client to smell and identify different odors.
② Ask client to shrug the shoulders.
③ Ask client to read a Snellen chart.
④ Ask client to stick out tongue and move from side to side.

13.49 Which plan is most appropriate for a client in septic shock?

① Administer Atenolol (Tenorim).
② Position in semi-Fowlers position.
③ Restrict dietary protein.
④ Increase IV fluids.

13.50 A client with a closed head injury has a nasogastric tube in place and begins to vomit. What is the highest priority?

① Check the nasogastric tube for appropriate placement.
② Reposition client in bed to a side-lying position.
③ Notify physician.
④ Remove the tube immediately.

13.51 The client has had an acute myocardial infarction and is on a cardiac monitor. She is beginning to have premature ventricular contractions (PVCs) at 10/minute. The nurse will administer which of these ordered drugs?

① Atropine
② Nitroglycerin
③ Propanolol (Inderal®)
④ Lidocaine

13.52 Organize these steps in chronological order with #1 being the first step for a client who is having a nasogastric tube removed.

① Assist client into semi-Fowler's position.
② Ask client to hold her breath.
③ Assess bowel function by auscultation for peristalsis.
④ Flush tube with 10 ml of normal saline.
⑤ Withdraw the tube gently and steadily.
⑥ Monitor client for nausea, vomiting.

13.53 Prior to administering Atenolol (Tenormin) and Digoxin (Tanoxin), which assessment would be most important to report and document?

① Bradycardia
② Tachycardia
③ Hypertension
④ Serum potassium-3.8 meq/l

13.54 A psychiatric client with the diagnosis of schizo-phrenia tells the nurse that he is the President of the United States. What would be the priority action for the nurse?

① Confront the client regarding this delusion and bring him back to reality.
② Reflect this statement back to the client to encourage therapeutic communication.
③ Respond with an open-ended response to get client to further discuss his thoughts.
④ Verify identify of the client prior to administering his medication.

13.55 A client is experiencing septic shock and the provider wants dosing of medications to be regulated so that a mean arterial pressure (MAP) between 65 and 75 mm Hg is maintained. Which of the client's blood pressure readings meet this goal?

① 135/90
② 125/80
③ 115/70
④ 105/60

13.56 What would be most important to monitor on a client who is taking Lisinopril (Zestril)?

① Serum potassium
② Serum pH
③ Serum calcium
④ Heart rate

13.57 Following an automobile accident, a client is admitted to the hospital with a head injury. Which clinical finding would indicate the cerebral edema is increasing and the client is deteriorating?

① Increase in pain
② Irregular respiratory pattern
③ Narrowing of the pulse pressure
④ Increase in heart rate

13.58 The physician orders heparin 7,000 U S.C. q8h for a client with deep vein thrombosis. The heparin available is 20,000 units per 1 ml. How many milliliters of heparin should the nurse administer?

① 0.2 ml
② 0.3 ml
③ 0.35 ml
④ 3.5 ml

13.59 Which interventions would be most appropriate for a 3-month-old infant in a right hip spica cast?

① Palpate the left radial artery and compare it to the right.
② Check cast for tightness by inserting fingers between skin and cast.
③ Blanch the skin of areas proximal to the casted right leg.
④ Medicate frequently for pain.

13.60 The nurse is caring for a female client in the ER who was attacked and raped 6 hours ago. What initial nursing action would be most important?

① Clean wounds immediately.
② Obtain written informed consent for examination.
③ Determine if the woman has bathed or douched.
④ Obtain laboratory specimens.

Category Analysis – CGFNS™

1.	Psycho-Social	21.	Sensory-Perception-Mobility	41.	Psycho-Social
2.	Safe Effective Care	22.	Sensory-Perception-Mobility	42.	Basic Care & Comfort
3.	Pharmacology	23.	Safe Effective Care	43.	Basic Care & Comfort
4.	Nutrition	24.	Safe Effective Care	44.	Psycho-Social
5.	Safe Effective Care	25.	Safe Effective Care	45.	Pharmacology
6.	Fluid-Gas	26.	Safe Effective Care	46.	Sensory-Perception-Mobility
7.	Safe Effective Care	27.	Pharmacology	47.	Elimination
8.	Basic Care & Comfort	28.	Health Promotion	48.	Sensory-Perception-Mobility
9.	Basic Care & Comfort	29.	Health Promotion	49.	Fluid-Gas
10.	Health Promotion	30.	Health Promotion	50.	Elimination
11.	Pharmacology	31.	Health Promotion	51.	Pharmacology
12.	Basic Care & Comfort	32.	Psycho-Social	52.	Elimination
13.	Elimination	33.	Fluid-Gas	53.	Pharmacology
14.	Safe Effective Care	34.	Fluid-Gas	54.	Psycho-Social
15.	Pharmacology	35.	Fluid-Gas	55.	Fluid-Gas
16.	Health Promotion	36.	Elimination	56.	Pharmacology
17.	Nutrition	37.	Fluid-Gas	57.	Sensory-Perception-Mobility
18.	Safe Effective Care	38.	Safe Effective Care	58.	Pharmacology
19.	Safe Effective Care	39.	Elimination	59.	Sensory-Perception-Mobility
20.	Nutrition	40.	Elimination	60.	Safe Effective Care

Directions

1. Determine questions missed by checking answers.
2. Write the number of the questions missed across the top line marked "item missed."
3. Check category analysis page to determine category of question.
4. Put a check mark under item missed and beside content.
5. Count check marks in each row and write the number in totals column.
6. Use this information to:
   - identify areas for further study.
   - determine which content test to take next.

We recommend studying content where most items are missed—then taking that content test.

Number of the Questions Incorrectly Answered

CGFNS™	Items Missed																														Totals
C Safe Effective Care																															
O Health Promotion and Maintenance																															
Psycho-Social Integrity																															
N Physiological Adaptation: Fluid Gas																															
T Reduction of Risk Potential: Sensory-Perception-Mobility																															
E Basic Care and Comfort: Elimination																															
N Physiological Adaptation: Nutrition																															
T Pharmacological and Parenteral Therapies																															

Answers & Rationales

13.1 ④ Option #4 is correct. Alcohol and drug use is a common unrecognized problem in the elderly in the United States. The client is exhibiting manifestation of substance withdrawal; and in recognizing this, the nurse should gather more data from the client. Option #1 is incorrect because it makes an unfounded assumption and ignores the client's symptoms. Option #2 is incorrect because it ignores the client's reported concerns. Option #3 is incorrect because it is asking the client for a diagnosis rather than the nurse using the information given by the client to formulate her own nursing diagnosis.

13.2 ③ Option #3 is correct.

13.3 ③ Option #3 is correct. The probable cause of the client's respiratory failure and Addison's is the cessation of prednisone. It is most vital that that drug be reinstituted. Therefore, the first drug that should be given is Methylprednisolone (Solu-Medrol). Because of its untoward cardiovascular effects, epinephrine should be avoided unless other more specific medications have failed. Albuterol (Proventil) is indicated in this instance but does not have the priority of Methylprednisolone (Solu-Medrol). Ipratropium is ineffective in emergencies.

13.4 ④ Option #4 is correct. Coffee and cola drinks are discouraged in GERD because the increased gastric motility and the likelihood of reflux. Drinking before bed is discouraged because it is preferred that the stomach be empty when reclining. High fiber and low fat diets are recommended in cases of GERD.

13.5 ① Option #1 is correct. When confronted with a fire, the most important response from a nurse is to rescue the client. In order of priority, the proper responses are: 1) rescue; 2) alarm; 3) confine the fire; and 4) evacuate.

13.6 ② Option #2 is correct. Rectal penetration such as a digital exam or rectal intercourse can cause a false high PSA result. If this has occurred, 48 hours must pass before the test can be done. Allergies to iodine or radiopaque dye, straining with voiding or defecation, and eating red meat are not contraindications for testing.

13.7 ④ Option #4 is correct. Focusing on the horizon level helps maintain the balance of a client with Parkinsonism who is having ambulation difficulties. The client should be taught to swing the arms when walking—not to keep them still. The feet should be widely spaced at shoulder width or greater. The patient should try to maintain an erect posture—not a forward-leaning one.

13.8 ③ Option #3 is correct. The client has thrombocytosis, which predisposes him to thrombus formation. Fluid intake reduces the risk of thrombus by maintaining an adequate amount of water in the serum. The other measures identified are associated with thrombocytopenia.

13.9 ② Option #2 is correct. When removing a dressing, the tape should be removed toward the wound, not away from it, as pulling away from the wound may disrupt healing. Home care of an abscess wound requires medical asepsis so clean gloves are acceptable during the procedure. It is standard practice to clean wounds with saline. Measuring the wound can give the provider information regarding the progress of the healing.

13.10 ② Option #2 is correct. This clinical finding is most indicative of Bronchophony. Option #1 is a finding for a client with a pneumothorax. Option #3—these breath sounds are auscultated over the majority of the lung fields.

13.11 ④ Option #4 is correct. Option #1 is not as inclusive as #4. Option #2—blood should be verified with another nurse. Option #3 should be actual volume versus projected amount since the infusion may need to be discontinued prior to total amount being infused.

13.12 ④ Option #4 is correct. This is a primary concern since it provides a baseline and an ongoing record of potential increase in the weight. Options #1, #2, and #3 are incorrect. Option #1 should read the patellar reflexes since they are more indicative of neurological problems with PIH or magnesium sulfate toxicity. Option #2 is not routinely done. Option #3 would be a decrease in urine output if assessing magnesium sulfate toxicity.

13.13 ③ Option #3 is correct. In the early postoperative period following a renal transplant, hematuria is an expected observation. The nurse should continue to observe the urine as increasing hematuria is not a normal finding and should be reported. Early hematuria is not a sign of transplant rejection. There is no evidence that the client needs increased fluid intake. Checking for proteinuria is not indicated in this incident.

13.14 ③ Option #3 is correct. Of the four clients described, the only one that must receive an assessment from the RN is the newly arriving client. An RN must perform the initial assessment of a client.

13.15 ③ Option #3 is correct. To ensure getting the full dose of the drug, after the dose has been taken, water should be added to the container, swished around to mix with the residue of the drug, and the water should then be drunk. Option #1 is incorrect because not all citrus juices should be mixed with the drug. Grapefruit juice is contraindicated. Option #2 is incorrect because the drug should be taken immediately after mixing. Option #4 is incorrect because the drug will adhere to the sides of a plastic or styrofoam cup. Only a glass container should be used.

13.16 ② Option #2 is correct. The nurse needs more information, more assessment, before optimal help can be given to the client. Therefore, it is ideal for the nurse to ask for clarification of the client's statement. Options #1, #3, and #4 are all incorrect because these responses bypass the necessary assessment. The client did not state that intercourse is painful so #1 is making an assumption. Option #3 is incorrect because in most cases, intercourse after a vaginal hysterectomy does not need to be postponed for 6 weeks. Option #4 is incorrect because it undervalues the nursing role and overlooks the opportunity to help the client in her dilemma.

13.17 ④ Option #4 is correct. One of the most reliable physical finding of deep vein thrombosis, a post-op complication, is edema of the affected leg. When discovered, a nurse should measure both legs at midthigh and midcalf so that the nurse's report to the provider is complete and accurate. Option #1 is incorrect because increased activity of the leg without concurrent treatment for deep vein thrombosis may actually dislodge the clot. Talk to the provider before instituting this strategy. Option #2 is incorrect because it does not address the immediate need of the client, and in renal failure and heart failure, edema is bilateral. Option #3 is incorrect because it does not address the immediate need of the client and will not help to resolve the problem of a deep vein thrombosis.

13.18 ④ Option #4 is correct. It provides the most inclusive and objective information.

13.19 ① Option #1 is correct. There is a significant difference in the skin assessment of the practical nurse and the registered nurse. The registered nurse is obligated to discuss the matter with the practical nurse. Option #2 is incorrect. One nurse should not alter the charting of another nurse. Option #3 is incorrect. The nurse should not make this assumption without talking to the practical nurse first. Option #4 is incorrect. As a matter of professional respect, it is preferred that the registered nurse speak to the practical nurse before involving the client in the matter.

13.20 ② The client has a symptom of compartment syndrome which is a complication of trauma and fractures. In this case, the best position for the arm is neutral or at heart level. Option #1 is incorrect because it reduces arterial flow to the arm and increases tissue ischemia. Option #3 is incorrect because it can increase swelling and further impair circulation to the extremity. Option #4 is incorrect because it both reduces arterial flow and increases swelling of the extremity.

13.21 ④ Option #4 is correct. A lower-than-normal PaCO² can actually benefit the client because it reduces intracranial pressure by preventing cerebral vasodilation. The results should be reported to the physician, and monitoring for signs of increased intracranial pressure should continue. Option #1 is incorrect. Instructing the client to slow his breathing rate is inappropriate because it could elevate the PaCO² which could increase intracranial pressure. Option #2 is incorrect. There is no evidence that suction is indicated. Suctioning elevates intracranial pressure and therefore should be avoided. Option #3 is incorrect. There is no evidence that supplemental oxygen is needed. An abnormal PaCO² does not indicate the need for supplemental oxygen.

13.22 ② Option #2 is correct. The Brudzinski sign indicates bacterial meningitis, a complication of sinusitis. The client's greatest need is a regimen of antibiotics to which the causative agent is sensitive. Option #1 is incorrect. Bacterial meningitis causes increased intracranial pressure, and it is important for the nurse to monitor for manifestation of increased intracranial pressure. However, in this circumstance, it is not the highest priority. Option #3 is incorrect. Because of the risk for seizures in bacterial meningitis, padded side rails are an important nursing intervention. However, this intervention does not have priority over instituting the client's antibiotic therapy. Option #4 data does not indicate the use of a hypotonic solution for hydrating the client.

13.23 ② Option #2 is correct. This is the most accurate form of documentation. Option #1 is incorrect due to the word "error." Options #3 and #4 contain unnecessary information.

13.24 ④ Option #4 is correct. Just remember, "RACE." (Rescue, Activate, Confine, and Extinguish)

13.25 ④ Option #4 is correct. Maintaining client confidentiality/privacy is most important to this situation. Options #1, #2, and #3 do not address this concern with privacy. These answers focus on the journalist and hospital. The correct answer is the answer that is client-focused.

13.26 ② Option #2 is correct. The L&D nurse provides care for clients with pregnancy induced hypertension. These assessments and plans of care would correlate with the nurse's skills. Options #1, #3, and #4 would not be appropriate for this nurse. L&D nurses do not routinely provide care for children. Options #3 and #4 require an understanding of cardiology.

13.27 ③ Option #3 is the most correct answer. Options #1 and #2 are appropriate but not as inclusive as Option #3. Option #4 should be included in the once-per-shift documentation. This question states "after establishing IV access."

13.28 ① Option #1 is correct. This change would be most indicative of a potential complication with (BPH) benign prostate hypertrophy. Options #2, #3, and #4 are incorrect. Option #4 would be indicative of an infection.

13.29 ③ Option #3 is correct since the newborn is only getting colostrum for the first few days. This screening may have a possible false negative result with the initial screening. Options #1, #2, and #4 are inaccurate and would not provide valid information.

13.30 ② Option #2 is correct because this is when the breasts are least congested. Option #1 is when the breasts are most congested. Option #3 is unnecessary. The recommended frequency is monthly. Option #4 is for post-menopausal women.

13.31 ④ Option #4—undescended testicles make the client high risk for testicular cancer. Mumps, inguinal hernia in childhood, orchitis, and testicular cancer in the contra lateral testis are other predisposing factors. Options #1, #2, and #3 are not factors that contribute to testicular cancer.

13.32 ① Option #1 is correct for the Hindu family. For an Islam family member death, only relatives or a priest may touch the body. The family washes the body and then turns it to face Mecca. Option #3 is appropriate for a Buddhist family. Option #4 is not true. Donation of organs may be done.

13.33 ② Option #2 is correct. As a result of the PEEP, the cardiac output may decrease. Options #1, #3, and #4 are incorrect for PEEP.

13.34   #4 would be done first.
#5 would be done second.
#1 would be done third.
#2 would be done fourth.
#3 would be done last.

13.35   ③   Option #3 is correct. ARDS is a form of pulmonary edema that is characterized by dyspnea, labored respiration, and low PaO_2. Option #3 indicates client's deterioration. Options #1 and #3 are incorrect. Option #4—increasing levels of CO_2 are generally not a problem.

13.36   ②   Option #2 is correct. Rebound pain is manifested by pressing firmly over the area known as McBurney's point. The rebound pain, decreased bowel sounds, tender abdomen, and fever, are all characteristic of appendicitis. Options #1, #3, and #4 are incorrect.

13.37   ③   Option #3 is correct. When the low alarm sounds, this usually indicates a leak. Options #1, #2, and #4 would result in a high volume alarm.

13.38   ④   Option #4 is correct. Options #1, #2, and #3 are incorrect. Option #1 should be in a sterile container. Option #2—client may be on a specific type of diet prior to test being done to minimize false results. Option #3 should be collected from various areas of stool.

13.39   ③   Option #3 is a priority. Within 24 hours client should be voiding normally. Options #1, #2, and #4 are incorrect. Option #1 should be increased. Option #2 is not totally correct. The size of the catheter should have been documented when it is placed. Option #4 is important but is not a priority for this question.

13.40   ③   Common causes of acute renal failure are renal ischemia precipitated by hypovolemia or heart failure and crush injury. Option #1 is incorrect because ileostomy clients do not experience hypovolemia to the extent that would lead to renal failure. Option #2 is incorrect because pancreatitis is not likely to cause renal failure. Option #4 is incorrect because femoral fractures are more likely to lead to fat embolism.

13.41   ④   Option #4 is correct. Most abused women eventually leave the situation. Interventions may not produce quick outcomes, but they can begin to facilitate the process of healing. Options #1, #2, and #3 are incorrect. Option #1—the husband will not change without identifying cause of anxiety and altering the manner he deals with it. Options #2 and #3 do not indicate counseling was effective.

13.42   ④   Option #4 is correct. Clinical manifestations from diabetes may result in severe dehydration. These manifestations may include: dry skin and mucous membranes; weight loss; decrease in blood pressure; decrease in central venous pressure; weakness; confusion; or speech difficulty in elderly. Options #1 and #3 are clinical manifestations of diabetes insipidus but not complications. Option #2 is normal range.

13.43   ①   Research indicates there is an increased growth of organisms after four hours. Options #2 and #3 are inappropriate due to increased organism growth. Option #4 is not a necessary action to maintain asepsis.

13.44   ②   This statement reflects the client's understanding of the side effects of chemotherapy. Option #1 may or may not occur. Option #3 is not realistic. It may be possible at times, but the question requests a "realistic perception." Option #4 is inaccurate and may reflect blame and guilt.

13.45   ③   Option #3 is correct. Option #1 is incorrect. It should be lubricated with a water-soluble lubricant. Option #2 should not be done because the tampon would absorb the medication and decrease its effectiveness. Option #4 should read to direct the applicator down initially (toward the spine), and then up and back (toward) the cervix.

13.46   ②   Option #2 is correct. The unaffected leg moves up first, followed by the crutches, and the affected leg. Options #1, #3, and #4 are incorrect. When going downstairs, affected leg and crutches move down first.

13.47   ③   Continuous bladder irrigation prevents the formation of clots which can lead to obstruction and spasm in the postoperative TURP client. Option #1 refers to a possible preoperative complication of infection due to the enlarged prostate. Option #2 will be ineffective. Option #4 is incorrect because medicine is not routinely administered via CBI in a first-day post op TURP.

13.48   ②   Option #2 is correct for the CNXI (spinal accessory). Option #1 is evaluation of the CNI (olfactory). Option #3 is evaluation of the CNII (optic). Option #4 is evaluation for the CNXII (hypoglossal).

13.49 ④ Option #4 is correct. Due to dilation of blood vessels from the overwhelming infection, the client experiences a decrease in venous return. To maintain adequate circulation, IV fluid replacement is essential. Position should be supine with legs elevated.

13.50 ② Option #2 is correct. It is done to decrease risk of aspiration. Options #1, #3, and #4 are incorrect. While the nurse may implement Option #1, it is not a priority to Option #2.

13.51 ④ Lidocaine decreases cardiac irritability and is the first line drug for treatment of PVCs. Option #1—atropine—is an anticholinergic drug used to treat bradycardia and heart block effect. Option #2—nitroglycerin—is primarily given for anginal pain. Option #3—Inderal—is used (primarily) to treat supraventricular dysrhythmias.

13.52 ③ #3 is the first step. #1 is the second step. #4 is the
① third step. Flushing will ensure that the tube doesn't
④ contain stomach contents that could irritate tissues
② during tube removal. #2 is the fourth step. This is
⑤ to close epiglottis. #5 is the fifth step. #6 is the sixth
⑥ step. For 48 hours, monitor client for GI dysfunction including nausea, vomiting, abdominal distention, and food intolerance.

13.53 ① Option #1 is correct. When clients take beta blockers concurrently with cardiac glycoside and/or calcium channel blockers, there is an increased risk for bradycardia. Options #2, #3 and #4 are not correct for this situation. Option #4 is therapeutic.

13.54 ④ Option #4 is correct. Safety is a priority in the clinical situation. Client identification is imperative since he is delusional. Option #1 is not a priority to #4. Options #2 and #3 include strategies for effective communication.

13.55 ④ Option #4 is correct. The formula for mean arterial pressure (MAP) is SBP + 2 DBP divided by 3. The blood pressure with mean arterial pressure between 65 and 75 is 105/60 (MAP = 75).

13.56 ① Option #1 is priority. This medication may cause retention of potassium. Options #2, #3, and #4 are incorrect.

13.57 ② Clients with increased intracranial pressure have Bradycardia, an irregular respiratory rate, and a widening of the pulse pressure. Option #1 is not a sign that a client with a head injury is deteriorating. The earliest sign of a change in the client's neurological status is an alteration in the level of consciousness. Option #3—There is a widening of pulse pressure with increased intracranial pressure. Narrowing of the pulse pressure indicates hypovolemic shock. Option #4—Bradycardia—is a sign of increasing intracranial pressure.

13.58 ③ Option #3 is correct.

$$\frac{20,000 \text{ U}}{1 \text{ ml}} = \frac{7,000 \text{ U}}{X}$$

$$20,000 \text{ X} = 7,000 \text{ U}$$

$$X = \frac{7,000 \text{ U}}{20,000 \text{ U}}$$

13.59 ② Option #2 is correct. Check the cast to make sure it is not constricting circulation. The child is not in traction; the arms are not part of the treatment; and the circulation is checked distal to the cast, not proximal. Medicating frequently is inappropriate.

13.60 ② Option #2 is correct. Consent must be a priority action before obtaining laboratory specimens and completing a specific interview or calling the police.

People learn in many different ways. We want to tell you about our stuff because our business is to help you PASS.
www.icanpublishing.com

NURSING MADE INSANELY EASY, 4th Ed. is a pocket-sized book, chock full of drawings and information, streamlining nursing and allied health education with an EASY, totally different bottom-line approach to concepts.

E essential concepts assist learners to prepare for exams, exit exams, and NCLEX®.

A assist nursing graduates to remember health and disease concepts.

S special images per page with essential concepts on the opposite page.

Y your learning is memorable and fun.

For example, one look at "Go Getter Gertrude" and you will remember the most important facts about the concept of hyperthyroidism and Graves' Disease *forever*.

★★

PHARMACOLOGY MADE INSANELY EASY, 2nd Ed. makes learning pharmacology INSANELY easy!

D drug-drug interactions easy to recall

R reviews HIGH ALERT medications

U unusually easy format

G gives memory tools

S simplifies key points

The perfect companion to complement the best-selling books *Nursing Made Insanely Easy!* and *NCLEX-RN® 101: How to Pass!* This book has over 1000 drugs in just 130 images to help you transform your journey in learning pharmacology by making it FUN and EASY!

★★

NCLEX-RN® REVIEW CDs. Pass your NCLEX® and CGFNS™ with confidence after this fun and easy listening program. This program is recorded in an actual live review course that includes the concepts listed in the NCLEX-RN® test plan on 12 CDs. We CAN help you prepare for the NCLEX® and CGFNS™ and you can listen at your convenience!

★★

NCLEX-RN® non-traditional live review, brought to your site for 50 participants or more, or call our office at **1-800-234-0575** for information and dates on our sites in many states. This course provides the SECRETS to NCLEX® success in a fun and easy 3-day format. The books–NURSING MADE INSANELY EASY, 4th ed. and NCLEX-RN® 101: HOW TO PASS, 6th ed. with a CD of a sample exam accompanying the book– are included in the cost of this review course.

★★

PHARMACOLOGY MADE INSANELY EASY REVIEW A 1-day live interactive review brought to your site for 50 participants or more. Call ICAN Publishing, Inc. at **1-866-428-5589** for information and dates on our sites in many states. If there is not a site in your state, we will be happy to establish one for you! This course provides the SECRETS to NCLEX® and clinical practice success regarding pharmacology in a FUN and EASY 1-day format. The book *Pharmacology Made Insanely Easy!*, 2nd Ed., a packet of pharmacology material and sample test questions evaluating pharmacology are included in the cost of this dynamic pharmacology review. Participants leave saying, *"Wow, I finally get it!"*

Order now!

To order call 1-866-428-5589 or mail to ICAN Publishing, Inc. P.O. Box 6192, Bossier City, LA 71171, or order online at **www.icanpublishing.com**. We accept Mastercard, Visa , Discover cards , American Express, money orders or personal checks. Please do not send cash in the mail.

Yes, I wish to order:

❏ **NCLEX RN® 101: HOW TO PASS, 6th edition** by Rayfield & Manning with a CD containing practice questions • **$35.00 plus $7.00 shipping* and handling**

❏ **NURSING MADE INSANELY EASY, 4th edition** by Rayfield & Manning • **$35.00 plus $7.00 shipping* and handling**

❏ **PHARMACOLOGY MADE INSANELY EASY, 2nd edition** by Manning & Rayfield • **$35.00 plus $7.00 shipping* and handling**

❏ **NCLEX-RN® Review Audio Program** by Sylvia Rayfield & Associates, Inc. • **$99.00 plus $8.00 shipping* and handling.**

❏ **SELF STUDY PACKET includes the audio CD program & all 3 books** • **$209.00 plus $12.00 shipping* and handling**

❏ **Register me for a Sylvia Rayfield & Associates Review Course • $280 of registration** (Includes NURSING MADE INSANELY EASY, 4th ed. and NCLEX-RN® 101: HOW TO PASS, 6th ed.).

* Prices for U. S. shipping only. International shipping rates will differ. Prices subject to change. U.S. shipping by Priority Mail.

Be sure and call to tell us where you want to take the review course. Discounts are given to groups of more than 50 participants!

WE KNOW IF YOU BELIEVE YOU CAN PASS, YOU WILL. WE DEVELOPED THESE TOOLS TO HELP!

Nursing Made Insanely Easy, Fourth Edition

and

NCLEX®-RN 101: HOW TO PASS, Sixth Edition

are used in

Sylvia Rayfield & Associates, Inc.
Review Courses
www.sylviarayfield.com

These non-traditional live reviews are nationally known and have a pass rate of 98%. Call **1-800-234-0575** for the review class nearest you, or to start one at your school.

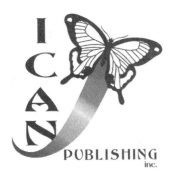

ICAN Publishing, Inc.
P.O. Box 6192
Bossier City, LA 71171
1-866-428-5589
www.icanpublishing.com

Feeling ANXIOUS About Learning Pharmacology?

A mount to remember is too much?

N CLEX-RN™ —Ready for the pharmacology changes?

X actly what you need to know.

I don't even know where to begin!

O verwhelmed?

U nsure of yourself?

S cared?

If your answer is YES, this program is for you! I CAN Publishing, Inc. can now bring to your school, nursing organization, or hospital the popular and most sought after one day program, **Pharmacology Made Insanely Easy**. We developed this program to make learning pharmacology fun, easy, and memorable. We want you to relax and laugh even while you are studying a challenging topic. Since the NCLEX-RN® has increased pharmacology, we want to provide you with a program to increase the confidence in answering questions successfully as well as to enhance clinical practice.

What are participants saying about the program?

"Wow! I finally understand pharmacokinetics and it was actually fun to learn!"

"This program saved me on the NCLEX-RN®! I was able to remember to prioritize my drugs."

"I will never forget cephalosporins thanks to "CEF/CEPH the GIANT"!

"I was always nervous about drug-drug interactions, but I am leaving this program with much more confidence."

"This has been the most interactive course I have ever experienced. Where were you when I was struggling to stay awake while reading my pharmacology text books?"

How Do I Register?

Call **866.428.5589** and register now. For additional information visit our web page at **www.icanpublishing.com**. Coordinate a program at your school for 40 or more participants and receive a **FREE** course. Members of the Student Nurses' Association will receive a discount.

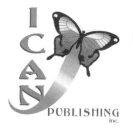

I CAN Publishing, Inc.
P. O. Box 6192
Bossier City, **LA 71171**
1.866.428.5589
www.icanpublishing.com

 *Notes*

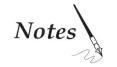

Notes

 *Notes*